MW01252999

Bhutani's
Color Atlas of
DERMATOLOGY

BHUTANI'S COLOR ATLAS OF DERMATOLOGY

Sixth Edition

Neena Khanna MD

Professor
Department of Dermatology and Venereology
All India Institute of Medical Sciences
New Delhi, India

Saurabh Singh MD DNB

Assistant Professor
Department of Dermatology and Venereology
Employees' State Insurance Corporation (ESIC)
Medical College and Hospital
Faridabad, Haryana, India

JAYPEE *The Health Sciences Publisher*

New Delhi | London | Philadelphia | Panama

Jaypee Brothers Medical Publishers (P) Ltd.

Headquarters
Jaypee Brothers Medical Publishers (P) Ltd.
4838/24, Ansari Road, Daryaganj
New Delhi 110 002, India
Phone: +91-11-43574357
Fax: +91-11-43574314
E-mail: jaypee@jaypeebrothers.com

Overseas Offices

J.P. Medical Ltd.
83, Victoria Street, London
SW1H 0HW (UK)
Phone: +44-20 3170 8910
Fax: +44(0)20 3008 6180
E-mail: info@jpmedpub.com

Jaypee-Highlights Medical Publishers Inc.
City of Knowledge, Bld. 237, Clayton
Panama City, Panama
Phone: +1 507-301-0496
Fax: +1 507-301-0499
E-mail: cservice@jphmedical.com

Jaypee Medical Inc.
The Bourse
111, South Independence Mall East
Suite 835, Philadelphia, PA 19106, USA
Phone: +1 267-519-9789
E-mail: jpmed.us@gmail.com

Jaypee Brothers Medical Publishers (P) Ltd.
17/1-B, Babar Road, Block-B, Shaymali
Mohammadpur, Dhaka-1207
Bangladesh
Mobile: +08801912003485
E-mail: jaypeedhaka@gmail.com

Jaypee Brothers Medical Publishers (P) Ltd.
Bhotahity, Kathmandu, Nepal
Phone: +977-9741283608
E-mail: kathmandu@jaypeebrothers.com

Website: www.jaypeebrothers.com
Website: www.jaypeedigital.com

Inquiries for bulk sales may be solicited at: jaypee@jaypeebrothers.com

Bhutani's Color Atlas of Dermatology

First Edition: 1982

Sixth Edition: **2015**

ISBN: 978-93-5152-302-4

Printed at: Replika Press Pvt. Ltd.

Dedicated to

Professor Lalit K Bhutani
and his parents

Foreword to the First Edition

It gives me great pleasure to contribute a foreword for this book, which has been written by an eminent teacher and research worker. Professor Lalit K Bhutani, who is the Head of the Department of Dermatology and Venereology at the All India Institute of Medical Sciences, New Delhi, is a renowned dermatologist, a teacher of repute and an internationally recognized research worker in the field of dermatology. He has been guest lecturer at many national and international universities and holds memberships of several international dermatological societies. His research interests have centered around such subjects as leprosy, pigmentary problems, mycological diseases and sexually transmitted diseases. He has made special contributions in the field of immunology of leprosy.

This book is the result of much painstaking work and reflects the vast experience of Professor Bhutani. Through the excellent reproduction of colored pictures of dermatological lesions, the author has provided a clear understanding of various dermatological disorders. His stress on dermatological problems seen in the tropics is praiseworthy. The material has been well planned and presented in a very lucid manner. The book will be useful to clinicians in general as well as specialists in this field. I congratulate Professor Bhutani for his praiseworthy attempt and wish this work all success.

1982

VTH Gunaratne FRCP DPH
World Health Organization
South East Asia Regional Office

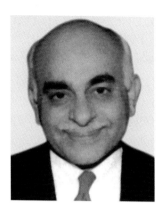

Late Professor Lalit K Bhutani (1936–2004)

Dr Bhutani, an eminent physician, and a dermatologist and venereologist of international repute, contributed immensely to the development of the discipline in India and placed it on the global dermatology map. He was deeply involved in the management of sexually transmitted diseases including HIV and AIDS besides development and progression of modern management of leprosy in India and beyond. His other fields of interest were dermatopathology and photobiology. He was the first to describe the condition *lichen planus pigmentosus*.

A graduate of University of Punjab (1958), he moved to join All India Institute of Medical Sciences (AIIMS), New Delhi. An almost reluctant entrant into the field of dermatology and venereology, he became one of its most brilliant teachers and took over the reins of the department of AIIMS in 1979. He eventually rose to become the Dean and Director of this prestigious institute from which he retired in 1996. He continued to provide invaluable service as an honorary consultant dermatologist at Sitaram Bhartiya Institute of Science and Research, New Delhi, until his death. He was appointed Honorary Physician to the President of India in 1983.

In recognition of his brilliant academic achievements, he was awarded Honorary Fellowship of the Royal College of Physicians (Edinburgh) in 1987 and received the prestigious BC Roy Award for excellence in teaching. His commitment to teaching was reflected in his authorship of two immensely popular (almost Biblical) atlases "Colour Atlas of Dermatology" and "Atlas of Sexually Transmitted Diseases". A keen researcher, he had to his credit nearly 150 publications in national and international journals of repute and contributed chapters to several books of Medicine and Dermatology.

He held several prestigious positions in his specialty and was elected President of Indian Association of Dermatology and Venereology (1979–80) and its General Secretary (1973–74). That he successfully hosted the VII International Congress of Dermatology and Venereology in New Delhi in 1994, (first ever for an Asian country) speaks volumes of his organizational skills.

He was invited to participate in and chair a number of national and international conferences and seminars. He was honored with a number of visiting professorships at various institutes internationally, such as Mayo Clinic, Rochester, USA, and King Faisal University, Dammam, Saudi Arabia, where he was the architect of its postgraduate residency program which is still being followed. He was associated in various capacities with a number of international and national professional bodies such as American Academy of Dermatology, British Association of Dermatology, American Society of Photobiology, International Society of Dermatopathology, American Venereal Disease Association, and European Society of Dermatologic Research. He also served on a number of WHO, sponsored consultancies and acted as an adviser on sexually transmitted diseases including HIV and AIDS in many countries around the world.

A brilliant orator, his talks were full of clarity and peppered with humor. He dotted his presentations with the most fascinating clinical pictures many of which are now part of this atlas. His well-catalogued collection of clinical photographs could easily be passed off as a 'Library of Dermatological Images'.

Dr Bhutani, much loved by his colleagues and friends, was an inspiration to those around him. Many a young doctors have been propelled to clinical excellence by his warm bedside manner and teaching abilities and many dermatologists will remain indebted to him.

Preface to the Sixth Edition

A classic is often known by the name of its creator rather than by the title given to it. This is so true for the Color Atlas of Dermatology. It is frequently referred to as Dr Bhutani's atlas or simply as LKB's atlas. One of the most popular books in dermatology, several batches of undergraduate and postgraduate students swear by it even today. It is also a 'must have' for general practitioners (GPs) and practicing dermatologists.

This atlas, like the previous editions, is intended for senior medical students, general practitioners and also entrants into the field of dermatology. The book is divided into 25 chapters: some diseases have been classified etiologically while others have been grouped conventionally; however, some groupings have been made morphologically to emphasize how dermatoses, with different etiogenesis, may simulate each other. Newer therapies have been incorporated (albeit briefly) to make the book comprehensive. Throughout the book, Professor Bhutani's inimitable and crisp style, which became very popular and identified with the atlas, has been retained.

Neena Khanna
Saurabh Singh

Preface to the First Edition

This atlas is intended primarily for senior medical students, general practitioners and residents in dermatology and internal medicine. Next to the actual patient, a color photograph is perhaps the most useful learning material in dermatology. Such atlases in the West have an understandable bias on locally important conditions. A certain emphasis on tropical dermatoses may be discernable here; other more cosmopolitan diseases have been given adequate coverage.

On account of the ease with which populations from one part of the world have moved to another, the physician is constantly faced with the challenge of diagnosing and treating exotic conditions. The projection in this atlas of skin lesions on a pigmented background will aid the physician in his diagnosis. A brief description has been given for an easy interpretation; selected photomicrographs are added for further help. Notes on treatment are brief and meant as a guideline. The book combines visual impression of morphologic lesions with factual information, and supplements the standard textbooks.

The book is divided into nineteen chapters with various diseases conventionally grouped; some unconventional grouping has also been made to emphasize close clinical simulation. A chapter on sexually transmitted diseases has been included since in many countries the specialities of dermatology and venereology are practised jointly.

All photographs including photomicrographs have been taken by myself. Most are from patients seen in India; some are from patients seen in Africa or South-East Asia. Acknowledgment is made for permission to reproduce my two fluorescent photographs on page 98 from *Arch. Derm*. 110:427, 1974, copyright 1974, American Medical Association.

Three persons played a dominant role in shaping my career in dermatology: Professor KC Kandhari, my teacher and mentor, initiated me into dermatology; Professor IA Magnus and Professor CD Calnan encouraged me to continue. This book is in a sense a tribute to them.

My colleague and friend Dr RK Pandhi generously gave his valuable time and suggestions at every stage; but for his inestimable help, this book would not have been completed. Other friends helped in different ways: Professor NC Nayak with advice on selection of photomicrographs and histologic description; Drs Roger Harman, R Bikhchandani, AS Kumar, Jose Thomas, Sharad Goel, Jasleen Kaur, Anuradha Kathpalia, Messfin Demisse with help in critical evaluation of the manuscript and galley proofs. Dr E Nair provided specimens of pediculi and mite. Professors RK Panja, BMS Bedi and Dr Dharam Pal gave useful suggestions. Professors YK Malhotra, R Patnaik and Dr Daljit S Nagreh permitted the use of their patients' photographs. Mr ML Bhalla and Mr Awasthy helped in the processing of photomicrographs. Mr Krishan Kumar rendered useful secretarial assistance.

I am most grateful to Mr SN Mehta, the publisher, and Mrs Susan Gale, the editor, for all their help. They displayed rare patience and understanding in handling the manuscript, the pictures and the entire work.

Professor V Ramalingaswami and Professor HD Tandon supported and encouraged me throughout. I am most thankful to them.

Nitin and Nishit, my sons, made some very useful and valuable suggestions.

Manorama, my wife, was a constant, unfailing source of encouragement, help and inspiration-a crutch which I could lean upon-any time and every time.

LK Bhutani

Acknowledgments

The present work would not have been possible without the contributions of several of my colleagues. Drs Riti, Kamal, Ajay, Gitika, and Tanir who nit-picked the manuscript to its culmination. Ms Tanu and Meenu who helped in correcting the manuscript in its initial stages.

I am grateful to Dr Somesh Gupta for permitting me to use pictures of his 'operated' patients (2 pictures on page 470 and 4 pictures on page 472). So also my gratitude to my faculty colleagues (many of whom are Dr Bhutani's students) for letting us photograph their 'in-patients'. I am also grateful to Dr Harsh Mohan for permitting me to use picture of histopathology of sarcoidosis (on page 199).

I express my appreciation and gratitude to Shri Jitendar P Vij (Group Chairman) and Mr Ankit Vij (Group President) of M/s Jaypee Brothers Medical Publishers (P) Ltd., New Delhi, India, which is one of the largest Medical Publishers in the world, for their assistance and help. Mr Tarun Duneja (Director-Publishing) has been instrumental in getting the final shape of the book. Also, my acknowledgments to Ms Samina Khan (Executive Assistant to Director-Publishing), Mr KK Raman (Production Manager), Mr Sunil Kumar Dogra (Production Executive), Mr Neelambar Pant (Production Coordinator), Mr Manoj Pahuja (Senior Graphic Designer), Mr Varun Rana (Typesetter), Mr Himanshu Sharma (Proofreader) and other members for their immense patience to bring out the book.

The task of completing the book would have been impossible, had it not been for the ever-encouraging presence of Mr Ranbir Singh, whose untiring efforts smoothened all obstacles during the production of the book. His patience and eye for detail are the reasons for the quality of this book.

I am indeed indebted to Dr (Mrs) Bhutani for again reposing faith in me and believing that I could carry out the herculean task of bringing out a book which had acquired 'Biblical status'. Her presence and perseverance were pivotal in helping us meet the targeted dates. She was always there as the guiding force and her unflinching encouragement brought out the best in the team.

I would be failing in my duty if I did not thank the 'behind the scene' people. Anil and my brats who put up with sharing my time with the laptop.

Neena Khanna

First of all, I am grateful to Dr Neena Khanna for entrusting me with this herculean task of carrying forward and being a part of Dr LK Bhutani's atlas, the work for which I had a desire since my undergraduate days at AIIMS, New Delhi, India. And I share and echo indebtedness to Dr Mrs Bhutani for giving this opportunity. The love and support of my parents and sisters have been my guiding force. The 'quartet' of you have always allowed me the liberty to be a 'parasite', take the honest utmost difficult path to success and to bask in the glory thence forth; Papa, Mummy and Didis', I dedicate this to you! My love to my tiny little nieces and nephews who had virtually labelled me 'laptop Mama', without expecting even an ounce of attention from my end. I would be failing in my duty if I do not thank Dr Shanta Passi (Dermatology Specialist, ESIC Hospital, Faridabad) for taking care of OPDs and my patients thus relieving me for book work whenever needed and allowing photography of few of her patients for the same purpose. I am grateful to Dr Asim Das, Dean, ESIC College, for allowing me to work on the book and to the office orderly. Mr

Shailender for keeping office open, when needed, beyond office hours. I am especially thankful to Drs Mayank, Piyush and Narendra, for they had been my 'official chariots', and all other faculty members of our college for providing a 'healthy' workplace. Finally, a toast to our MBBS teacher Dr Deorari (Prof. Neonatology, AIIMS, New Delhi) who mentioned once that I must also embark on writing an Atlas since I had joined a department of Dr Bhutani's repute!

Saurabh Singh

Contents

1

Pyodermas

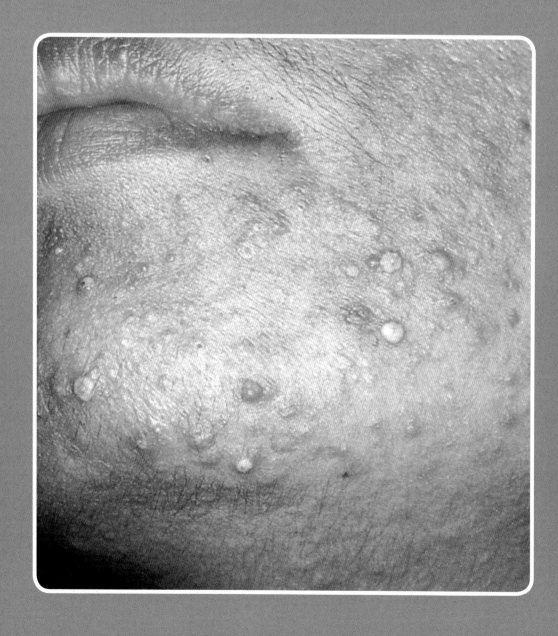

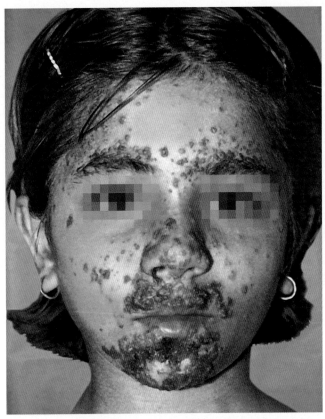

Impetigo contagiosa: lesions with dirty crusts and erythematous halo. Multiple lesions resulting from autoinoculation.

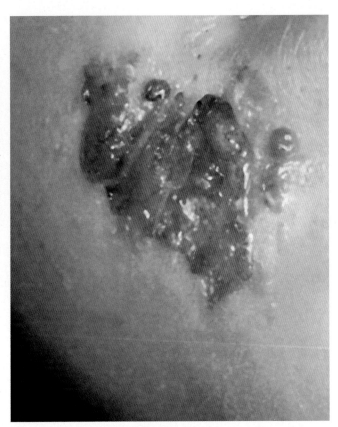

Impetigo contagiosa: close-up showing honey-colored 'stuck-on' crusts.

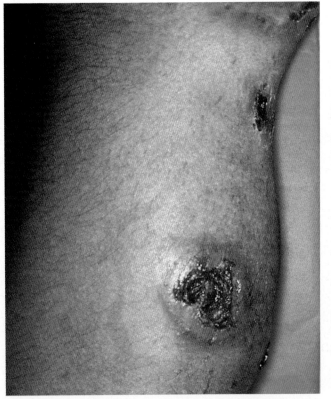

Ecthyma: hemorrhagic crusts which on removal reveal an ulcer.

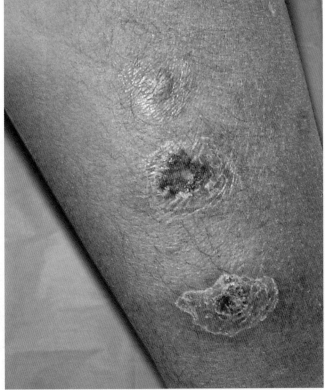

Ecthyma: heals with scarring.

Normal skin not sterile. Inhabited by:

- **Residents:** present permanently. Include bacteria (non-pathogenic staphylococci, micrococci and diphtheroids) and fungi (pityrosporum).
- **Transients:** pathogenic organisms which live only transiently on skin.

Skin infections caused by pyococcal (pus producing) organisms are called pyodermas. Organisms commonly incriminated include *Staphylococcus aureus* and *Streptococcus pyogenes.*

Pyodermas classsified as:

- **Nonfollicular:** when infection is not particularly folliculocentric. Nonfollicular pyodermas include **localized** infections which may be caused by staphylococci (impetigo contagiosa/bullous impetigo/ecthyma), or by streptococci (impetigo contagiosa/ecthyma). Or **spreading** infection which are usually caused by streptococci (erysipelas/cellulitis).
- **Follicular:** folliculocentric pyodermas are invariably caused by staphylococci and include superficial and deep folliculitis, furuncles and carbuncles.

Pyodermas also classsified as:

- **Primary pyodermas:** arise in normal (not diseased) skin; have a defined morphology.
- **Secondary pyodermas:** arise in diseased skin (scabies, pediculosis, insect bite hypersensitivity dermatophytic infection, atopic dermatitis, miliaria); have variable morphology.

IMPETIGO CONTAGIOSA

Etiology

Frequently caused by *Strep pyogenes.* Less often *Staph aureus* (phage group II). Often mixed. Poor personal hygiene, insect bites, trauma, infestations (scabies, pediculosis) predispose.

Epidemiology

Common; spreads amongst contacts. Auto-inoculable, infants and children prone.

Clinical Manifestations

Clinically, transient vesicules/pustules evolve into lesions with dirty yellow 'stuck on' crusts with an erythematous halo. Heal without sequelae. Regional lymphadenopathy frequent. Face, limbs and less frequently other parts of the body involved. Nephritogenic strains of streptococci cause acute glomerulonephritis, a serious but uncommon complication.

Investigations

Direct Microscopy

Gram stain shows either Gram positive cocci in chains (streptococci) or in clusters (staphylococcus). Helps in immediate institution of appropriate empirical therapy.

Culture

Culture and antibiotic sensitivity done in appropriate situations.

Histopathology

Histology reveals a subcorneal split containing polymorphs.

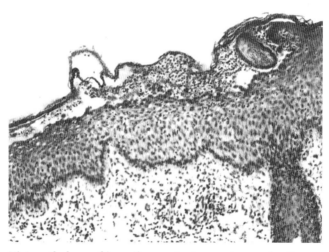

Histopathology of impetigo contagiosa: subcorneal split containing polymorphonuclear leukocytes.

ECTHYMA

Etiology

Strep pyogenes or *Staph aureus.* Or mixed etiology. Children with poor personal hygiene, malnutrition, skin infestations affected.

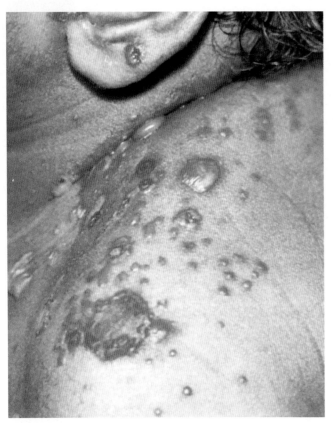

Bullous impetigo: large vesiculo-pustular lesions. Heal in center and spread centripetally.

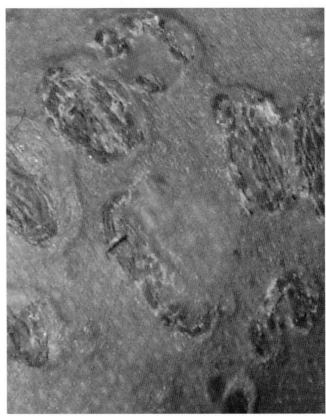

Bullous impetigo: central healing with peripheral extension resulting in circinate lesions.

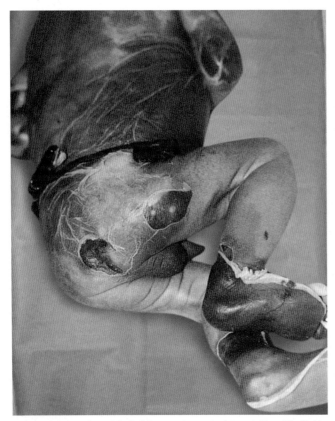

Staphylococcal scalded skin syndrome: sheets of 'scalded' skin peeling off.

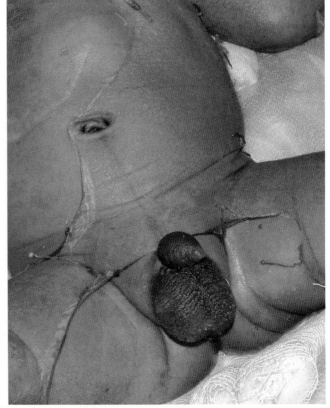

Staphylococcal scalded skin syndrome: sheets of peeling skin. Note denudation is superficial.

Clinical Manifestations

Uncommon. Similar to but deeper than impetigo contagiosa. Ulcers covered with thick, adherent, dirty greyish brown crusts and red edematous halo. Removal reveals punched out ulcers with indurated margins. Heal slowly with scars. Lower extremities commonly affected.

Diagnosis

Direct Microscopy

Gram stain shows either Gram positive cocci in chains (streptococci) or in clusters (*Staphylococcus*). Helps in institution of appropriate empirical therapy.

Epidemiology

Infants and children affected. May spread as epidemic in nurseries with serious and sometimes fatal results.

Clinical Manifestations

Clinically bullae soon turn into large pustules that burst to form crusted lesions. Central healing with peripheral extension. Circinate lesions characteristic. Face, neck, perineum frequently affected. Moderate to severe constitutional symptoms.

Investigations

Direct Microscopy

Gram stain of exudate reveals Gram positive cocci in clusters.

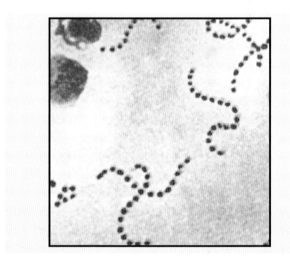

Histopathology of Gram stain from lesion of ecthyma: shows Gram positive cocci in chains, suggestive of streptococcal infection. May also show Gram positive cocci in clusters.

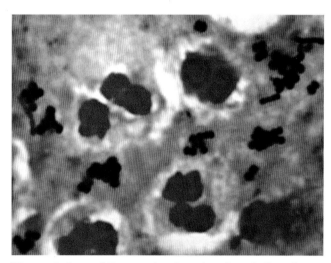

Histopathology of Gram stain of exudate from bullous impetigo: shows Gram positive cocci in clusters suggestive of staphylococcal infection.

Culture

Culture and antibiotic sensitivity done in appropriate situations (non-responsive disease). And recurrent infection.

BULLOUS IMPETIGO

Etiology

Staph aureus (phage group II, type 71). Bullae caused by staphylococcal epidermolysin.

Culture

Culture (if done) grows *Staph aureus* (phage group II).

STAPHYLOCOCCAL SCALDED SKIN SYNDROME (SSSS)

Etiology

Serious toxin-mediated (epidermolysin) manifestation of staphylococcal infection.

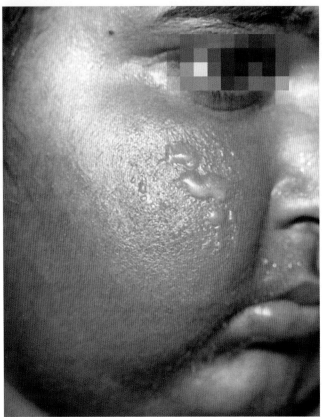

Cellulitis: ill-defined, edematous lesion with vesiculation.

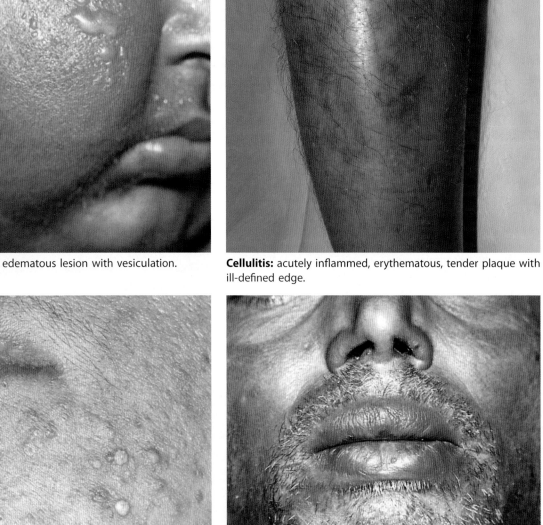

Cellulitis: acutely inflammed, erythematous, tender plaque with ill-defined edge.

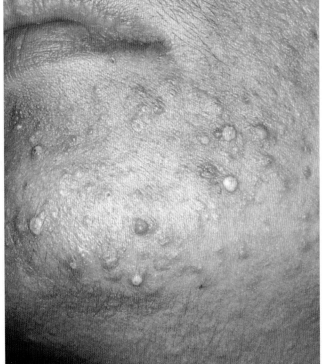

Superficial folliculitis: follicular pustules on the face. Deep folliculitis.

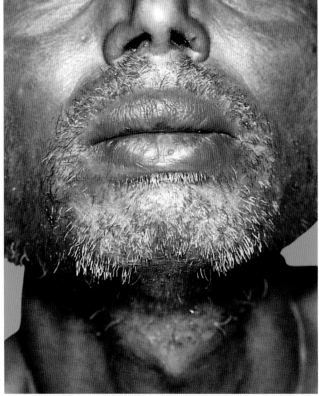

Sycosis barbae: scaly and crusted plaque surmounted by pustules.

Focus of *Staphylococcus* either cutaneous or extracutaneous.

Clinical Manifestations

Infants and children affected. Skin appears scalded-red, tender, discolored and denuded. Patient toxic. Potentially fatal condition unless treated energetically and promptly with appropriate antibiotics.

CELLULITIS

Etiology

Strep pyogenes. Less frequently *Staph aureus.* Infection of the subcutaneous tissue. Often follows an antecedent skin pathology (lymphedema common predisposing factor; so also interdigital fungal infection). Or wound. Diabetes mellitus and immunosuppressives also predispose.

Clinical Manifestations

Acute, intensely painful, red, warm, tender, edematous swelling of the affected part. Erythematous ill-defined edge. May be surmounted by vesicles. Or undergo necrosis and gangrene. Lymphangitis and regional lymphadenopathy present. Leg and foot most frequently involved. Constitutional symptoms pronounced.

Erysipelas: similar to, but more superficial than cellulitis. Edge well-defined. Serious in infants and children.

Investigations

Diagnosis usually clinical.

Direct Microscopy

Gram stain from surmounting vesicle/exudate from necrotic area shows Gram positive cocci in chains most frequently.

Culture

Strep pyogenes

Less frequently others.

Histopathology

Of doubtful value in subacute infections.

FOLLICULITIS

Superficial Folliculitis (Follicular Impetigo of Bockhart)

Common. *Staph aureus* infection of follicular ostia. Commonly seen in children or young adults. Discrete, superficial dome shaped pustules around a hair. Heal with no residue.

Deep Folliculitis (Sycosis)

Common. *Staph aureus* infection of the whole follicle. Adult males affected. Scattered or grouped perifollicular pustules on an edematous, scaly and crusted plaque. Recurrent and chronic. Often heal without scarring. Certain forms, though heal with scars (lupoid sycosis; folliculitis decalvans).

Common sites: beard, upper lip, scalp.

Pustular Dermatitis Atrophicans of the Legs

Not uncommon in India. Superficial and deep follicular pustules with scaling. Recurrent and chronic. Heal with atrophy and scarring. Often bilateral and symmetrical. Shins (common), thighs (occasional). No definite predisposing factor determined-vegetable oils; sometimes implicated.

BOIL (FURUNCLE)

Folliculitis with perifolliculitis.

Etiology

Staph aureus. Recurrent in diabetics or predisposed individuals (malnutrition, on systemic corticosteroids or immunosuppressive therapy, obesity, lymphomas). However, generally most patients even with recurrent boils—otherwise healthy—recurrences probably related to carrier state.

Clinical Manifestations

Common. Single or multiple. Painful, red, firm, tender nodules that develops a pustular top and becomes fluctuant. Points, ruptures and discharges a necrotic core. Heals with scar. Hairy parts of the body subject to friction such as buttocks, face, commonly affected. Fever and other constitutional symptoms often present.

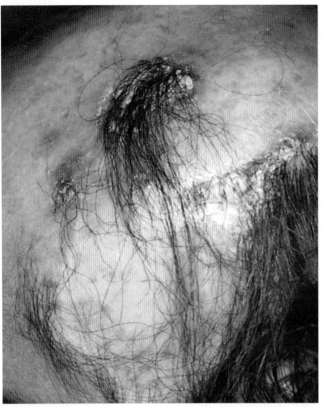

Folliculitis decalvans, scalp: follicular pustules leading to scarring alopecia.

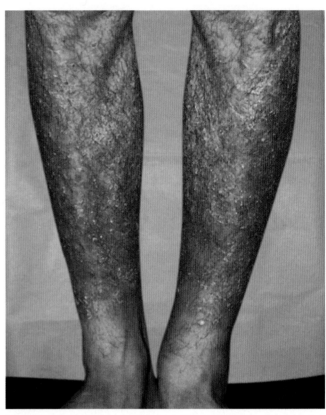

Pustular dermatitis atrophicans of legs: follicular pustules with loss of hair and atrophy of skin.

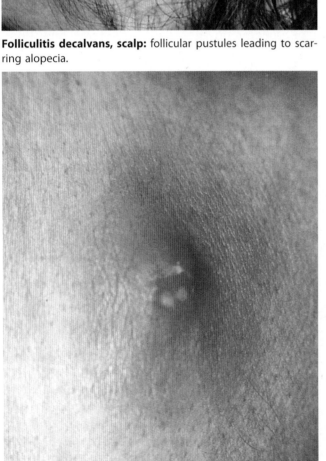

Furuncle: two adjoining follicles involved. Firm, erythematous nodule, surmounted with pustule. Very painful.

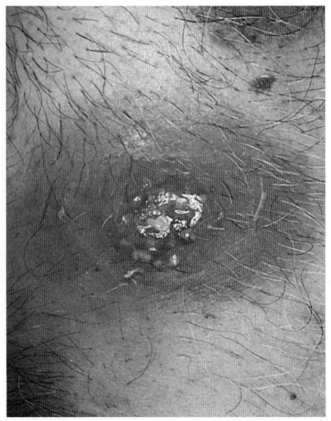

Carbuncle: painful, erythematous, dome shaped indurated swelling that pours out pus and necrotic material from several opening. Seen on back, buttocks and neck.

Stye (hordeolum): A furuncle of the eyelash. Common, sometimes recurrent. Painful red nodule on the lid margin with swelling of the eyelid.

Investigations

Direct Microscopy

Gram stain shows Gram positive cocci in clusters suggestive of staphylococci.

Culture

Often needed, mainly for antibiotic sensitivity.

CARBUNCLE

Cluster of boils.

Etiology

Staph aureus. Abscesses of adjoining hair follicles. Adults, often obese, diabetics.

Clinical Manifestation

Painful, erythematous, dome-shaped, tender and indurated swelling that becomes pustular and necrotic with pus pouring out from several openings. Back, buttocks, nape of neck commonly affected. Spontaneous healing rare. Moderate to severe constitutional symptoms.

Investigations

Vide supra, under furuncle.

PRINCIPLES OF MANAGEMENT OF PYODERMAS

Evaluation

Gram Stain

Gram staining, a quick side lab test which gives immediate clue to empirical antibiotic therapy to be instituted.

Culture

Usually not done unless infection resistant to treatment. Or recurrent.

Rule Out Underlying Disease

Especially in recurrent infections. Systemic diseases like diabetes, immunocompromised states (HIV infection, malignancies, iatrogenic). Or underlying skin diseases (infestations, dermatophytic infections, atopic states). Also exclude carrier state in recurrent infection.

Treatment

General Measures

Scrupulous personal hygiene of paramount importance. Soap and water wash most helpful—prevents spread and recurrences. Keep skin dry. Treatment of underlying predisposing conditions. Remove crusts with warm compresses (saline, potassium permanganate). Or simply soap. Immobolization and elevation of affected limb in cellulitis. Fluid and electrolyte maintenance for SSSS. Incision and drainage for boils and carbuncles. Recurrent infections need measures to reduce carrier state of *Staph aureus*.

Specific Treatment

Topical agents used for few/superficial lesions. Systemic therapy needed for widespread lesions, deeper infections (furuncles carbuncle ecthyma, cellulitis/erysipelas). Or in presence of lymphadenopathy and constitutional symptoms. Always for SSSS and cellulitis/erysipelas where aggressive even parenteral therapy often warranted.

Topical Treatment

Topical agents used include 2% framycetin sulfate, 1% neomycin, polymyxin B-bacitracin combination, 2% mupirocin, 2% sodium fusidate, 1% retapamulin, 5–10% povidone–iodine.

Systemic Therapy

Choice of antibiotic governed by organisms suspected. Or antibiotic sensitivity determined. As a rule of thumb, bullous impetigo and follicular pyodermas caused by *Staph aureus*. Cellulitis and erysipelas caused by *Strep pyogenes.* And impetigo contagiosa and ecthyma caused by either.

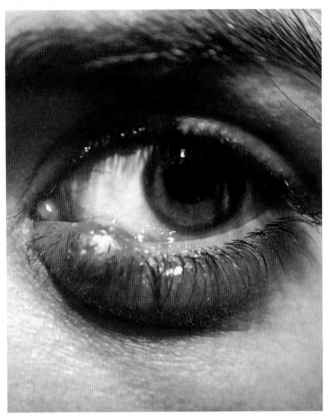

Stye: red nodule on the lid margin.

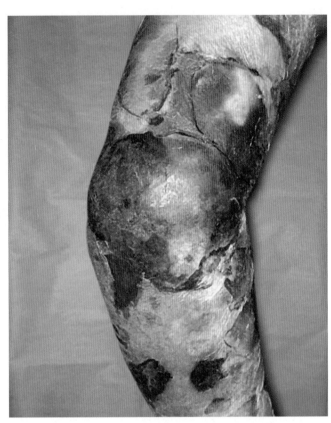

Anthrax: hemorrhagic necrotic crusts with several large bullae. Severe constitutional symptoms.

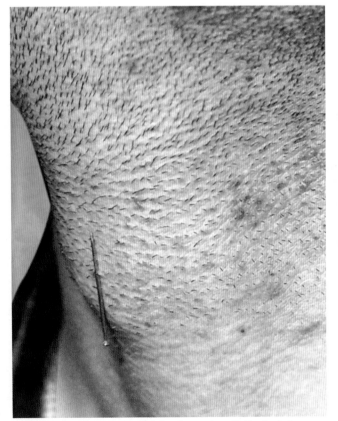

Pseudofolliculitis: multiple follicular and perifollicular inflammatory papules; needle held by the loop formed by ingrown hair.

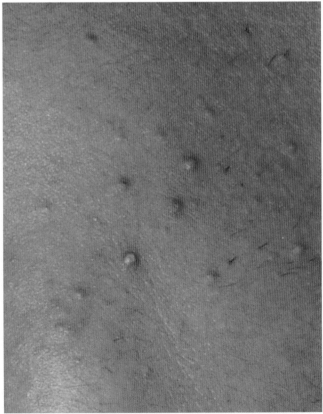

Post waxing folliculitis: follicular erythematous papules and pustules. Occur 2–3 weeks after waxing. A pseudofolliculitis.

Streptococcal infections: in general, treated with penicillins (benzyl penicillin/amoxicillin) cephalosporins and macrolides.

Staphylococcal infections: treated with penicillinase resistant penicillins (cloxacillin, methicillin). Or a combination of penicillin with β-lactamase inhibitors (clavulanic acid). Or macrolides. Or cephalosporins.

ANTHRAX

Etiology

Bacillus anthracis, a Gram-positive rod. Acquired from animals. Threatened use, as an agent of biological warfare.

Clinical Manifestations

Rare. Clinically, presents as pustules or bullae, on an erythematous, edematous base. Pustules rupture to form a hemorrhagic crust, surrounded by vesicles and bullae. Severe constitutional symptoms. Lymphadenopathy variable.

Treatment

Urgent. Large doses of parenteral benzyl penicillin G (4–6 million units/day). Or tetracyclines. Or ciprofloxacin for 2 weeks.

NON-PYOCOCCAL DERMATOSES SIMULATING PYODERMAS

Pseudofolliculitis (Pili Incarnati)

Etiology

Foreign body reaction to beard or pubic hair. In curly haired, black adult males who shave. Either due to penetration of follicular wall by sharp tip of growing hair (transfollicular) or by re-entry of curly hair into skin (extrafollicular). Close shaving (by pulling skin taut and using double/triple-bladed razors) predisposes—the sharp tip of growing hair easily pierces follicular wall resulting in inflammation. Also after epilation of hair (post waxing folliculitis).

Clinical Manifestations

Manifest as painful follicular or perifollicular erythematous, papules with central hair shaft. Free

end of hair released (out of the papule) on gently lifting hair shaft. Chronic and recurrent. Pustules or abscesses may complicate. Beard/pubic area. And areas waxed.

Treatment

Preventive measures include hydration of hair before shaving. Using single-edged, foil guarded safety razors. Or using chemical depilation. In active lesions, avoid shaving for 3–4 weeks. Topical retinoids (remove thin epidermis covering of regrowing follicle) and mild topical corticosteroids (reduce inflammation). Severe cases (pustules/abscesses) need topical and oral antibiotics (erythromycin or clindamycin).

Folliculitis Keloidalis (Acne Keloidalis)

Rare. Adult male blacks. Cause unknown. Asymptomatic, keloidal, follicular papules or irregular plaques present on the lower margin of the scalp hair line.

Treatment

Unsatisfactory. Topical potent fluorinated or intralesional corticosteroids. Excision if necessary.

INFECTIONS CAUSED BY RESIDENT FLORA

Erythrasma

Etiology

Corynebacterium minutissimum. More frequent in warm and humid climate; tends to clear in winter. Obesity and hyperhidrosis predispose.

Clinical Manifestations

Common. Asymptomatic or mildly pruritic. Reddish-brown, sharply defined, irregular macules mainly in the axillae and groins. And interdigital spaces of feet (perhaps the most common, but seldom manifests clinically in an uncomplicated form). Relapses common in summer.

Investigations

Coral-red fluorescence under Wood's UV lamp diagnostic.

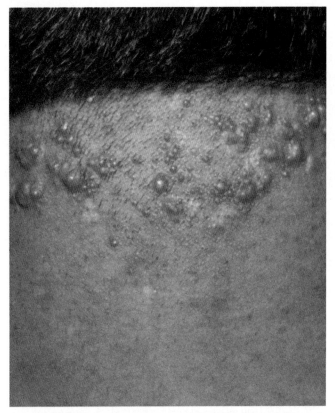

Acne keloidalis: hypertrophic papules on the nape of the neck.

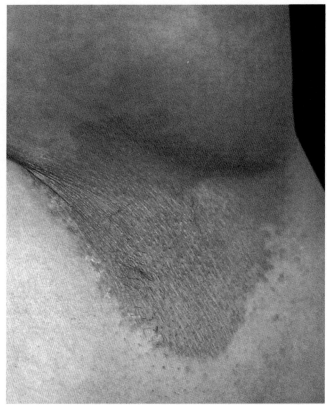

Erythrasma: non-inflammatory brownish irregular macule in axilla.

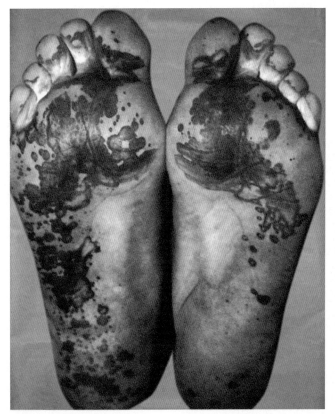

Pitted keratolysis: brownish superficial erosions-discrete and confluent.

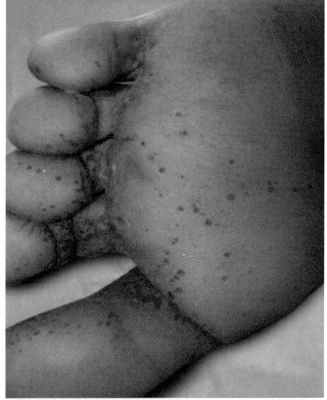

Pitted keratolysis: close-up of crateriform pits. Note interdigital intertrigo.

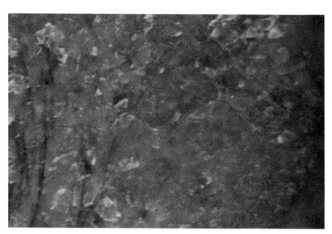

Wood's lamp examination of erythrasma: shows coral-red fluorescence.

Treatment

Keep area dry. Apply topical 2–5% erythromycin lotion/gel. Or 1% imidazole lotion/powder. Systemic erythromycin therapy perhaps not necessary.

Pitted Keratolysis

Etiology

Micrococcus sedentarius. And also *Corynebacterium spp.* Plantar hyperhidrosis and wearing of occlusive footwear predispose.

Epidemiology

Uncommon.

Clinical Manifestations

Young adult males more susceptible. Asymptomatic, well-defined, circular or irregular, discrete and confluent superficially pitted lesions (crateriform pits) on the soles; may be associated with interdigital intertrigo. Bilaterally symmetrical.

Treatment

Preventable condition by keeping area dry. Avoid occlusive footwear. Treat hyperhidrosis (with 20% aluminium chloride hexahydrate). Specific treatment includes benzoyl peroxide 5% gel. Or an imidazole powder/cream.

2

Fungal Infections

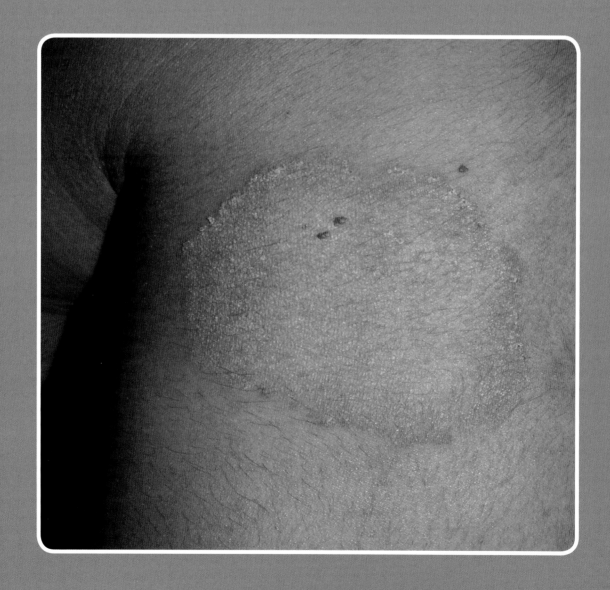

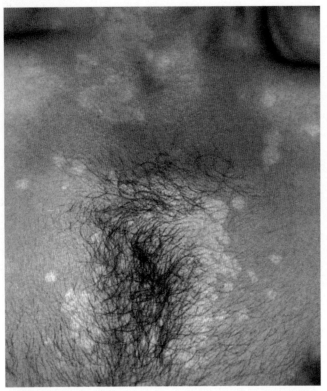

Pityriasis versicolor: hypopigmented, discrete and confluent macules with branny scales.

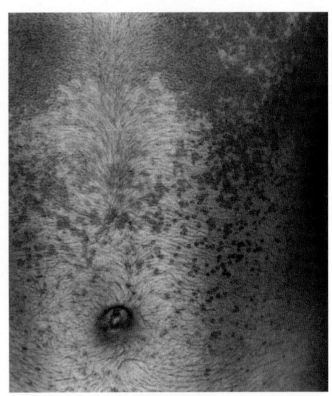

Pityriasis versicolor: hyperpigmented, scaly macules—discrete and confluent. Note many lesions perifollicular.

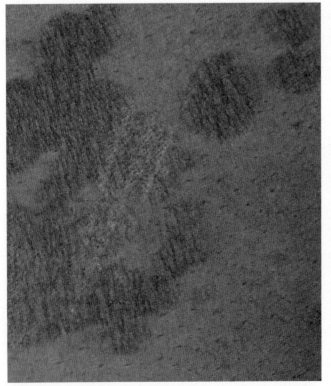

Pityriasis versicolor: hyperpigmented macules with scaling accentuated by scratching. With permission of Elsevier, Illustrated Synopsis of Dermatology and Sexually Transmitted Infections.

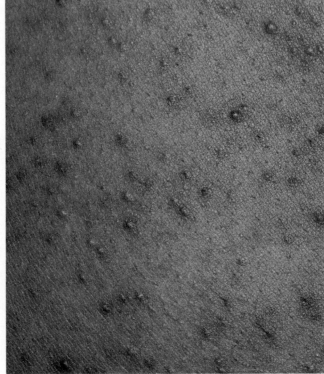

Pityrosporum folliculitis: follicular papules and pustules on trunk. With permission of Elsevier, Illustrated Synopsis of Dermatology and Sexually Transmitted Infections.

Fungi broadly classified as moulds (e.g. dermatophytes), yeasts (e.g. *Candida spp*), and dimorphic fungi (Malassezia, histoplasmosis, coccidioidomycosis).

Fungal infections of skin either superficial or deep (subcutaneous). Or skin involved incidentally in systemic fungal infections.

- **Superficial:** three groups of fungi relevant in superficial fungal infections–dermatophytes (*Trichophyton, Epidermophyton, Microsporum spp*), *Candida spp* and *Pityrosporum spp* Humidity, occlusion, diabetes, immune deficiency states predispose to superficial fungal infections.
- **Deep:** variable geographic distribution of subcutaneous fungal infection. Mycetomas and sporotrichosis common in India and the tropics.
- **Incidental involvement in systemic mycoses:** immune deficiency states predispose to infections such as cryptococcosis, histoplasmosis and candidosis.

PITYROSPORUM INFECTION

Etiology

Malassezia furfur, a saprophytic dimorphic, resident fungus.

Epidemiology

Very common in warm humid climates. Usually affects adolescents and adults.

Clinical Manifestations

Pityriasis Versicolor

Cosmetically objectionable asymptomatic, hypopigmented (on dark skin) and/or hyperpigmented (on white skin), well-defined, perifollicular, small macules with fine branny scales (accentuated by scratching). Confluence may produce large lesions. On the front and back of the chest, neck, upper arms. Recurrences frequent.

Pityrosporum (Malassezia) Folliculitis

Itchy, erythematous, small follicular papules/pustules. Back, chest, proximal extremities.

Investigations

Wood's Lamp

Yellow fluorescence.

Direct Microscopy

Potassium hydroxide (KOH) mount of scales (pityriasis versicolor)/pustule (pityrosporum folliculitis) shows typical meat ball and spaghetti appearance—short septate hyphae and thick walled spores.

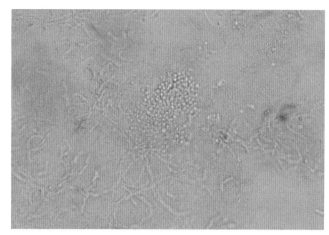

Potassium hydroxide mount of scale of pityriasis versicolor: shows typical spaghetti and meat ball appearance. (short septate hyphae and thick walled spores).

Culture

Usually not required.

Treatment

General Measures

Keep skin dry. Avoid use of synthetic occlusive garments that prevent evaporation of sweat.

Specific Therapy

Topical therapy

Indicated for limited disease. Several choices available—ketoconazole, 2% shampoo, used twice a week for 4–6 weeks. Lathered on affected skin and left for 5–10 minutes for 3 consecutive days. Alternatively, 2.5% selenium sulphide

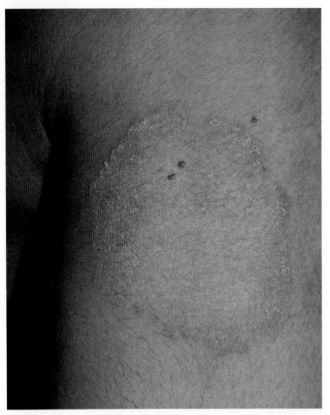

Tinea corporis: well-defined, annular lesion with erythematous scaly border with papulovesicles and relatively, clear center.

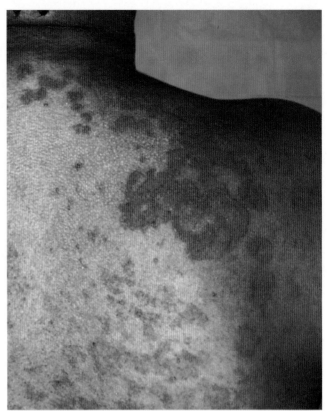

Tinea corporis: circinate lesions; note 'active' erythematous elevated border.

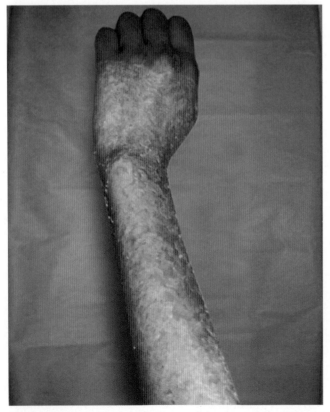

Tinea imbricata: concentric lesions with brown scales and almost clear intervening skin.

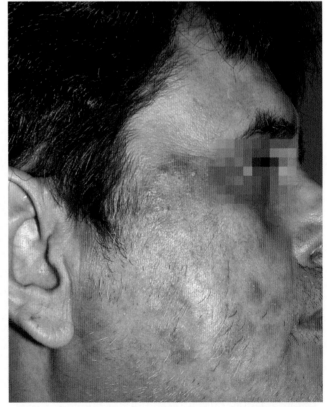

Tinea faciei: circinate lesions. This one has incomplete central clearing.

suspension applied overnight, 2–3 times a week and less frequently as improvement occurs. Other antifungals such as 1% tolnaftate, imidazole compounds (2% miconazole, 1% clotrimazole, 1% econazole) and 1% terbinafine equally effective.

Systemic therapy

Indicated in extensive lesions. Or recurrent disease. Ketoconazole, 400 mg single dose. Or itraconazole 400 mg single dose. Fluconazole, 400 single dose. Terbinafine orally not effective.

DERMATOPHYTOSES (RINGWORM)

Etiology

Infections caused by dermatophytes (species *Trichophyton, Epidermophyton* or *Microsporum*).

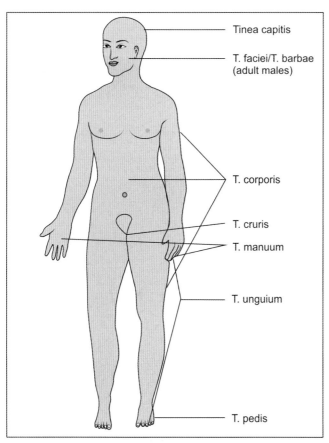

Sites of predilection: Tinea.

Nomenclature

Designated as tinea (to indicate ringworm) followed by the name of the affected part, hence tinea capitis for infection of scalp, tinea cruris for ringworm of groins, thighs and buttocks, tinea corporis (trunk and limbs), tinea barbae (beard), tinea faciei (face), tinea pedis (feet), tinea manuum (hands) and tinea unguium (nails).

Clinical Manifestations

Tinea Corporis

Classic ringworm. All age groups, but generally adults, affected. Any dermatophyte species. Single or multiple, small or large, itchy, well-defined, circinate or annular plaques. Papulovesicles and scales at the active border. Central portion relatively clear; spread peripherally. Heal with hyperpigmentation. Trunk, extremities involved.

Variants

Tinea imbricata

Uncommon variant of tinea corporis confined to certain geographical areas. Caused by *Trichophyton concentricum*. Extremely itchy concentric rings of brownish scales attached at one edge. And clear intervening skin.

Tinea faciei

Tinea of face.

Tinea incognito

Tinea infection modified by steroids. Manifests as ill-defined scaly lesions with minimal inflammation. Diagnosis often based on a positive KOH mount.

Tinea Cruris

Common. Adults affected more frequently. And males due to regional anatomical differences and type of apparrel. Itchy, often bilaterally symmetrical, large half-moon shaped or multiple small, well-defined, oval or circinate scaly plaques with papulovesicles at the active border. Central clearance often incomplete. Groins, thighs, buttocks and scrotum involved.

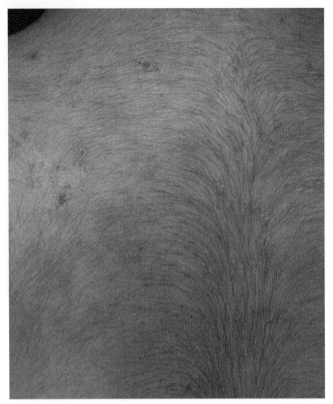

Tinea incognito: ill-defined scaly lesions with minimal scaling. Patient was using topical steroids. With permission of Elsevier, Illustrated Synopsis of Dermatology and Sexually Transmitted Infections.

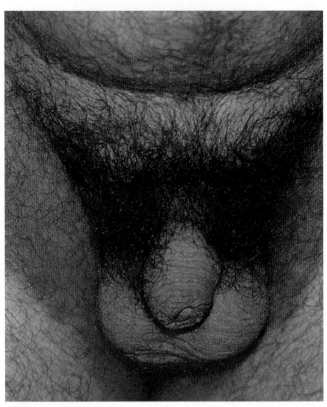

Tinea cruris: bilateral well-defined half moon-shaped lesions with 'active' borders.

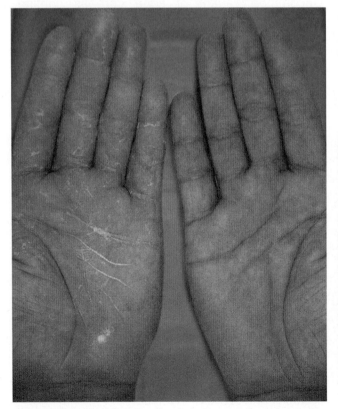

Tinea manuum: well-defined scaly lesions on the palm; unilaterality conspicuous.

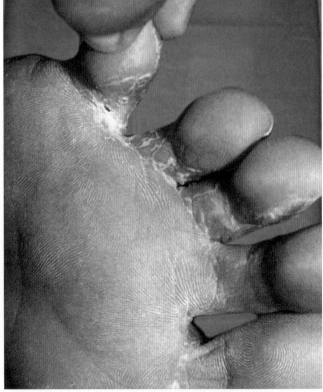

Tinea pedis, intertriginous variant: scaly lesions in between the lateral toe spaces.

Tinea Manuum

Relatively uncommon. Adults affected. Diffuse hyperkeratosis with fine white scales. Or well-defined, circular, scaly patches on the palm. Often unilateral.

Tinea Pedis (Athlete's Foot)

Commonly affects 'shoe-wearing' adult population. Armed forces personnel and athletes particularly affected, hence called 'athlete's foot'. Hyperhidrosis predisposes. Nail infection a frequent association. Three variants:

- *Intertriginous type:* itchy maceration, scaling and fissuring particularly in the lateral toe web spaces (3rd and 4th).
- *Hyperkeratotic type:* diffuse hyperkeratosis with fine scales on soles and heels.
- *Vesicular type:* multiple (often painful) blisters or pustules.

Tinea Capitis

Children, boys more often. Degree of inflammation variable:

- *Non-inflammatory type:* circular or oval scaly, mildly inflammatory partially alopecic areas with broken-off, dull-grey hair or black dots. Hair break off or can be pulled out easily.
- *Inflammatory type:* follicular pustules. Or inflamed, boggy, painful swellings, studded with exudative folliculopustules-kerion. Cervical lymphadenopathy frequent.
- *Favus:* special variant; characterized by hair surrounded by yellowish, cup-shaped crusts called scutula. Results in extensive cicatricial alopecia. Common in Kashmir and the Middle East.

Tinea Barbae

Adult males affected. Inflammatory swellings with follicular pustules—similar to kerion. Occasionally well-defined alopecic patches with scaling and dull broken-off hair. Affected hair either break or can be pulled out painlessly with relative ease.

Tinea Unguium

Caused by dermatophytes *c.f.*, onychomycosis which is caused by any fungus. Adults affected. Cosmetic problem and a reservoir of infection (so association with tinea of other sites). Asymmetric involvement; all nails seldom affected. Toe nails more frequently involved. Several subtypes recognized:

- *Distal lateral subungual onychomycosis (DLSO):* manifests as yellow-white subungual hyperkeratosis and onycholysis.
- *White superficial onychomycosis (WSO):* manifests as small, white, speckled or powdery patches on surface of nail plate which becomes roughened and crumbles easily.
- *Proximal subungual onychomycosis (PSO):* manifests as area of leukonychia in proximal nail plate that moves distally with nail growth. Seen in HIV-infected.
- *Endonyx onychomycosis (EO):* manifests as milky white discoloration of the nail plate with no subungual hyperkeratosis or onycholysis.

Investigations

Diagnosis often clinical. In doubtful cases, KOH mount, Wood's lamp examination (in tinea capitis), culture (in tinea unguium), and rarely biopsy necessary.

Wood's Lamp Examination

Helpful in screening epidemics of tinea capitis. Typically green fluorescence, though not all species fluoresce.

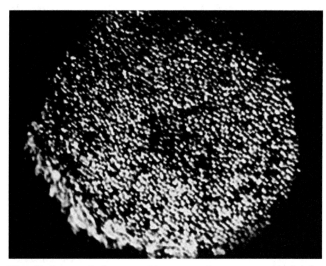

Wood's lamp of tinea capitis: green fluorescence. Useful for screening epidemics, though not always positive.

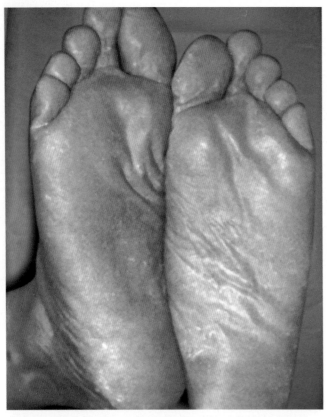

Tinea pedis, hyperkeratotic variant: diffuse scaling of the soles of the feet.

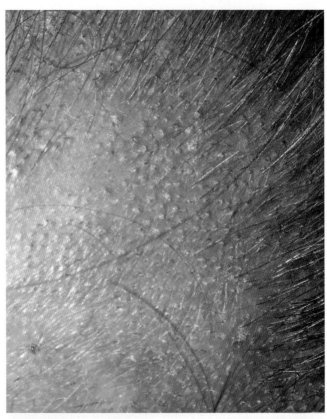

Tinea capitis, non-inflammatory variant: alopecic areas with black dots. With permission Elsevier.

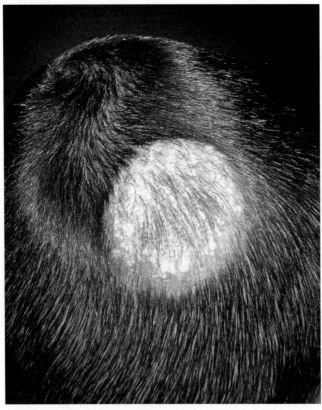

Tinea capitis, kerion: solitary boggy plaque, studded with follicular pustules, overlying hair sparsening.

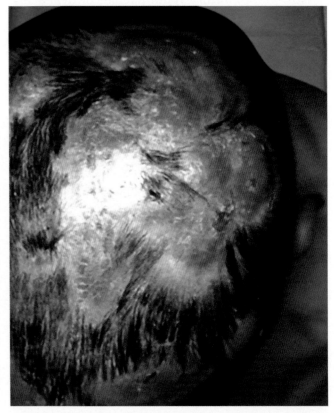

Tinea capitis, kerion: alopecic areas with multiple inflammatory swellings.

Direct Microscopy

Samples include skin scrapings, nail clippings or plucked hair dissolved in KOH. Area cleaned and active edge of skin lesion superficially scraped with scalpel. Or hair pulled. Or nail clippings and subungual debris collected and treated in a drop of 10–20% KOH solution, on a glass slide for half an hour or longer (hair and nails require several hours). Viewed under microscope with subdued

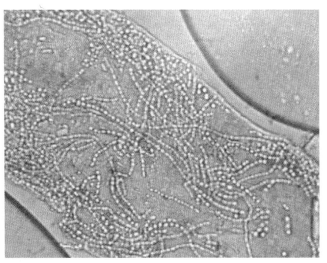

Potassium hydroxide mount of tinea capitis, endothrix: spores inside hair shaft. With permission Macmillan Fungal infections.

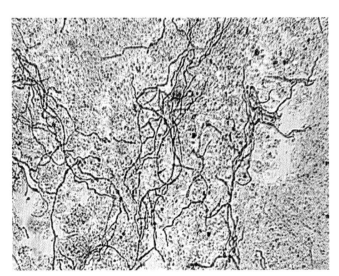

Potassium hydroxide mount of tinea corporis: septate hyphae of dermatophytes.

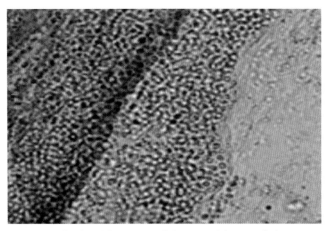

Potassium hydroxide mount of tinea capitis, ectothrix: spores on surface of hair shaft.

light. Fungal elements seen as long septate, branching filaments (hyphae) in dermatophytoses. In tinea capitis 2 patterns seen—endothrix (infection within hair shaft) and ectothrix (infection outside hair shaft).

Culture

Necessary for onychomycosis to differentiate dermatophytic (tinea unguium) from non dermatophytic infections to optimize treatment. Culture media used include Sabouraud's dextrose agar and dermatophyte culture medium.

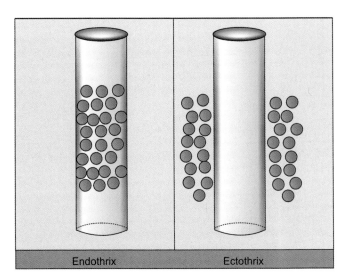

Endothrix | Ectothrix

Tinea capitis: diagrammatic representation of endothrix and ectothrix. In endothrix, organisms (spores or arthroconidia) inside the hair shaft while in ectothrix they are outside the shaft.

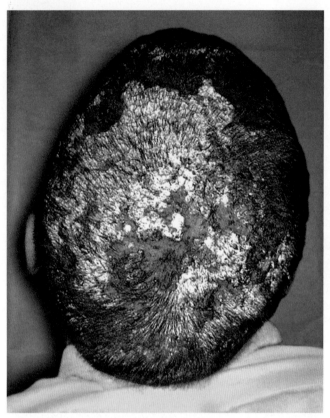

Tinea capitis, favus: depressed crusted lesions with cicatricial alopecia.

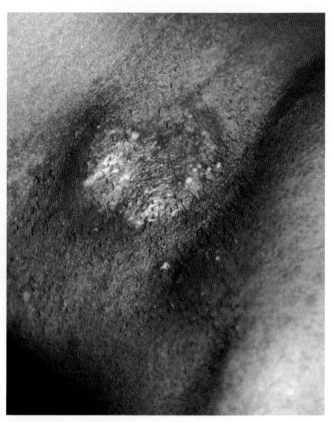

Tinea barbae: inflammatory boggy swelling with pustules, in beard area of adult male.

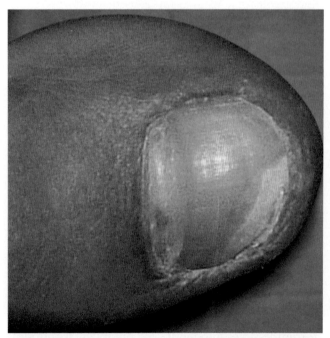

Tinea unguium, distal lateral subungual onychomycosis: manifests as distal and lateral yellow white subungual hyperkeratosis and onycholysis.

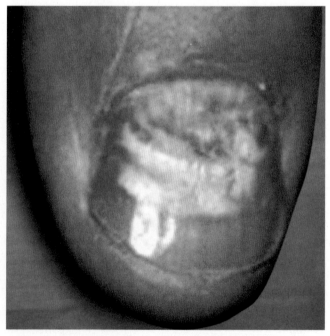

Tinea unguium, proximal subungual onychomycosis: area of leukonychia in proximal part of nail plate.

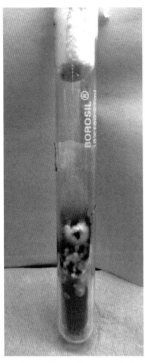

Culture of dermatophyte: Growth occurs in 7–14 days. Speciation based on culture characteristic and morphology of micro and macroconidia on microscopy.

Courtesy: Dr Immaculata Xess, Department of Microbiology, All India Institute of Medical Sciences (AIIMS), New Delhi.

Histopathology

Rarely required. Fungal elements best visualized using special stains like PAS.

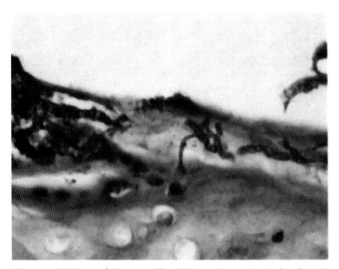

Histopathology of tinea pedis: PAS positive septate hyphae in stratum corneum.

Treatment

General Measures

Keep area dry and areated.

Tinea capitis: Use antifungal shampoos. Do not share combs/brushes.

T. pedis: Avoid occlusive footwear.

T. cruris: Avoid synthetic underclothes.

Specific Therapy

Topical therapy

Topical therapy adequate for localized lesions (except tinea unguium. And tinea capitis and barbae). Regular application of any of the several antifungal agents (creams, gels, lotions, powders) of imidazoles (1% clotrimazole, 2% miconazole, 1% econazole, 2% ketoconazole, 0.5% fluconazole), 1% tolnaftate, 1% ciclopirox olamine, 1% haloprogin, 1% naftifine hydrochloride, 1% terbinafine, 1% butenafine, 20% undecylinic acid and its salts. Continue treatment for a couple of weeks, after clinical subsidence. Distal involvement of single nail plate may be treated with 1% amorolfine lacquer once a week. Or 8% ciclopirox lacquer daily for 8–9 months.

Systemic therapy

Invariably needed for tinea unguium, tinea capitis and tinea barbae. And extensive tinea corporis or resistant tinea cruris infections.

Terbinafine: fungicidal. Treatment of choice (except for some forms of tinea capitis, where griseofulvin preferred). Given as 250 mg daily for 2 weeks (tinea corporis, cruris, pedis, manuum) to 6 weeks (finger nail infection) to 12 weeks (toe nail infection). Cost a limiting factor.

Itraconazole: Broad spectrum. Preferred to terbinafine in onychomycosis which has not been speciated by culture. Given as 400 mg × 7 day pulses every month for 2 (finger nail infection)-3 (toe nail infection) cycles.

Griseofulvin: Treatment of choice for tinea capitis (caused by *Microsporum spp*). Given as 10 mg/kg, after a fatty meal for 6–12 weeks.

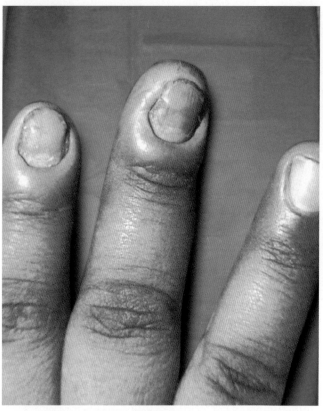

Candidal paronychia: subacute inflammation of the posterior and lateral nail folds with detachment from nail plate. Deformity of the nail plate secondary to involvement of nail matrix.

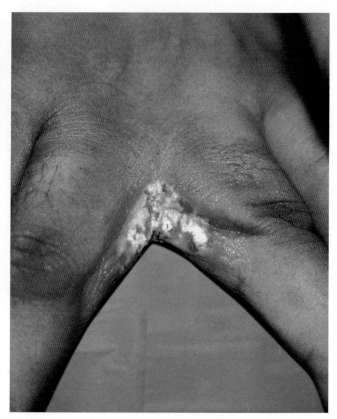

Candidal intertrigo: macerated and eroded interdigital space.

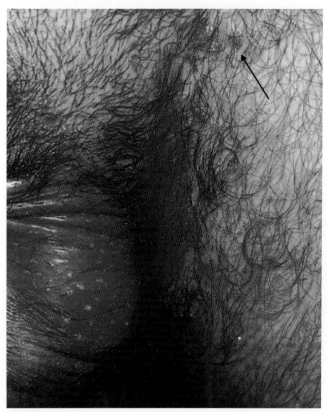

Candidal intertrigo: acutely inflamed erythematous lesions in the folds of skin. Note satellite vesiculo-pustules.

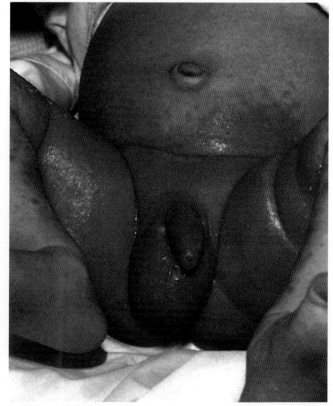

Napkin candidiasis: acutely inflamed intertriginous areas with satellite vesiculo-pustules.

CANDIDIASIS (CANDIDOSIS)

Etiology

Candida albicans, a yeast-like fungus. Also *C. glabrata, C. tropicalis* or other species. Candida a normal commensal of gastrointestinal tract and vagina. Systemic broad spectrum antibiotics, corticosteroid therapy, diabetes mellitus, HIV infection and malignancies and their chemotherapy predispose.

Clinical Manifestations

Several parts of body affected.

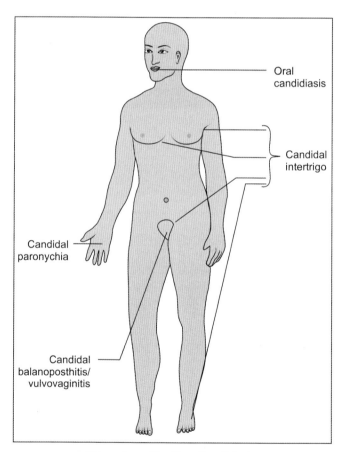

Sites of predilection: Candidiasis.

Paronychia

Infection of posterior and lateral nail folds. Seen in adults. Housewives, washermen, cooks, bartenders or people engaged in 'wet' work prone. Nail folds red, swollen, tender and detached from the nail plate. Occasionally a bead of pus can be expressed. Nail plate deformed and discolored secondary to involvement of the matrix (under the posterior nail fold). No mass under the nail plate. Many or all finger nails may be involved (*c.f.* tinea unguium).

Candidal Intertrigo

Common. Obesity and diabetes mellitus predispose. Erythematous, raw, moist, macerated and eroded areas with well-defined fringed edges and satellite superficial vesiculo-pustular lesions. Itching or burning present. Interdigital spaces, groins, axillae or area under pendulous breasts.

Napkin Candidiasis

Infants or young children. Occlusive diapers, poor local hygiene, use of topical steroids and systemic broad spectrum antibiotics predispose. Acute diaper eruption with angry looking intertriginous denuded areas with or without fringed borders and satellite vesiculopustules.

Genital Candidiasis

Predisposed by diabetes, intake of broad spectrum antibiotics, oral contraceptives and pregnancy (in women). Sometimes sexually transmitted:
- *Candidal balanoposthitis:* macerated glans and prepuce; lesions with fringed margin.
- *Candidal vulvovaginitis:* thick white curdy vaginal discharge. And extremely itchy, erythematous vulvitis.

Oral Candidiasis

Disease of diseased generally. Several variants described:
- *Acute pseudomembranous candidiasis:* most common variant. Neonates. And in diseased mucosa (pemphigus vulgaris, oral lichen planus). Discrete plaques surmounted by creamy/curdy membrane. On buccal mucosa, palate, gums.
- *Acute atrophic candidiasis:* use of broad spectrum antibiotics and immunosuppression predisposes. Atrophic erythematous areas.
- *Chronic atrophic candidiasis:* in denture wearing elderly. Sharply demarcated erythematous atrophic area on palate.

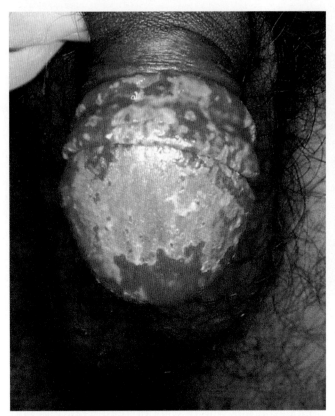

Candidal balanoposthitis: macerated glans and prepuce; eroded lesions have fringed margins.

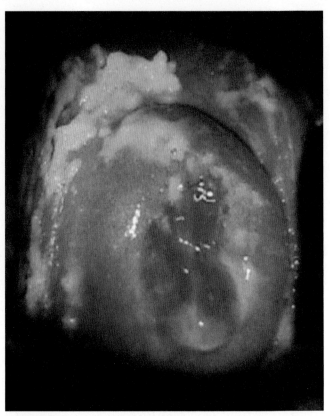

Vaginal discharge due to candida: Curdy white discharge coating the vaginal walls and cervical os.

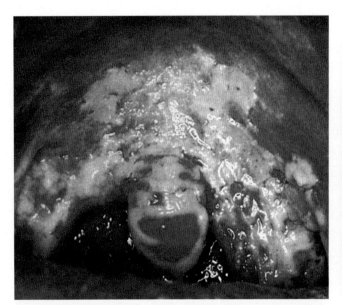

Oral candidiasis, acute pseudomembranous: discrete and confluent 'curdy' lesions in a patient with widespread metastatic malignant lesions.

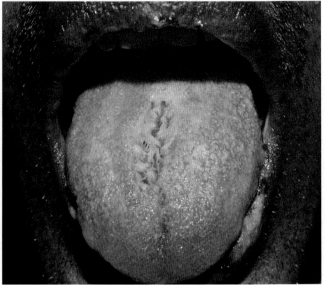

Oral candidiasis, chronic hyperplastic variant: adherent white plaque on tongue of a smoker. With permission Elsevier. Khanna N. Illustrated Synopsis of Dermatology and STDs.

- *Chronic hyperplastic candidiasis (candidal leucoplakia):* in smokers. Adherent firm plaques on tongue and buccal mucosa.
- *Angular cheilitis (perleche):* raw angles of mouth with curdy membrane.

Investigations

Direct Microscopy

Clinical diagnosis of candidiasis to be substantiated by demonstration of fungi (budding yeasts and pseudohyphae) in 10% KOH solution. Mycelial filaments (hyphae) suggest a pathogenic role.

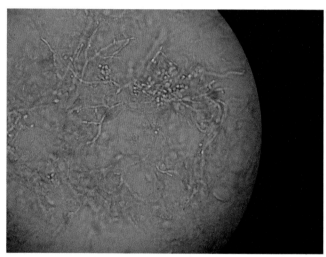

Potassium hydroxide mount of candida: showing budding yeasts and pseudohyphae.

Culture

Usually not necessary. Except for speciation in treatment of poorly-responsive patients.

Treatment

General Measures

Maintain scrupulous dryness of involved part. Rinse off soap thoroughly. Diabetes mellitus, obesity, other endocrinopathies or immunodeficiency states should be corrected.

Specific Therapy

Topical therapy

For localized infection. Imidazole or nystatin preparations-creams, lotions, oral paints effective. Oral nystatin not absorbed, helps in eradicating the intestinal reservoir; of no direct therapeutic value.

Systemic therapy

Systemic therapy for extensive infection. And for recurrent disease. Fluconazole 50–150 mg daily for 5–7 days. Given weekly for recurrent infection.

MYCETOMA (MADURA FOOT)

Mycetoma, literally a fungal tumor.

Etiology

Caused by:
- *Fungi:* called **eumycotic mycetoma**. Common organisms include *Madurella mycetomatis, M. grisea*.
- *Actinomycetes:* called **actinomycotic mycetoma**. Common organism include *Actinomadura madurae, A pelletieri*.

Epidemiology

Adults, often males.

Clinical Manifestations

Ill-defined, firm to woody-hard, subcutaneous swelling that develops sinuses discharging seropurulent fluid containing white or colored granules (microcolonies of organisms). Affected part irregularly enlarged and deformed. Underlying muscles and bone(s) may be involved. Insidious progression over years; simultaneous healing with scars and deformities. Foot (so **Madura foot**) or other parts of the body. No lymphadenopathy. No systemic involvement.

Investigations

Direct Microscopy

Fungi (or bacteria) demonstrable on direct microscopy of granules in a 10–20% KOH preparation or using Gram stain.

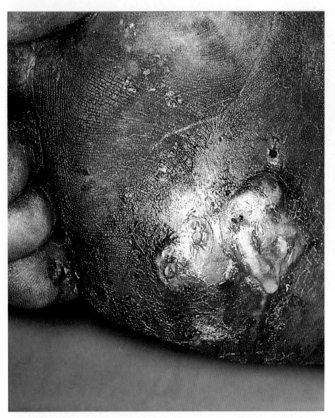

Mycetoma foot: woody-hard subcutaneous swelling with multiple nodules and sinuses.

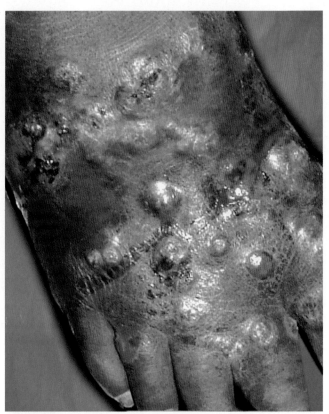

Mycetoma: multiple nodules with discharging sinuses on foot–so called madura foot.

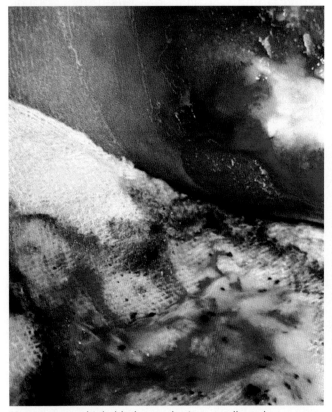

Mycetoma: multiple black granules in pus collected on a gauze piece, left covering the sinus for 24–48 hours.

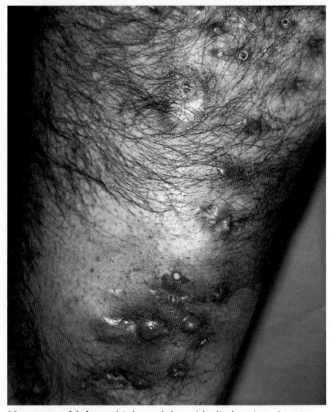

Mycetoma thigh: multiple nodules with discharging sinuses.

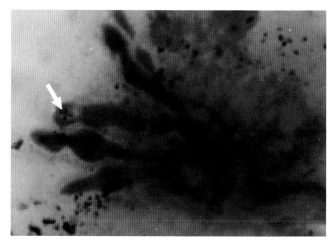

Gram stain mount of mycetoma granule: shows fungal hyphae.

Courtesy: Dr Immaculata Xess, Department of Microbiology, All India Institute of Medical Sciences (AIIMS), New Delhi.

Culture

To differentiate actinomycotic and eumycotic mycetoma.

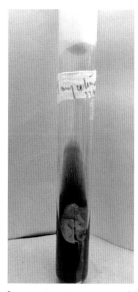

Culture of grain from mycetoma: growth of *M. mycetomatis* from a patient with eumycotic mycetoma.

Courtesy: Dr Immaculata Xess, Department of Microbiology, All India Institute of Medical Sciences (AIIMS), New Delhi.

Histopathology

Histological sections using hematoxylin and eosin stains and preferably PAS or Gram's stain. Shows chronic inflammatory reaction with neutrophilic abscesses and scattered giant cells and grains in center.

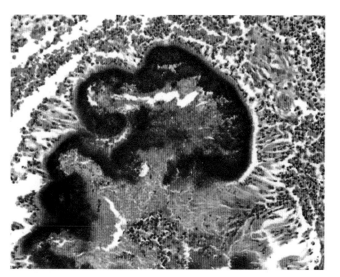

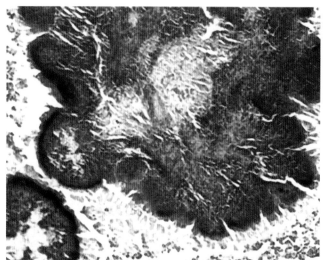

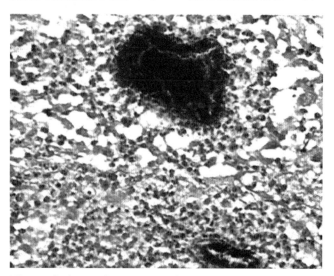

Histopathology of mycetoma: hematoxylin and eosin stain (top); Gram's stain (middle); Ziehl-Neelsen stain (bottom).

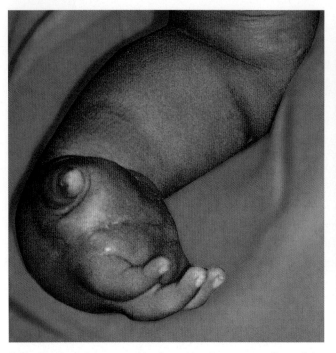

Subcutaneous zygomycosis: firm subcutaneous swelling of the arm with an erythematous halo.

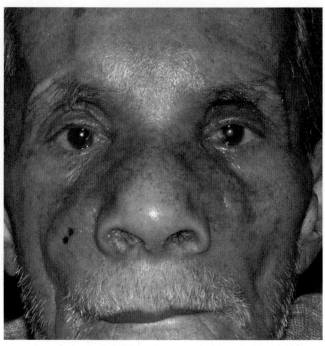

Subcutaneous zygomycosis: firm subcutaneous swelling of central face, with well-defined margin.

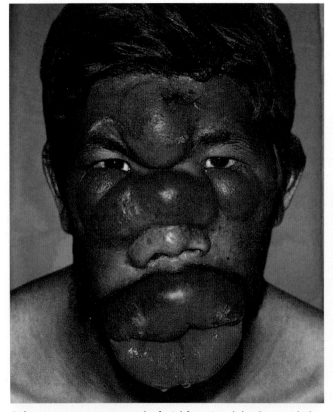

Subcutaneous zygomycosis: facial form in adults. Responded to potassium iodide dramatically.

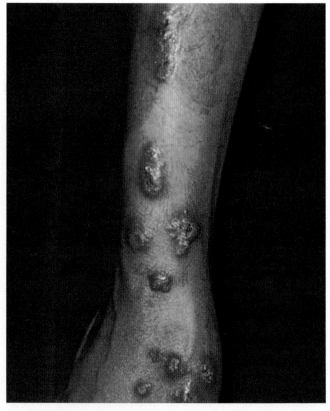

Sporotrichosis, lymphangitic variant: granulomatous, lesions, arranged linearly due to lymphatic spread. Permission with Elsevier.

Treatment

Actinomycotic Mycetoma

High doses of dapsone (200 mg/day) or cotrimoxazole preferably combined with another antibiotic such as tetracycline for 6 months or longer. Rifampicin and amikacin also useful in some patients. Often given as a 2 step regime.

Eumycetoma Mycetoma

Generally not amenable to chemotherapy. Dapsone or newer antifungals of imidazole (ketoconazole) or triazole (itraconazole, fluconazole) group or amphotericin B (highly toxic) may be tried. Unresponsive mycetomas require surgical intervention, even amputation.

SUBCUTANEOUS ZYGOMYCOSIS

Etiology

Caused by *Basidiobolus haptosporus* (in children) or *Conidiobolus coronatus* (in young adults).

Clinical Manifestations

Rare. Asymptomatic, gradually progressive, firm subcutaneous swelling, freely movable over deeper structures but adherent to overlying skin. Well marginated mass characteristically lifted up by inserting the fingers underneath. Erythematous periphery. No lymphadenopathy. On buttocks, limbs in children. And face, paranasal areas in adults.

Investigations

Direct Microscopy

Not usually helpful.

Culture

Organisms readily cultured on SDA.

Histopathology

Chronic granuloma with large number of eosinophils. Fungus presents as large strap like fungi without cross walls, often surrounded by refractile eosinophilic material (Splendore-Hoeppli phenomenon).

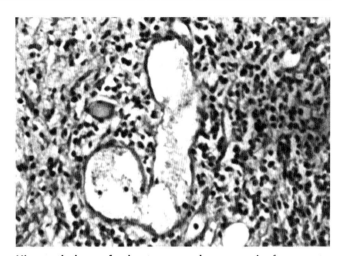

Histopathology of subcutaneous phycomycosis: fungus present as large strap-like elements without septae. Note eosinophils.

Treatment

Drug of choice, saturated solution of potassium iodide. Most lesions respond (almost dramatically) to 15–45 drops/day for several weeks. Iodism temporary and reversible. Treat resistant or relapsed cases with itraconazole 400 mg/day orally for several weeks.

SPOROTRICHOSIS

Etiology

Sporothrix schenckii. Natural habitat, wood and soil.

Epidemiology

Wide geographic distribution. Common in North Eastern parts of India and foot hills of Himalayas.

Clinical Manifestations

Infection preceded by an injury, often a wood prick. Two variants recognized:
- *Lymphangitic:* initial noduloulcerative lesion; spreads in a linear fashion along the lymphatics. Intervening lymphatic cord between two lesions, pathognomic.
- *Fixed:* single noduloulcerative plaque. Regional lymph nodes may be enlarged. Exposed parts of body affected.

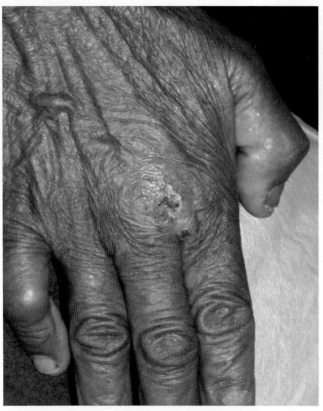

Sporotrichosis, fixed variant: single noduloulcerative plaque on hand (exposed parts). Face another common site.

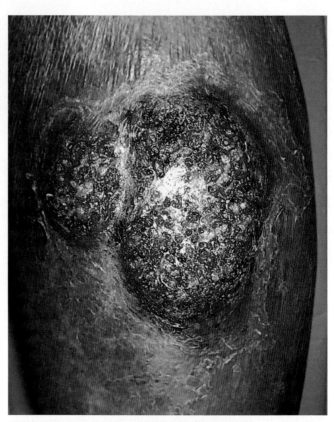

Chromomycosis: early superficially ulcerative and vegetative lesions.

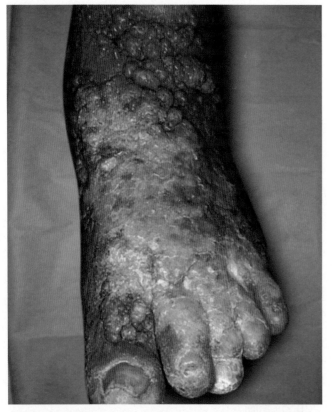

Chromomycosis: multiple vegetative lesions on the lower leg.

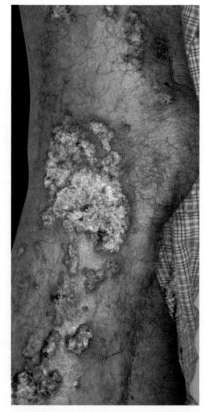

Chromomycosis: multiple vegetating nodules with black dots.

Investigations

Direct Microscopy

KOH mount rarely positive.

Culture

Ready isolated on SDA.

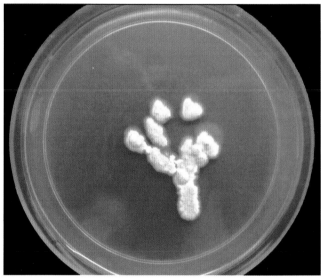

Culture of *Sporothrix schenkii*: leathery moist cream colonies which darken with age.

Courtesy: Dr Immaculata Xess, Department of Microbiology, All India Institute of Medical Sciences (AIIMS), New Delhi.

Histopathology

Mixed granuloma with neutrophil microabscesses. Sometimes small cigar shaped/oval yeast cells with surrounding asteroid body demonstrated.

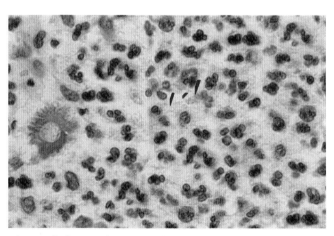

Histopathology of sporotrichosis: cigar shaped organisms usually very scanty. Conspicuous asteroid bodies representing a foreign body tissue reaction.

Treatment

Potassium iodide (KI) is almost specific. Five drops of saturated KI gradually increased to 15 drops orally, three times a day. Treatment continued for several weeks after clinical cure. Itraconazole 100–200 mg/day and terbinafine 250–500 mg/day, useful alternatives. Local application of heat useful in some patients.

CHROMOMYCOSIS

Etiology

Caused by several saprophytic, pigmented pathogens of species of *Phialophora*, *Fonsecaea* and *Cladophialophora*.

Clinical Manifestations

Adult males. Multiple, hyperkeratotic, warty, rough, dry plaques or cauliflower-like hard tumors with healthy intervening areas. May assume massive proportions (mossy foot). Black dots often surmount plaques. Satellite lesions along lymphatics. Feet and legs commonly affected. General health unaffected.

Investigations

Direct Microscopy

Skin scraping taken from skin surface. Best to take a black dot. Shows cluster of pigmented cells.

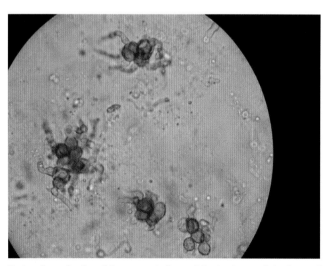

Potassium hydroxide mount from black dots of lesion of chromoblastomycosis: shows cluster of pigmented cells.

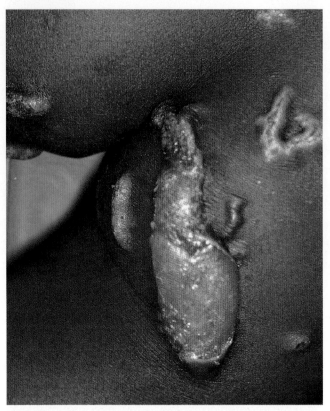

Lobomycosis: keloidal and ulcerative plaques, generally on exposed parts.

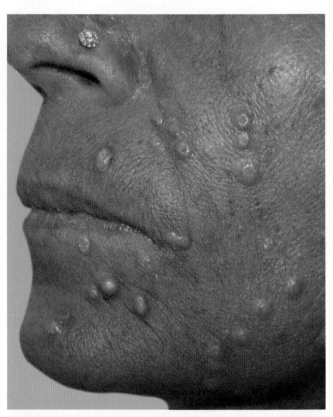

Cryptococcosis, in an HIV-positive patient: multiple skin colored papules with umbilication, resembling molluscum contagiosum on the face. Confirmed on biopsy.

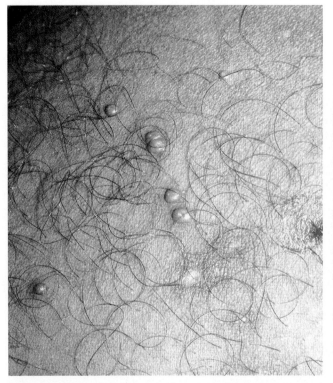

Cryptococcosis: close up of molluscum-like lesion. Note central crater.

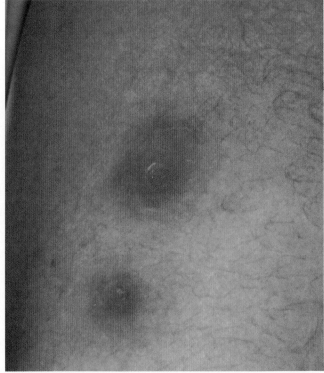

Cryptococcosis: sharply marginated, ulcerated plaques.

Culture

Black colonies.

Histopathology

Histopathology confirmatory. Foreign body granuloma with microabscesses. And brown fungal cells, in giant cells or in microabscesses.

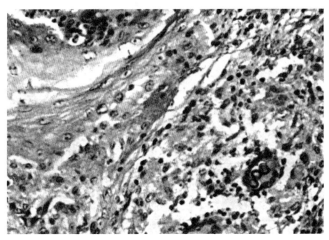

Histopathology of chromomycosis: foreign body granuloma with microabscesses and brown fungal cells.

Treatment

Systemic itraconazole or terbinafine combined with oral flucytosine often successful. Flucytosine with amphotericin B, an alternative. Ketoconazole not effective. Surgical removal of small lesions, preferably in combination with antifungal therapy. Treatment given till clinical resolution (several months).

LOBOMYCOSIS (KELOIDAL BLASTOMYCOSIS)

Rare. Caused by *Lacazia loboi*. Cutaneous lesions include nodules or plaques that progress insidiously to keloids/hypertrophic scars. May ulcerate. On exposed sites (face, legs, arms). No lymphadenopathy. No systemic involvement.

Treatment

Unsatisfactory. Excision of localized lesions an option.

CRYPTOCOCCOSIS

Etiology

Caused by *Cryptococcus neoformans*—a fungus of low virulence. Immunocompromised individuals predisposed. Portal of entry, respiratory tract.

Epidemiology

Rare. Widespread geographic distribution.

Clinical Manifestations

Central nervous system involvement, a dominant feature. Skin lesions infrequent and nonspecific—acneiform papules, molluscum contagiosum–like lesions, crusted/vegetating plaques. Rarely primary cutaneous cryptococcosis.

Investigations

Culture

Easy to culture.

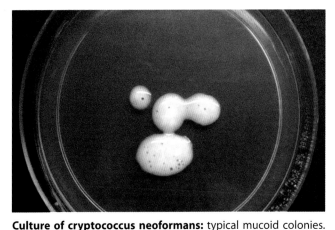

Culture of cryptococcus neoformans: typical mucoid colonies. Confirmed by microscopy and biochemical tests.

Courtesy: Dr Immaculata Xess, Department of Microbiology, All India Institute of Medical Sciences (AIIMS), New Delhi.

Histopathology

Skin lesions non-specific, so require histopathological confirmation. Pauci inflammatory or granulomatous lesion. Organisms visible as encapsulated budding yeasts. Special stain mucicarmine, Indiana ink, Nigro stain.

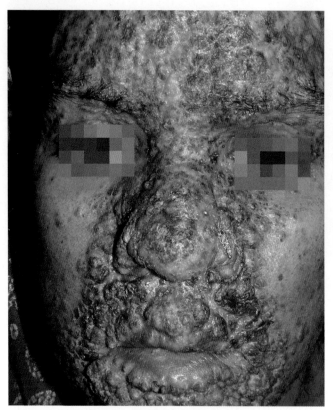

Histoplasmosis, disseminated in an HIV positive patient: multiple, disseminated crusted nodules and plaques. Diagnosis often made histopathologically.

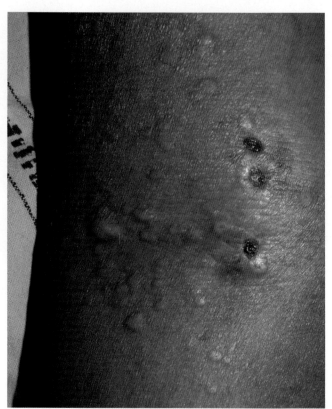

Histoplasmosis, disseminated: multiple papular lesions.

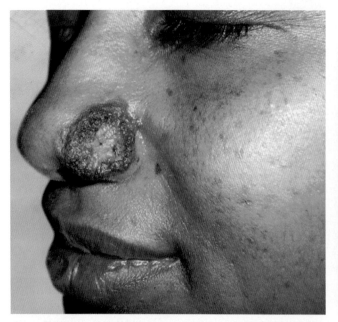

Histoplasmosis, primary cutaneous: well-defined erythematous scaly nodule which on biopsy revealed histoplasmosis.

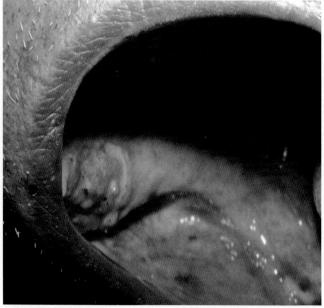

Histoplasmosis, disseminated: oral ulcers in a patient with disseminated histoplasmosis. Always rule out Addison's disease in patients with disseminated histoplasmosis.

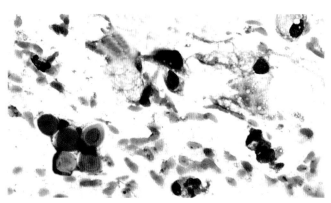

Smear of cryptococcosis: characteristically thick capsuled *Cryptococcus neoformans.*

Giemsa stained smear of *H. capsulatum*: shows intracellular small budding yeasts.

Courtesy: Dr Immaculata Xess, Department of Microbiology, All India Institute of Medical Sciences (AIIMS), New Delhi.

Treatment

Systemic involvement treated with amphotericin B, preferably combined with flucytosine. If cutaneous involvement alone, treat with fluconazole, 400–600 mg/day for 2 weeks. In patients with AIDS, treat with amphotericin B combined with flucytosine, followed by long term use of fluconazole.

HISTOPLASMOSIS

Etiology

Histoplasma capsulatum, an environmental saprophyte. Immunosuppressed individuals predisposed. Acquired by inhalation of spores.

Epidemiology

Widespread geographic distribution.

Clinical Manifestations

Spectrum of asymptomatic infection, benign symptomatic infection to progressive symptomatic infection. Respiratory infection either acute, or chronic. Acute disseminated infection in AIDS patients. Skin lesions non-specific—small papules (molluscum-like) to warty/ulcerated lesions. Chronic disseminated infection presents with oral ulcers and Addison's disease. Rare primary cutaneous infection.

Investigations

Direct Microscopy

Most frequently from sputum and blood.

Culture

Confirmed by culture. Always warn the lab, as highly infectious.

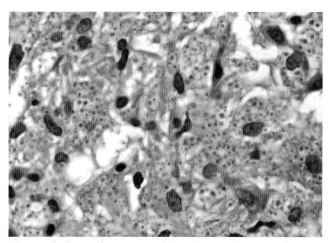

Histopathology of cutaneous histoplasmosis: *H. capsulatum* is seen packed in macrophages as tiny yeast forms.

Courtesy: Prof M Ramam, All India Institute of Medical Sciences (AIIMS), New Delhi.

Histopathology

Histopath confirmation often necessary. *H.capsulatum* appears as intracellular yeast cells. Special stains include GMS with which the organism stains black.

Serology

Serological tests available both for antibody as also antigen detection. Latter especially useful in AIDS patients.

Treatment

For localized forms, itraconazole. And for disseminated forms, amphotericin B.

3

Viral Infections

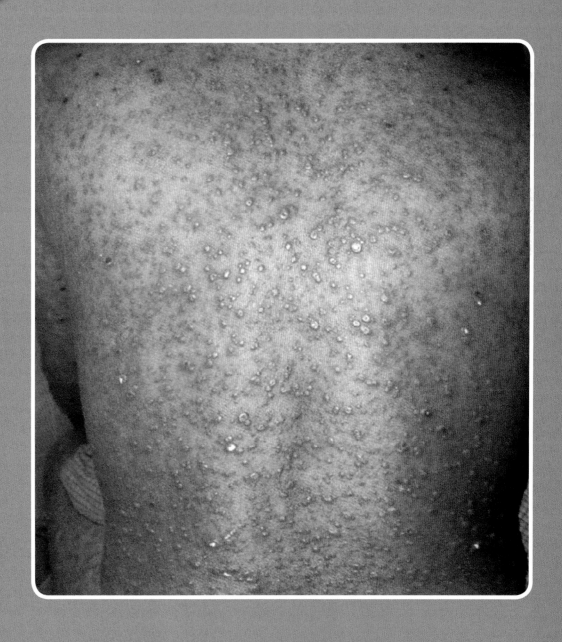

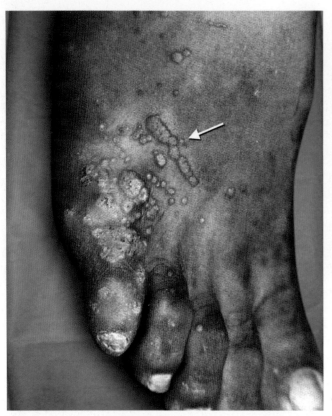

Verruca vulgaris foot: flat-topped and verrucous lesions. Linear spread due to auto inoculation.

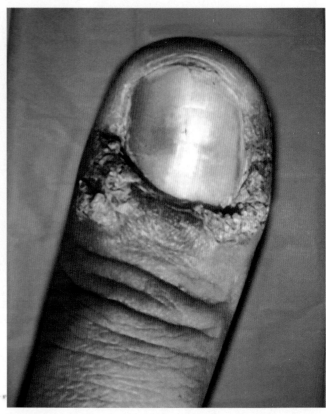

Periungual warts: variant of verruca vulgaris which often distorts the nail.

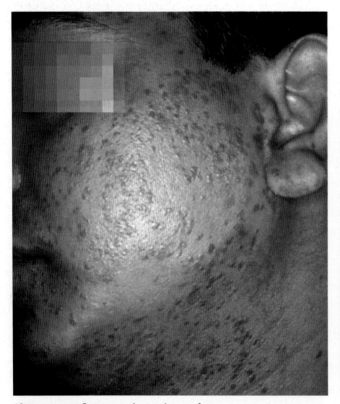

Plane warts: flat-topped papules on face.

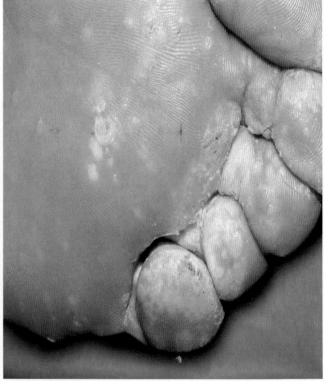

Superficial plantar warts (mosaic warts): painless, warts, often confluent.

Viral infections of the skin may be purely cutaneous such as warts and molluscum contagiosum. Or be part of an exanthem of a systemic viremia such as variola, measles and varicella. Since viruses multiply within living cells, skin infections generally confined to the epidermis.

WARTS

Etiology

Caused by human papilloma viruses (HPV). Several types of HPV. Good correlation between HPV type and clinical manifestations.

Epidemiology

Common. Children and young adults affected. Larger in size and number in immunocompromised individuals.

Clinical Manifestations

Verruca Vulgaris

Common warts. Children or young adults. Firm, irregular verrucous papules. Vary in number, size and shape. Distributed anywhere on the body, but more particularly on the exposed trauma prone sites.

Variant: periungual warts which often distort nails.

Verruca Plana

More frequent in children. Asymptomatic. Smooth, skin-colored, flat-topped papules. Trauma (such as caused by shaving the beard) promotes spread by autoinoculation (erroneously termed Koebner's isomorphic phenomenon). On the face or hands.

Plantar Warts

Two variants described:
- **Mosaic warts**: painless, superficial warts often confluent.
- **Myrmecia:** painful, deeper keratotic papules with a central depression.

Anogenital Warts

Sexually transmitted. Several variants described:
- **Condyloma acuminata:** erythematous fleshy lesions with finger like projections. On mucosal surface.
- **Plane and common warts:** typical lesions; penile shaft.
- **Bowenoid papulosis:** velvety brown papules.
- **Buschke Lowenstein tumor:** giant condyloma acuminata or verrucous carcinoma.

Filiform Warts

Keratotic protruberances. In beard region.

Epidermodysplasia Verruciformis

HPV infection in genetically predisposed. Two types of lesions flat scaly pityriasis versicolor-like lesions. And plane wart-like papules. May develop malignancy in photoexposed parts.

Investigations

Diagnosis clinical. Rarely biopsy resorted to. Shows large keratinocytes with eccentric pyknotic nucleus surrounded by perinuclear halo (koilocytes).

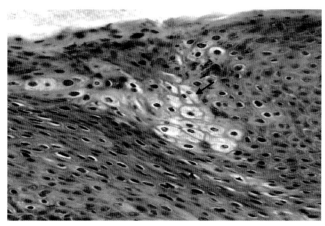

Histopathology of warts: shows koilocytes which are epidermal cells with hyperchromatic irregular nuclei and a perinuclear halo.

Treatment

Spontaneous resolution of warts not uncommon. Several treatment modalities available. Destroy mechanically, with cryotherapy or chemical or electric cautery or surgically. Or treat with immunotherapy.

Cryotherapy: with liquid nitrogen using a cotton tip applicator/spray. Or carbon dioxide slush or stick.

Chemical cautery: scrape with a curette and cauterize with 50–100% trichloroacetic acid or phenol. Deep curetting results in avoidable scars.

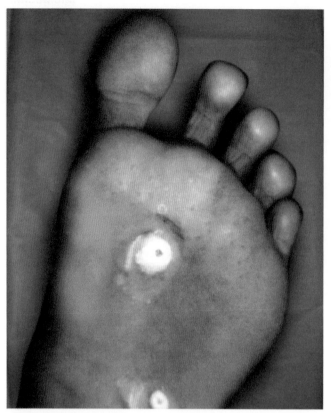

Deep plantar warts (myrmecia): paring off of the keratotic plaque will reveal a central irregular core.

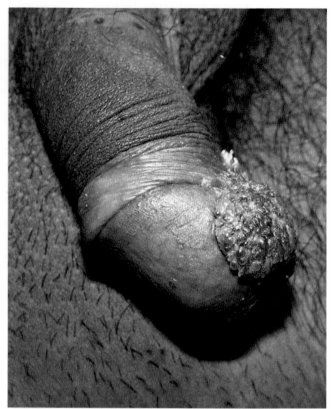

Condyloma acuminata: verrucous, fleshy plaque on glans. With permission.

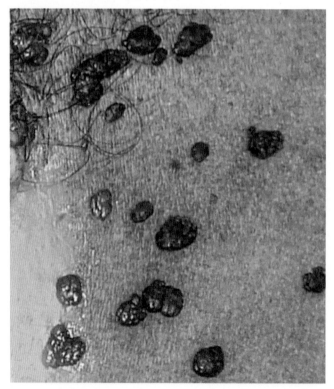

Bowenoid papulosis: multiple, small hyperpigmented papules with a velvety surface on upper thigh. Diagnosis confirmed histopathologically-shows carcinoma *in situ*.

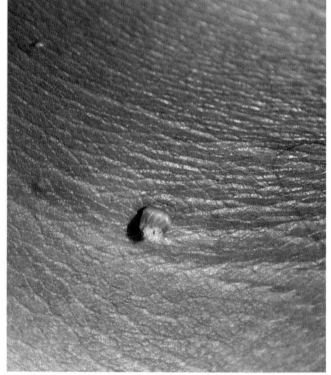

Filiform warts: keratotic protruberance in the neck.

Electrodessication: followed by curettage also useful.

Keratolytics: salicylic acid, 10–20%, alone or combined with lactic acid often gainfully employed.

Anogenital warts vaccine: by avalent and tetracycline vaccines available for imiquimod (5%)—an immune response modifier, treatment of choice. Self-applied thrice a week; preferable to achieve contact period of 4–6 hours for at least 12–16 weeks. Also podophyllin resin, 25% in alcohol or tincture benzoin co. effective in condylomata acuminata. Should be physician-applied strictly to the lesions (adjoining areas protected with vaseline application) and washed off after 2–4 hours to avoid irritation. Podophyllotoxin, a patient-applied alternative.

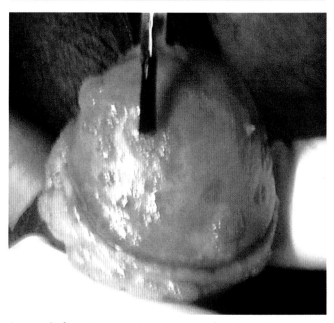

Anogenital warts: topical application of podophyllin (using a brush) after protecting adjacent normal skin with petroleum.

MOLLUSCUM CONTAGIOSUM

Etiology

Caused by a pox virus *Molluscum contagiosum virus*. Possibly transmitted by direct contact, including sexual. Or by fomites. Incubation period variable, 2 weeks to 2 months.

Epidemiology

Common in children.

Clinical Manifestations

Glistening pale-white, umbilicated, dome-shaped papules. Pinhead to 1 cm in size. Multiple, asymptomatic—often auto-innoculated lesions (pseudoisomorphic phenomenon). Distributed anywhere. Sexually transmitted lesions present on or around the genitals. Sometimes perilesional dermatitis (molluscum dermatitis). Occasional secondary infection. Giant, extensive lesions in HIV positive patients.

Investigations

Usually clinical. In doubtful/atypical cases, investigations assist diagnosis.

Dermoscopy

Central core conspicuous. Variety of blood vessel patterns described, including corona of blood vessels.

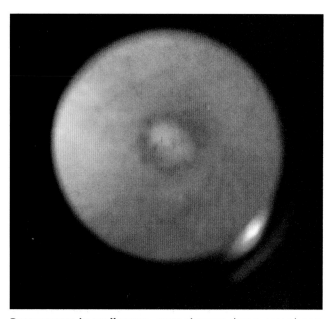

Dermoscopy in molluscum contagiosum: shows central core and corona of blood vessels.

Cytopathology

Giemsa Stain

Giemsa stained extruded material shows intracytoplasmic molluscum inclusion bodies.

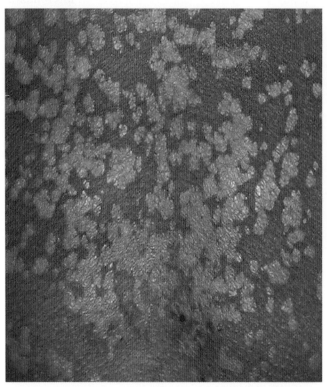

Epidermodysplasia verruciformis: extensive pityriasis versi-color like lesions. Patient also had plane wart like papules.

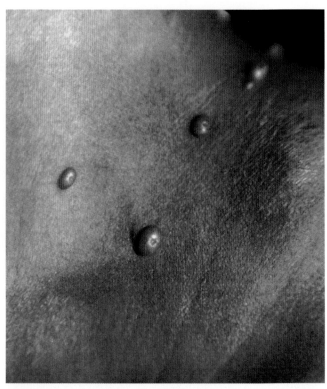

Molluscum contagiosum: umbilicated dome-shaped papules and nodules.

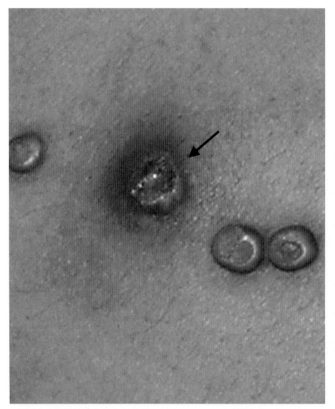

Molluscum contagiosum: with secondary infection.

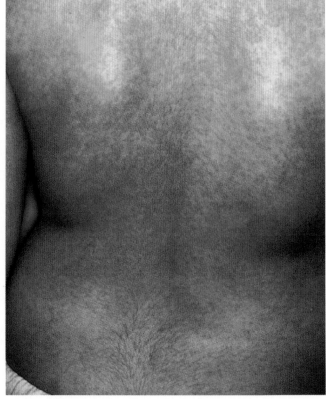

Measles: pink macular rash on the trunk.

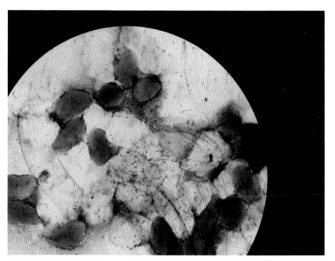

Giemsa stain of extruded material from molluscum contagiosum lesion: shows intracytoplasmic bodies.

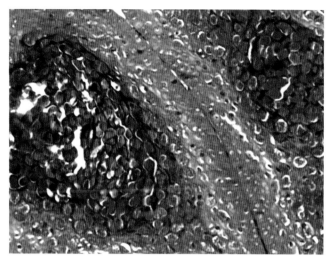

Histopathology of molluscum contagiosum: shows eosinophilic intracytoplasmic bodies (Henderson-Patterson bodies) pushing nucleus to periphery (signet ring appearance).

Normal Saline Mount

Crush smear of extirpated material mounted in normal saline shows ballooned keratinocytes stuffed with round intracytoplasmic molluscum bodies.

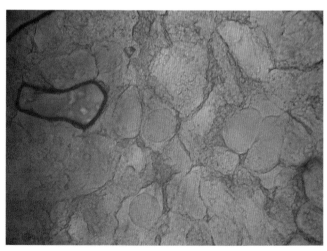

Normal saline mount of crush smear of molluscum body: shows multiple ballooned up keratinocytes stuffed with round intracytoplasmic molluscum bodies.

Biopsy

Histopathology confirmatory. Shows typical intracytoplasmic eosinophilic bodies (**Henderson-Patterson bodies**) pushing nucleus to periphery (signet ring appearance).

Treatment

Specific Measures

Needle extirpation, often followed by trichloroacetic acid (20–30%) application. Or curettage. Or cryotherapy. Or topical application of imiquimod, 5% or cidofovir, 3%.

MEASLES

Etiology

A paramyxovirus, measles virus.

Epidemiology

Common exanthem seen in children. Infants protected because of maternal antibodies.

Clinical Manifestations

Incubation period about 10 days.

Two phases of infection:
- ***Prodromal/catarrhal phase:*** accompanied with malaise and respiratory catarrh; second day, bluish white spots surrounded by erythematous halo in the buccal mucosa near the premolars-**Koplik's spots**.
- ***Exanthematous phase:*** disease infectious in this phase. Fourth day, pink macular rash, spreads in 24 hours from face to trunk and limbs. Later papules, discrete or confluent. Desquamates in about 10 days.

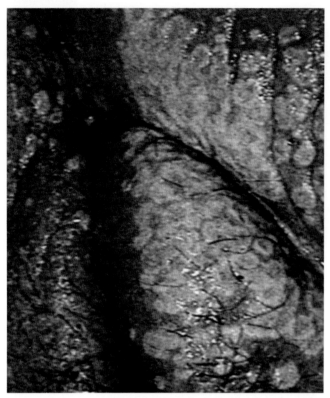

Primary genital herpes: closely grouped vesicles (some umbilicated) on the vulva, almost appearing as a white plaque. This patient is pregnant.

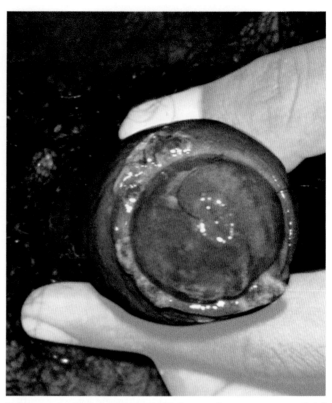

Primary genital herpes: multiple, erythematous superficial erosions, present circumferentially on prepuce and on glans. Difficult to retract the prepuce. Patient had bilateral tender lymphadenopathy and constitutional symptoms.

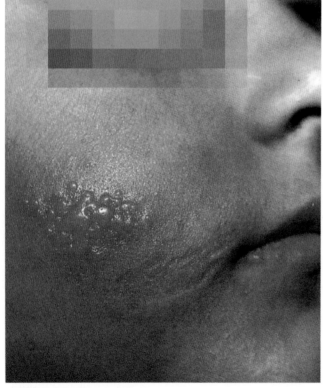

Recurrent herpes simplex: grouped vesicles; the adjoining scar is indicative of a previous attack.

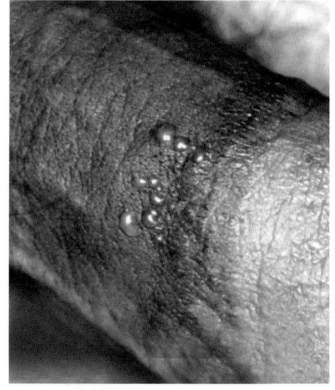

Recurrent genital herpes: grouped tiny vesicles on shaft of penis. No lymphadenopathy or constitutional symptoms.

Complications

High mortality in malnourished children.

Treatment
General Measures

Rest, antipyretics. Antibiotics, if secondary infection.

Prevention

Live attenuated virus vaccine.

HERPES SIMPLEX

Etiology

Herpes simplex virus (HSV): type I commonly causes extragenital and type II sexually transmitted genital infections.

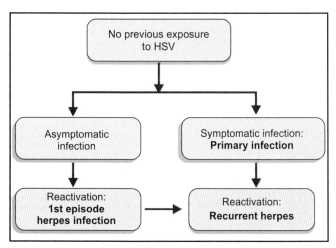

Classification of herpes simplex infection

Epidemiology

Primary infection, generally subclinical (so uncommon) but florid in immunodeficient or atopic subjects. Recurrent herpes simplex common. Extragenital infection seen in all age groups, while genital infection, seen in sexually active patients.

Clinical Manifestations

Primary episodes

Present as acute gingivostomatitis, pharyngitis or genital infection. More symptomatic, severe than recurrent infection. Confluent vesicles and aphthae like ulcers often covered with pseudomembrane on diffuse area of erythema. Lymphadenopathy and constitutional symptoms conspicous.

Recurrent episodes

Triggered by fever, exposure to sunlight and mental and physical stress. Small, grouped, closely-set vesicles, present on the face, particularly around the lips (**herpes labialis**). Or on genitalia (**herpes genitalis**). Local discomfort but no constitutional symptoms. Heal without residue and only occasionally with scars. Recurrences at the same (or proximate) sites.

Herpes and Human Immunodeficiency Virus Infection

- Initially similar features as in HIV negative.
- Prolonged and severe episodes of genital, perianal or oral herpes. Chronic non-healing perianal ulcer with herpetiform margin suggestive of underlying HIV infection.
- ↑ asymptomatic shedding.
- Atypical lesions.

Complications

- ***Eczema herpeticum (Kaposi's varicelliform eruption):*** generalized HSV infection in patients with underlying skin disease like pemphigus and atopic dermatitis. Diagnosis often needs cytopathologic/culture confirmation.
- ***Erythema multiforme:*** herpetic infection may be followed, weeks later, by targetoid lesions.

Investigations

Diagnosis generally clinical. Sometimes needs evaluation, especially in genital lesions.

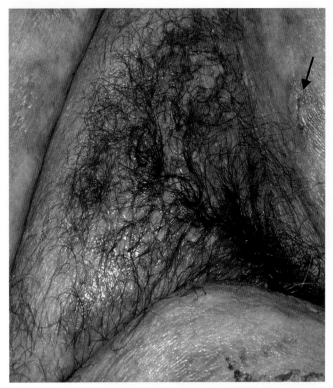

Genital herpes in HIV positive patient: widespread polycyclic lesions on the vulva, mons and lower abdomen. Note grouped lesions on thighs.

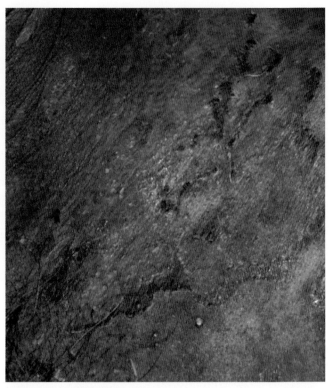

Eczema herpeticum: polycyclic lesions in a patient with underlying pemphigus. Other conditions which predispose include atopic dermatitis.

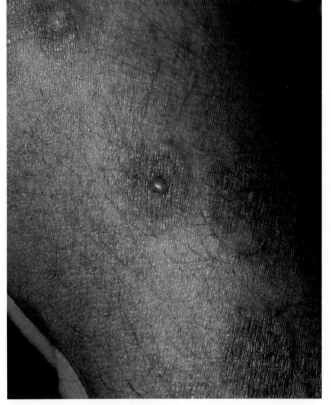

Complication of genital herpes: recurrent erythema multiforme associated with recurrent GH.

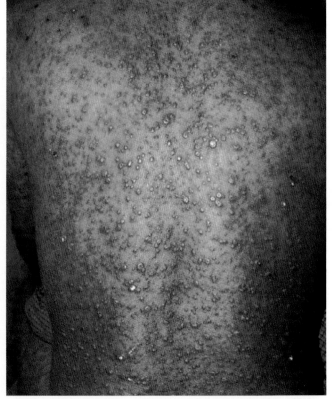

Chicken pox: papules and umbilicated vesicles in different stages of evolution.

Cytopathology

Tzanck smear done in doubtful cases. Stained with Giemsa (shows multinucleated giant cells). Or by direct fluorescent antibodies (apple green fluorescence).

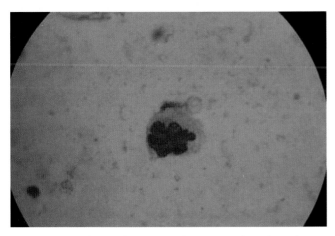

Giemsa stained Tzanck smear in herpes: multinucleated giant cells. Enlarged cell with multiple clustered nuclei-containing eosinophilic bodies.

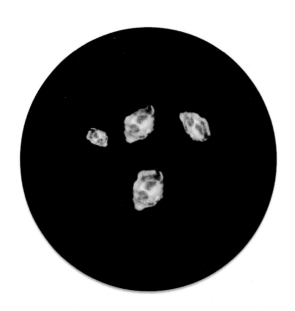

Direct immunofluoresence test on Tzanck smear in herpes: showing apple green intracellular fluorescence.

Culture and PCR

Confirmation by culture (cytopathic effect) and polymerase chain reaction.

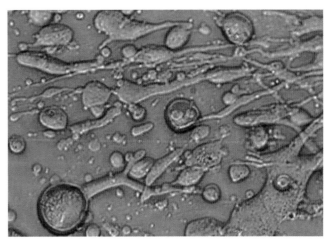

Tissue culture of herpes simplex virus: cytopathic effect usually within 48 hours. Further typed to determine whether HSV-1 or HSV-2.

Courtesy: Prof Lalit Dhar, Department of Microbiology, All India Institute of Medical Sciences (AIIMS), New Delhi.

Treatment
General Measures

Counselling. Inform about recurrences. Barrier sex in herpes genitalis.

Specific Therapy

Topical therapy of little (no) value. Systemic therapy needed only if infection severe (primary herpetic gingivostomatitis) or genital infection. And in HIV coinfected. Or as suppressive therapy in frequent recurrent infection. Or if severe psychosocial impact. Acyclovir, famciclovir, valacyclovir.

VARICELLA-ZOSTER VIRUS INFECTION

Chickenpox (Varicella)

Etiology

Varicella-zoster virus (VZV).

Epidemiology

Common. Spread via droplet infection. Commoner in children, severe in adults.

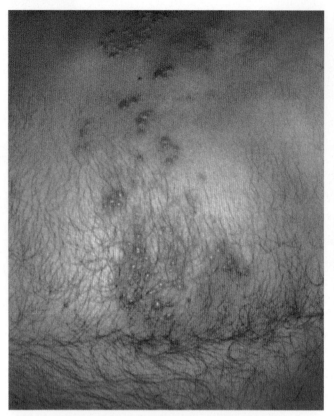

Herpes zoster: groups of vesicles on an erythematous background; dermatomes T6 and T7 affected; unilateral distribution.

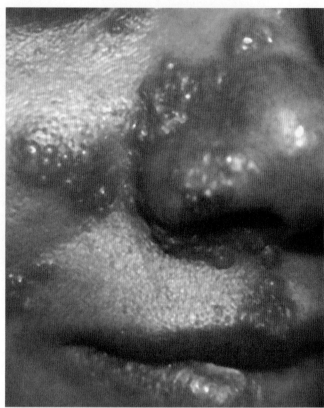

Trigeminal zoster: only mandibular division of the nerve involved.

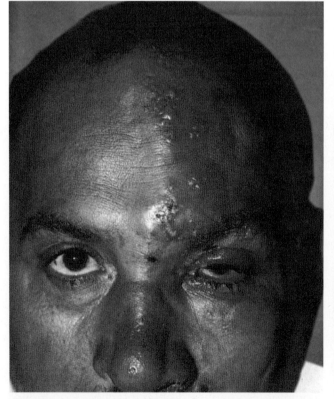

Trigeminal zoster: only ophthalmic division of trigeminal nerve involved.

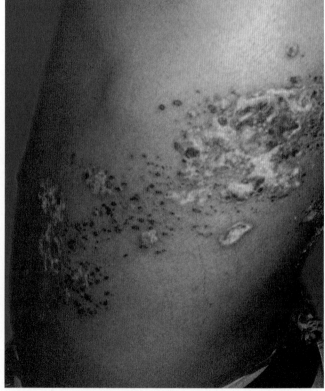

Herpes zoster in an HIV-positive patient: involvement of trunk in dermatomal pattern. Deeper ulcers with necrotic slough a clue to test for underlying HIV infection.

Clinical Manifestations

Incubation period about 2 weeks. Fever followed by a transient macular rash, rapidly evolving through papules to vesicles (occasionally hemorrhagic) and pustules; form crusts and heal with hyperpigmentation or minimal scarring. Lesions in different stages of evolution (*c.f.* smallpox). Centripetal distribution (trunk and proximal parts of the extremities), later spread to the peripheral parts; mucosae may be involved. Constitutional symptoms generally mild; occasionally severe, particularly in the adults. Itching variable, at times severe. Disease self limiting; rarely fatal outcome. An overt attack confers almost permanent immunity.

Investigations

Usually clinical. In doubtful cases Tzanck smear, culture and biopsy done.

Tzanck smear

Reveals multinucleated giant cells.

Biopsy

Reticular and ballooning degeneration of epidermal cells.

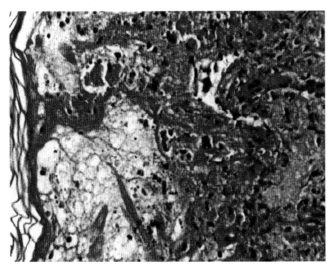

Histopathology of varicella: reticular and ballooning degeneration of epidermal cells.

Herpes Zoster

Etiology

Reactivation of latent VZV infection in a cranial nerve or posterior root ganglia long after an overt or sub-clinical varicella infection.

Clinical Manifestations

Pain, unilateral, may precede (by a couple of days), the appearance of skin lesions. Grouped vesicular lesions; distributed unilaterally on an erythematous base in a single or a few adjacent somatic or cranial dermatomes; lesions continue to appear for a week or so. Regional lymphadenopathy present. Constitutional symptoms mild. Heal with hyperpigmentation, depigmentation or occasionally with scarring. Trunk, face (trigeminal nerve distribution most frequent). Or extremities affected. Patients with AIDS and lymphomas develop florid (necrotic) or disseminated zoster.

Complications

Persistence of severe pain after healing of lesions, post herpetic neuralgia, a debilitating complication in elderly. Trigeminal zoster may result corneal ulcers and opacities. Ocular or facial palsies rarely.

Treatment

General Measures

Antihistamines for relief of itching (varicella) and analgesics for pain (zoster).

Specific Treatment

For chicken pox in children, no treatment. For adult and immunocompromised-acyclovir, famciclovir or valaciclovir. For zoster acyclovir (2–4 g/day), famciclovir (250 mg, 3 times a day) or valaciclovir (500 mg, twice a day) for 5–7 days given, within the first couple of days, may abort an attack of zoster and prevent post herpetic neuralgia. Amitriptyline (25 mg, thrice a day) or gabapentine (1,800–3,600 mg/day) effectively control post herpetic neuralgia.

4

Leprosy

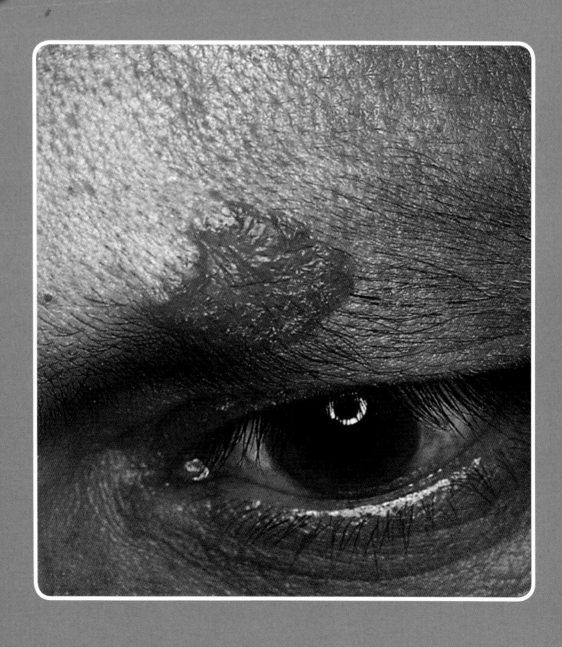

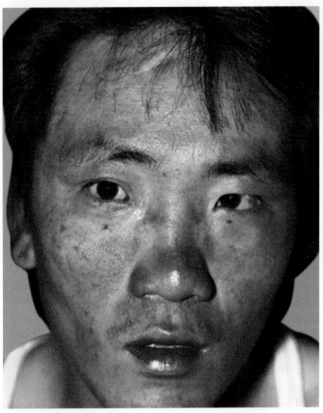

Lepromatous leprosy: mild diffuse cutaneous infiltration.

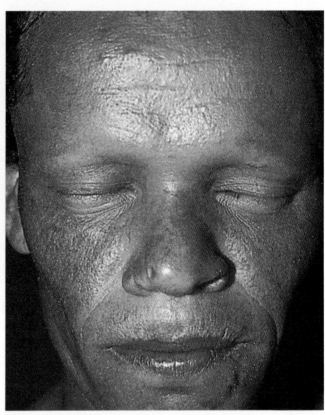

Lepromatous leprosy: infiltration of the skin with complete loss of eyebrows.

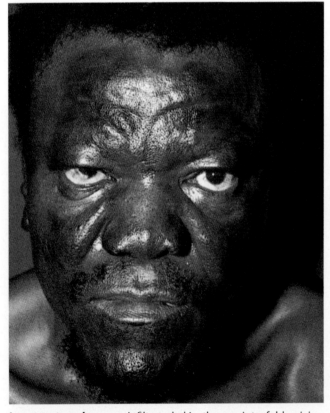

Lepromatous leprosy: infiltrated skin thrown into folds giving leonine facies.

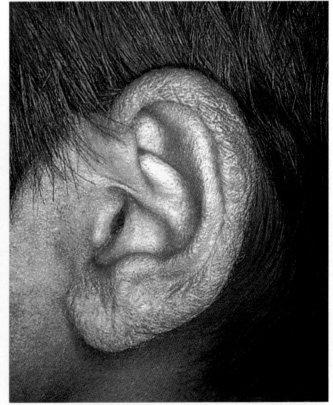

Lepromatous leprosy: diffuse ear lobe infiltration with nodulation.

ETIOLOGY

Mycobacterium leprae—an obligate intracellular acid and alcohol fast bacillus, 1–5 µ × 0.1–0.5 µ; not cultured *in vitro* so far. Animal models: mouse and nine banded armadillos; the latter a rich source of *M. leprae*.

EPIDEMIOLOGY

Transmission

Mode of acquisition of disease ill understood; nose an important portal of exit; millions of bacilli sprayed with each nose blow or on coughing by a lepromatous patient. Route of entry of *M. leprae* uncertain-possibly skin or respiratory mucosa.

Prevalence

Rare in affluent countries. Also prevalence of different types of leprosy varies geographically. Lepromatous leprosy predominant in South East Asia, tuberculoid in African continent, and pure tuberculoid universally infrequent. In India, various types fairly uniformly distributed. An important public health problem in the developing world. Eighty percent of global leprosy load in India; current prevalence (2014):0.68/10,000.

SPECTRUM

Varied spectral manifestations of leprosy possibly a result of differences in the specific cell mediated immunity (CMI) of the host. Two polar forms: lepromatous (LL) and tuberculoid (TT), and a broad intermediate borderline group. Also an early 'indeterminate' and a pure neural form.

Skin and nerves—common targets for the bacilli; several other organs and tissues also affected. A simplified concept of pathogenesis:
- *Lepromatous leprosy (LL):* highly bacillated, low host resistance, so systemic, infectious form.
- *Tuberculoid leprosy (TT):* high host resistance, poorly bacillated so localized, non-infectious disease.
- *Borderline group (BT, BB, BL):* intermediate host resistance, so variably bacillated. BT closer to TT; BL nearer to LL pole. BB truly midway.
- *Indeterminate leprosy:* early non-classifiable disease. May self resolve or transform to defined forms.
- *Primary neuritic leprosy:* neural involvement without any skin lesions.

CARDINAL FEATURES OF LEPROSY

In an endemic area, suspect leprosy if patient shows ONE of following cardinal signs:
- Skin lesion(s) consistent with leprosy with definite sensory loss, + thickened nerves. Skin lesion(s) either single or multiple. Usually hypopigmented (sometimes reddish or copper-colored). Macules (flat), papules (raised), or nodules common. Lesional sensory loss (to temperature, pin prick, light touch) typical feature of leprosy. Thickened nerves, mainly peripheral nerve trunks with loss of sensation in distribution of nerve. And motor weakness (nerve thickening in absence of sensory/motor deficit not reliable sign of leprosy).
- Positive acid-fast bacilli (AFB) in skin smears.

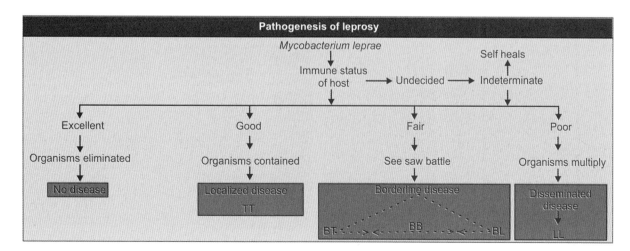

Pathogenesis of leprosy

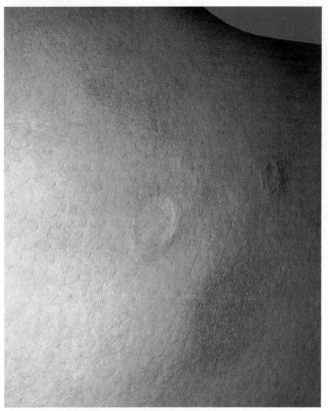

Lepromatous leprosy: nodules flatten with anetoderma.

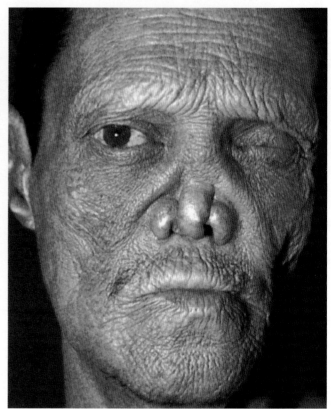

Lepromatous leprosy: healed with gross mutilation, including depressed nose.

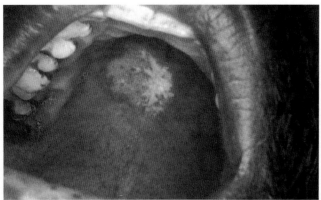

Lepromatous leprosy: oral lesions note ulcerations on the palate and infiltrated upper lip.

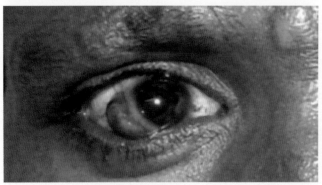

Lepromatous leprosy ocular involvement: uveitis and corneal opacities.

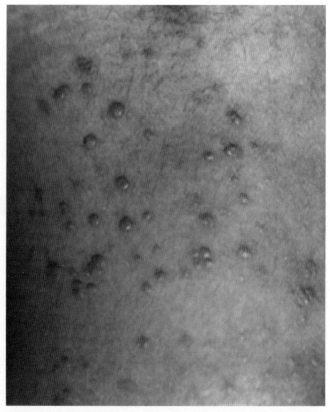

Histoid leprosy: succulent nodules on an apparently normal skin.

CLINICAL MANIFESTATIONS

Skin lesions either macular or infiltrated (papules/ nodules/plaques). Nerve involvement (thickened and/or tender) in all forms—late in LL and early in TT/BT. Major nerve trunks commonly clinically involved: facial, ulnar, median, lateral popliteal and posterior tibial. Rarely radial. Other nerves clinically examined—greater auricular and radial cutaneous.

Lepromatous Leprosy (LL)

Poor immune status of the host (negative lepromin skin test). Highly bacillated, disseminated, systemic disease. Multiple, bilaterally symmetrical, ill-defined, hypopigmented macules or diffusely infiltrated shiny, wrinkled, atrophic skin with or without papules and nodules. Degree of infiltration variable; severely infiltrated facial skin thrown into convoluted folds may give '**leonine** (lion-like) **facies**'. Diffusely infiltrated earlobes and eyebrow region, with loss of lateral eyebrows. Nasal and buccal mucosa infiltrated and inflamed; epistaxis not uncommon. Depressed bridge of the nose or perforated nasal septum or palate—now infrequent. Nerve involvement uniform but clinically manifests late, as acral (glove and stocking) anesthesia, predisposing to painless burns and injuries. And as neuropathic ulcers, resorbed digits and osteomyelitic changes. Also as muscle wasting, weakness and deformities. Autonomic involvement causes loss of sweating and edema of hands and feet.

Systemic involvement due to bacillemia. Generalized lymphadenopathy, hepatosplenomegaly, testicular atrophy, gynecomastia. Ocular lesions due to direct infiltration. Or secondary to sensory/motor deficits—conjunctivitis, keratitis, iridocyclitis.

Untreated, disease runs an indolent downhill course; interspersed with acute exacerbations called 'lepra' reactions; rarely 'burns' itself out after prolonged periods; rarely fatal due to secondary complications-infections, renal amyloidosis and renal failure.

Histoid Leprosy

A variant of LL. Infiltrated succulent, cutaneous nodules or plaques 'sitting' on an apparently uninfiltrated skin with or without other features of LL or BL; may appear *de novo* or in relapsed patients of BL/LL.

Tuberculoid Leprosy (TT)

Rarely seen. Good immune status of host (strongly positive lepromin skin test). Localized disease. Skin and nerves predominantly affected. Solitary or few lesions—sharply delineated, hypopigmented, dry, scaly, anesthetic or hypoesthetic macule(s) or infiltrated plaque(s). Edge elevated and most conspicuous part of the lesion with hair and sweating diminished or absent. Local (including feeder) nerve(s) thickened. Runs a relatively benign stable course. Often heals by itself.

Borderline Group

Unstable, intermediate forms between the two polar types. Subdivided into three types: borderline tuberculoid (BT), borderline (BB) and borderline lepromatous (BL), so designated based on whether clinical, histological and bacteriological features closer to TT, midway between TT and LL, or nearer to LL leprosy respectively.

Borderline Tuberculoid (BT)

Much like TT, with tuberculoid features less prominent: lesions more in number, not as sharply delineated; edge slightly sloped outwards. Satellite lesion(s) present around a large lesion (indicating spread). Loss of hair, sweating and sensations less pronounced than TT. Neural involvement less localized; larger nerve trunks thickened. Distribution of cutaneous lesions and neural involvement still asymmetrical. Lepromin skin test positive or negative.

Borderline (BB)

Most unstable form. Uncommon. Numerous skin lesions—macules or infiltrated plaques; some resemble BT, others BL and some have features peculiar to BB: an '**inverted saucer**' appearance (a flat center with broad infiltrated edge sloping peripherally). Nerve involvement and loss of sensations relatively late. Lepromin skin test negative.

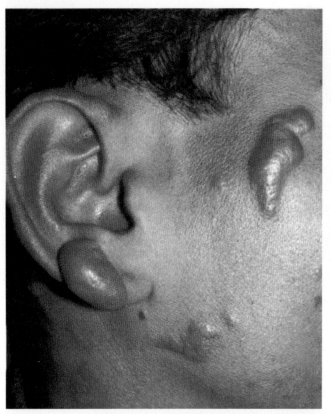

Histoid leprosy: succulent, firm nodules on earlobe and face.

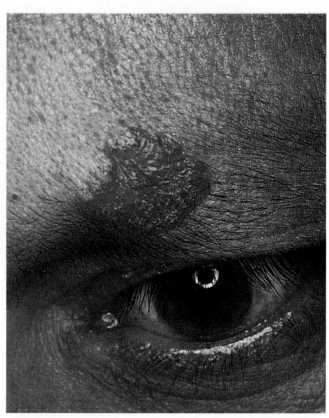

Tuberculoid leprosy: well-defined infiltrated plaque. Note decreased hair.

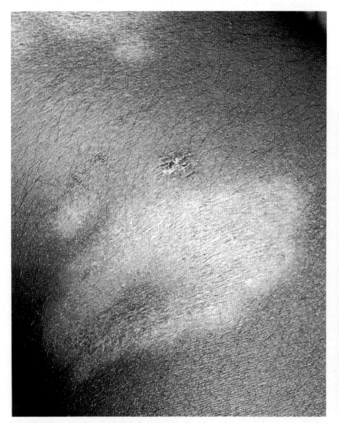

Borderline tuberculoid leprosy: lesion shows alopecia, infiltrated edge and a satellite lesion.

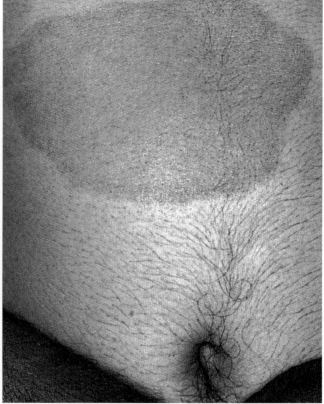

Borderline tuberculoid leprosy: uniformly infiltrated plaque.

Borderline Lepromatous (BL)

Much like LL. Most lesions small macules, plaques or nodules with ill-defined edges; some lesions are large and simulate BB or BT. Face and earlobes often infiltrated with or without nodulation and madarosis. Sensory loss late and less pronounced. Nerve trunk thickening relatively late and bilaterally symmetrical. Systemic involvement less prominent. May upgrade to BT or BB. Lepromin skin test negative.

Primary Neuritic Leprosy

Nerve involvement without a skin lesion. Spectral classification difficult; most patients possibly borderline. Peripheral nerve(s) thickened (and sometimes tender); unilateral or bilateral. Any nerve, though sometimes generally ulnar, radial, lateral popliteal, trigeminal and facial affected. Gradual sensory loss or motor deficit: paralysis, deformities, painless thermal burns or mechanical injuries, trophic changes and non-healing ulcers.

Indeterminate Leprosy

Non-classifiable early lesion suggestive of leprosy. Ill-defined, often a solitary hypopigmented macule (always) on the face. Or thigh or any other part of the body. Doubtful or minimal loss of sensations. Variable course: transforms into any of the polar forms or borderline group. Or more often spontaneously resolves without any residue; nerve thickening not definite. Demonstration of bacilli or damage to nerves on histology confirmatory.

REACTIONS IN LEPROSY (LEPRA REACTIONS)

Acute exacerbations in course of the disease, due to immunological changes. Triggered by specific chemotherapy, emotional/physical stress, pregnancy or intercurrent infections. Two types recognized: Type I and Type II.

Type I

Seen in BT, BB, BL (borderline forms). Acute exacerbations due to rapid alteration of leprosy-specific CMI of the host. Skin lesions acutely inflamed–red, edematous and tender; may desquamate or ulcerate. Nerves painful and tender; may develop nerve abscesses or palsies with increase in anesthesia, loss of motor function

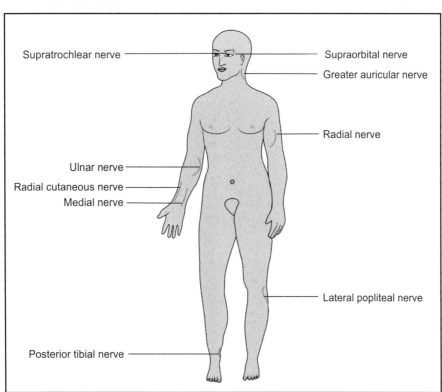

Peripheral nerve involvement in leprosy

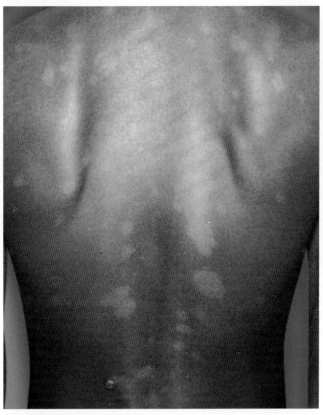

Borderline lepromatous leprosy: multiple, small lesions on a shiny infiltrated background.

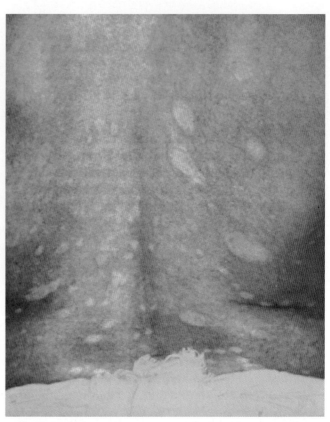

Borderline leprosy: multiple large and small lesions; bilaterally symmetrical.

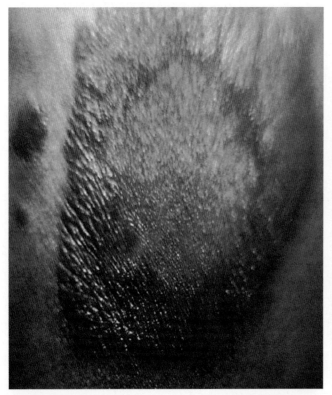

Borderline leprosy: 'inverted saucer' lesion with elevated sloping border.

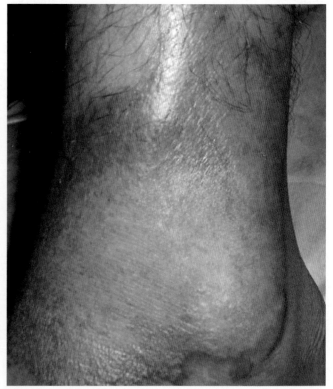

Borderline leprosy: 'inverted saucer' lesion with elevated sloping border.

Difference between late type 1 lepra reaction and relapse		
	Late type 1 lepra reaction	*Relapse*
Spectrum	Borderline leprosy	All types (TT-LL)
Onset	Sudden (<15 months after treatment)	Slow (1–5 years after treatment)
Old lesions	Show swelling, erythema and scaling	Show increase in size
New lesions	Rarely appear	Frequently appear
Acral lesions	Common	Uncommon
Nerve involvement	Previously involved nerves tender with sudden deterioration of function (motor/sensory)	Fresh nerves involved. Sudden deterioration in function not seen
Slit-skin smear	Usually negative	May become positive
Response to steroids	Good	Leads to progression of disease

or sudden paralysis. Constitutional symptoms mild or absent in BT, variable, sometimes moderate, in BB/BL.

Type I reaction of two types: upgrading (reversal) and downgrading. Upgrading reaction more common, in patients on treatment; with shift towards tuberculoid end and decrease in BI. Needs to be differentiated from relapse. Downgrading reactions less common, seen in untreated patients with shift towards lepromatous pole and increase in BI.

Type II (Erythema nodosum leprosum, ENL)

Common in LL or BL. An immune complex syndrome (Arthus reaction); no change in CMI. Recurrent crops of evanescent, acute, painful, tender, dusky red nodules and plaques that resolve in less than a week with hyperpigmentation. Occasionally sterile pustules that ulcerate and heal with scarring. Face, extremities and less often trunk involved. Neuritis, lymphadenopathy, arthritis, iridocyclitis, epididymoorchitis, proteinuria and varying constitutional symptoms. Leprosy lesions and the disease status unchanged. May relapse and remit for months/ years. Complete recovery; rarely eventuates in death due to secondary amyloidosis (very rare) or intercurrent infections.

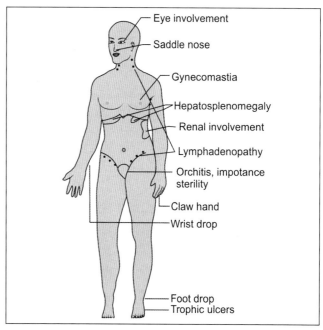

Complications of leprosy

INVESTIGATIONS

Leprosy suspected by the character of skin lesions; thickened, ± tender nerves, loss of cutaneous sensations and motor function. Confirmed by histological features and/or demonstration of bacilli in skin-slit smear or histologically.

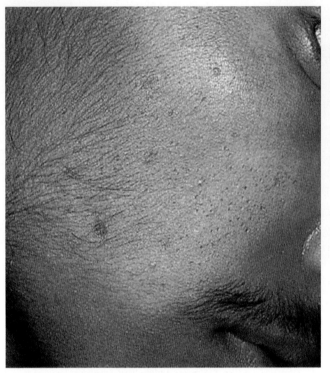

Indeterminate leprosy: note atrophic hypopigmented lesion on the face.

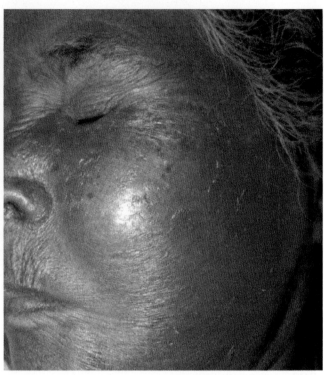

Type I reaction in borderline tuberculoid leprosy: well-defined lesion in type I reaction.

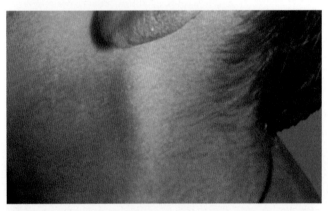

Nerve involvement in leprosy: visible thickened greater auricular nerve.

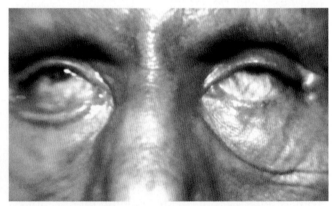

Nerve involvement in leprosy: bilateral facial palsy.

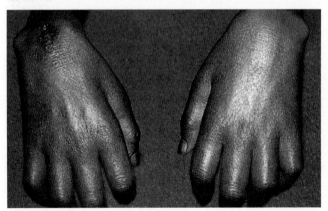

Nerve involvement in leprosy: claw hands due to bilateral ulnar and median nerve palsy.

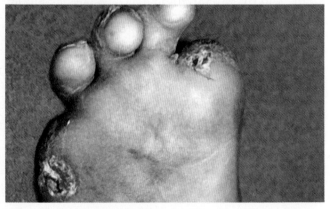

Nerve involvement in leprosy: trophic ulcer. Note hyperkeratotic edge.

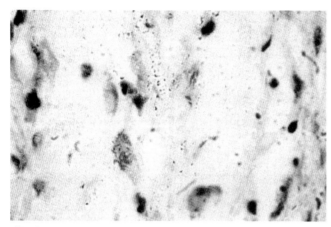

Slit-skin smear: BI of 6+ in a patient with lepromatous leprosy showing globi.

Skin-slit Smear Technique

Clean the lesion, incise 2–3 mm and 5 mm length deep, scrape edges and make a smear. Stain by **Ziehl-Neelsen** method and examine for AFB under 100x objective. Negative in TT/BT, progressive positivity towards lepromatous end. Bacteriological index (BI) a logarithmic scale, 0–6.

Histopathology

Often variable morphology of lesions in a single patient. Take multiple biopsies if necessary. Biopsy best taken from most infiltrated part of lesion (usually the edge).

All types of leprosy show epidermal atrophy and all but TT, a free subepidermal or **grenz zone** (papillary dermis devoid of infiltrate). Granulomatous infiltrate distributed around appendages and nerves—in lepromatous form tends to be rather diffuse while compact in tuberculoid. Nature of infiltrate and quantum of bacilli variable: lymphocytes and epithelioid cells and few bacilli in tuberculoid leprosy. Vacuolated macrophages (laden with bacilli) and few lymphocytes in the lepromatous form. Nerves and appendages often damaged or destroyed in TT/BT forms and preserved in BL/LL. Borderline forms intermediate histological features.

Lepromatous Leprosy

Diffuse monomorphic infiltrate of vacuolated, foamy, macrophages laden with AFB often in clumps, called globi. Lymphocytes conspicuously few. Overlying atrophic epidermis separated by a grenz zone.

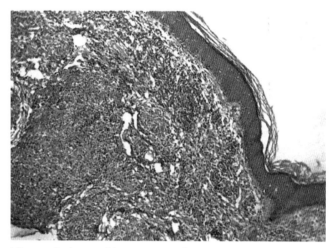

Histopathology of lepromatous leprosy: atrophic epidermis and diffuse dermal infiltrate with vacuolated macrophages sparing the subepidermal zone.

Histoid Leprosy

Pseudoencapsulated whorled collection of elongated, non-vacuolated histiocytes loaded with acid-fast bacilli. Vacuolated histiocytes may also be present.

Tuberculoid Leprosy

Well-defined, tuberculoid, often elongated/curvilinear granulomas, (epithelioid cells and giant cells; with peripheral rim of lymphocytes) around nerves

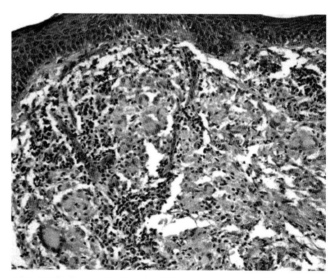

Histopathology of tuberculoid leprosy: tuberculoid curvilinear granuloma consisting of epitheliod cells and giant cells with a rim of lymphocytes at the periphery. Note granuloma encroaching epidermis.

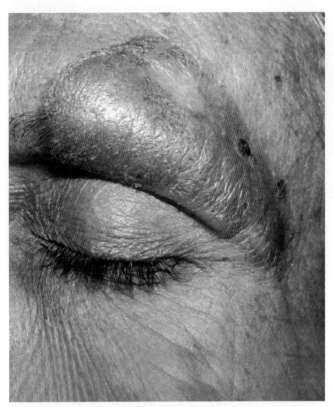

Type I reaction in borderline tuberculoid leprosy: erythematous, edematous and scaly plaque.

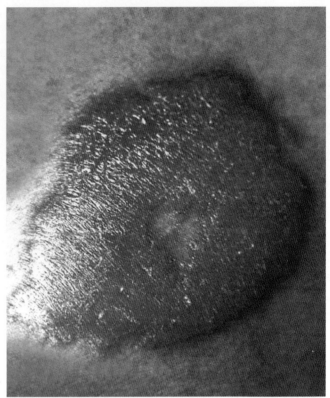

Type I reaction in borderline tuberculoid leprosy: erythematous edematous plaque.

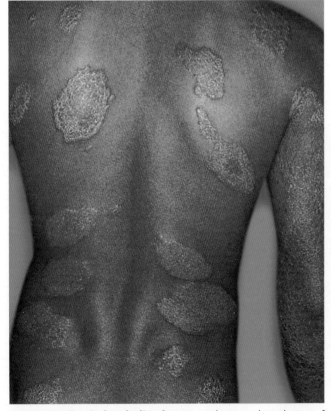

Type I reaction in borderline leprosy: edema and erythema of pre-existing lesions.

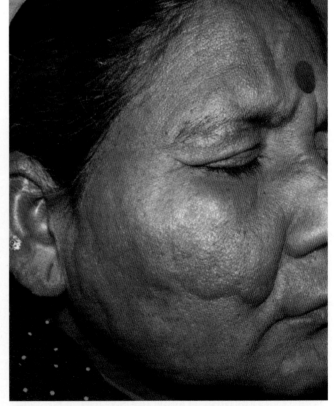

Type I reaction in borderline lepromatous leprosy: large plaque with erythema and edema. Patient has infiltration of ear lobes.

and appendages, which are often damaged or absent. Subepidermal zone infiltrated (absent Grenz zone), with granuloma encroaching epidermis. Bacilli not detected by conventional methods.

Borderline Tuberculoid Leprosy

Tuberculoid granuloma; subepidermal zone free; few bacilli.

Borderline Leprosy

Midway between lepromatous and tuberculoid leprosy; subepidermal zone free; acid-fast bacilli often demonstrable.

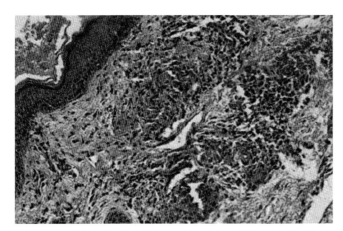

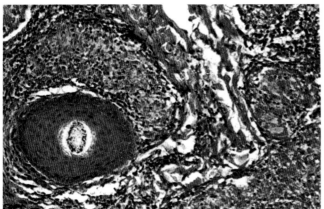

Histopathology of borderline tuberculoid leprosy: tuberculoid granulomas with free subepidermal zone and perifollicular location.

Borderline Lepromatous Leprosy

Picture closer to that of LL, but with many lymphocytes in the granuloma. Large number of acid-fast bacilli.

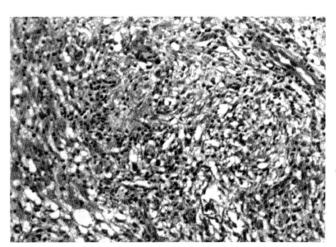

Histopathology of borderline lepromatous leprosy: granuloma of vacuolated histiocytes with numerous lymphocytes in the middle.

Reactions in Leprosy

Reversal type 1 reaction

Disorganization of granuloma with edema and infiltration with polymorphs.

Type 2 reaction

Lepromatous granuloma superimposed with acute inflammation in form of polymorphs and edema.

Treatment

For purpose of treatment all patients classified into paucibacillary (≤5 lesions, usually bacteriologically negative). Or multibacillary (bacteriologically positive) now defined by WHO as >5 lesions. Monotherapy with sulfones absolutely inadequate. Administer combination therapy with dapsone and rifampicin in paucibacillary types; add clofazimine in multibacillary types.

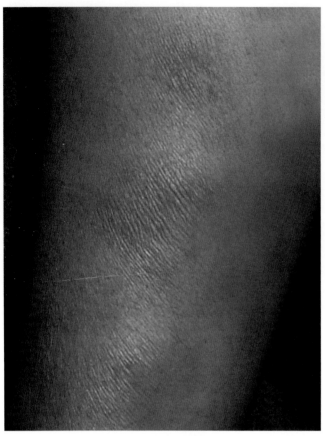

Type II reaction in lepromatous leprosy: erythema nodosum leprosum, erythematous, edematous plaques.

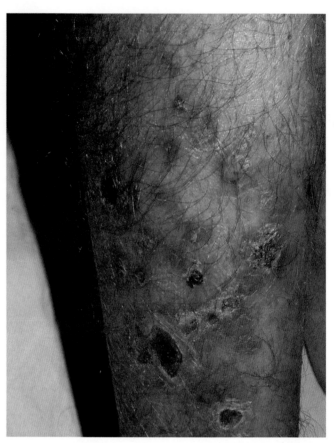

Erythema nodosum leprosum necroticans in lepromatous leprosy: erythematous tender nodules of erythema nodosum leprosum which have necrosed.

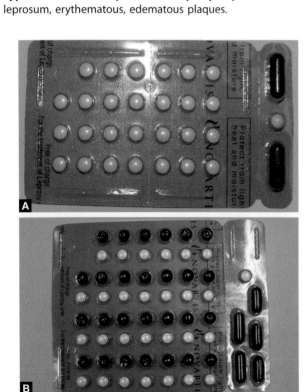

Multidrug therapy of leprosy: WHO supplied blister packs: A. for paucibacillarly leprosy (adult); B. for multibacillary leprosy (adult).

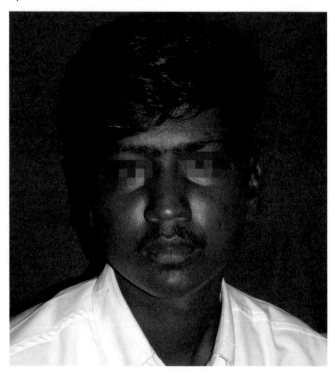

Side effect of treatment: clofazimine pigmentation.

For Paucibacillary Disease

Treatment for 6 months (can be taken by the patient over a period of 9 months) with:

- **Rifampicin:** 600 mg once a month (adult dose), given empty stomach; supervised.
- **Dapsone:** 100 mg/day (adult dose); self-administered daily.

For Multibacillary Leprosy

Treatment for a period of 12 months (can be taken by patient over a period of 18 months) with:

- **Rifampicin:** 600 mg once a month; supervised.
- **Dapsone:** 100 mg/day; self-administered.
- **Clofazimine:** 50 mg/day; self-administered. And 300 mg, once a month; supervised.

For Single Lesion Leprosy

Rifampicin 600 mg, ofloxacin, 400 mg and minocycline 100 mg given as single dose.

Newer Anti-leprosy Drugs

Clarithromycin, sparfloxacin, ofloxacin and levofloxacin; used as alternate regimens. In patients harboring resistant *M. leprae*. And intolerance to conventional therapy.

Reactions

Always continue antileprosy therapy. Rest, appropriate splints or other physiotherapeutic measures for the affected part.

Type I reaction

Depends on severity:

- **Mild type I reactions:** Non-steroidal anti inflammatory drugs (NSAIDs).
- **Severe type I reactions:** Oral steroids drugs of choice, particularly in patients with severe

Treatment of complications in leprosy	
Trophic ulcers	Rest Antibiotics—Surgical debridement Non-weight-bearing splint
Motor deficits	Physiotherapy Splints Surgical correction transfer
Iridocyclitis	Topical steroids Oral steroids
Orchitis	Oral steroids

neuritis, nerve abscesses or impending paralysis. Or extensive and acutely inflamed skin lesions. Prednisolone 1 mg/kg/day, tapered over 12–24 weeks.

Type II reaction

- **Mild reaction:** NSAIDs.
- **Severe reaction:** Thalidomide (300–400 mg/d), used under supervision, drug of choice. Corticosteroids used in severe neuritis, recent onset motor weakness, eye complications, orchitis and necrotic ENL. Clofazimine (200–300 mg/d), chloroquine, azathioprine, methotrexate, cyclosporine, antimonials, alternatives.

Immunotherapy

MDT kills *M. leprae*, but does not upgrade immune response. Additional immunotherapy induces faster bacterial clearance and decreases incidence, frequency and severity of reactions. Agents used include BCG, *Mw*, killed *M. leprae*, *ICRC strain*, *M. vaccae* and *M. habana*. Role in prophylaxis debatable.

Other Measures

Complications need to be treated.

5

Cutaneous Tuberculosis

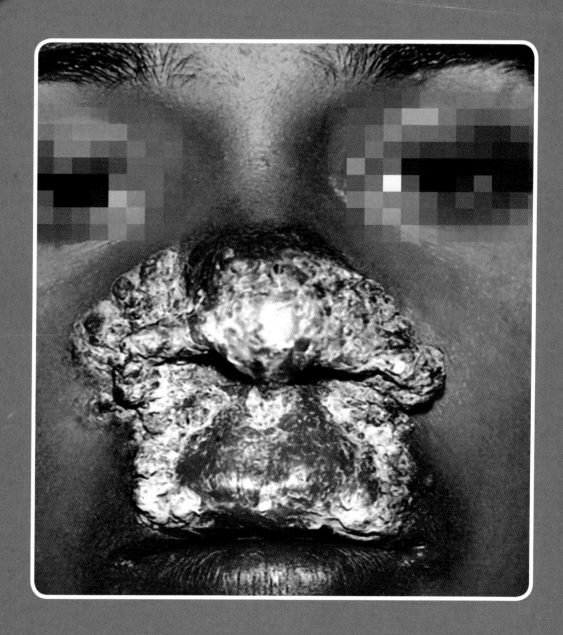

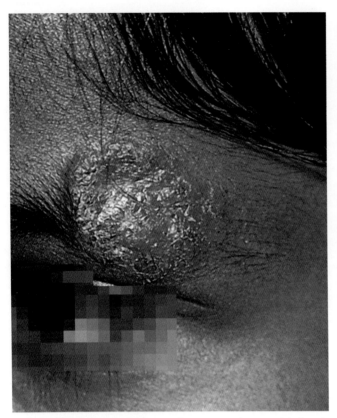

Lupus vulgaris: early lesion-erythematous plaque with barely discernable scarring. Face a common site.

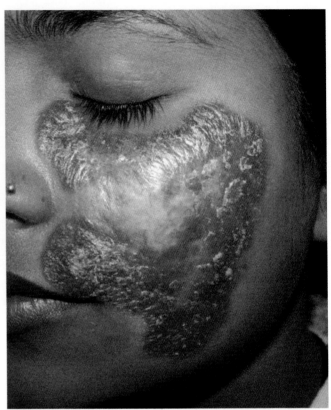

Lupus vulgaris: erythematous scaly plaque showing progression at one edge and scarring at the other. The edge is studded with papules which on diascopy presents an apple jelly appearance.

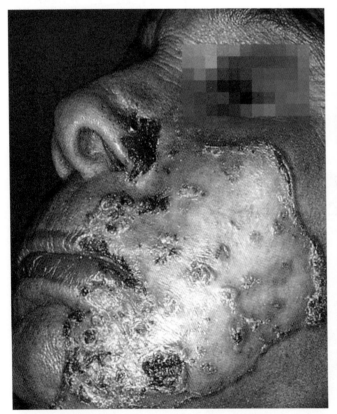

Lupus vulgaris: infiltrated annular plaque with central scarring. Note development of nodules in the scarred area.

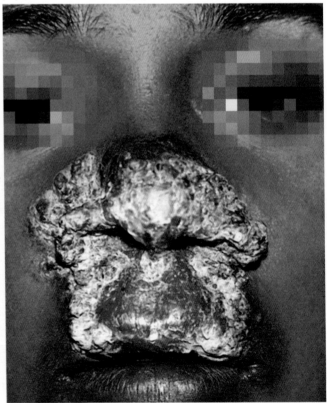

Lupus vulgaris: infiltrated plaque with central scarring. Lesions sometimes become hypertrophic and verrucous.

ETIOLOGY

Causative Agent

Skin infection caused by *Mycobacterium tuberculosis*, *M. bovis*, and rarely Bacillus Calmette-Guérin (BCG).

Pathogenesis

The bacilli reach the skin through exogenous inoculation. Or by hematogenous route. Or by contiguous spread from an underlying focus. Clinical manifestations depend on the mode of infection and immune status of the host particularly cell mediated immunity (CMI) which is a function of previous exposure to mycobacteria.

EPIDEMIOLOGY

Rare in the developed world; not uncommon in developing countries.

CLINICAL MANIFESTATIONS

Infection may be:
- *Primary:* First exposure
- *Secondary:* Post primary or subsequent exposures.

The clinical manifestations depend on the mode of entry of the bacteria in the skin and the immunity of the host.
- *Exogenous inoculation*

  ➢ In a non immune host manifests as tuberculous chancre.
  ➢ In an immune host manifests as tuberculosis verrucosa cutis.
- *Endogenous infection*
  ➢ In a host with low immunity manifests as acute miliary tuberculosis, orificial tuberculosis, tuberculous gumma.
  ➢ In host with good immunity manifests as lupus vulgaris and scrofuloderma.

Lupus Vulgaris

Most common form of tuberculosis of skin. Post-primary infection in children or adults with or without evidence of an extracutaneous tuberculous focus. Endogenous infection generally. Occasionally exogenous inoculation. Or results from BCG vaccination. Immune status of the host is good; tuberculin skin test is positive.

Morphology

Single, occasionally multiple lesions. Initial erythematous–brown papule evolves into infiltrated plaque(s) with atrophic scarring in the center and peripheral extension. Typically nodules appear in healed areas. Edge sharply defined, shows skin colored papules/nodules which show apple jelly appearance on diascopy. Varying degree of hyperkeratosis and verrucosity.

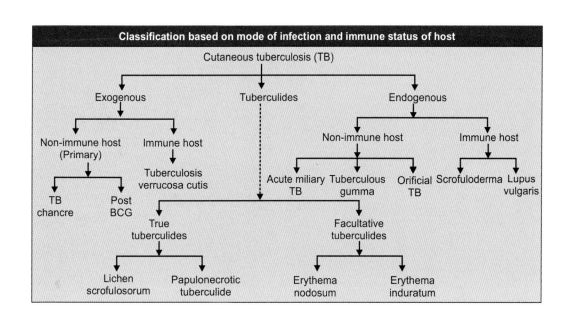

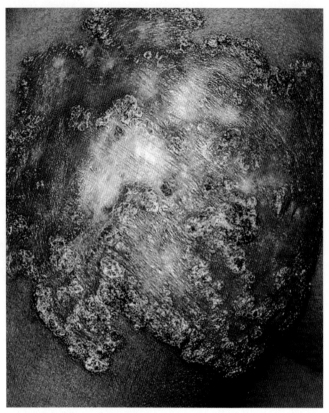

Lupus vulgaris: large plaque on the buttock with peripheral extension, central scarring and depigmentation.

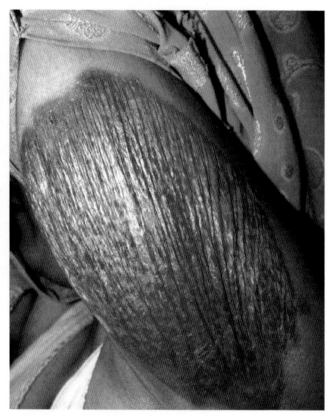

Lupus vulgaris: following BCG vaccination.

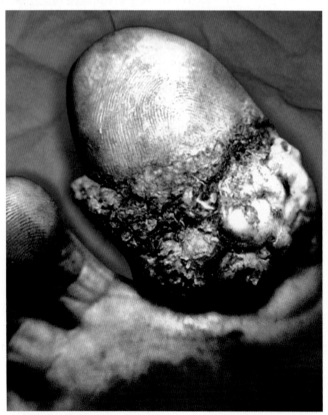

Tuberculosis verrucosa cutis: irregular hyperkeratotic lesion on the sole.

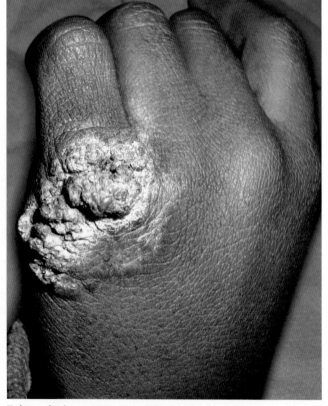

Tuberculosis verrucosa cutis: thick, hyperkeratotic plaque. Scarring seen below the plaque, suggestive of centrifugal spread.

Sites of Predilection

On the buttocks, face, extremities or trunk. May involve nasal mucosa.

Course

Extension with simultaneous spontaneous healing. Long standing patients may eventuate in severe mutilation. Or develop cutaneous horn or squamous cell carcinoma.

Tuberculosis Verrucosa Cutis (Warty Tuberculosis)

Relatively uncommon. Exogenous inoculation of skin in tuberculin positive children or young adults with good immune status.

Morphology

Single, irregular, brown or grey, warty, hyperkeratotic, papillomatous plaque with an erythematous border. Fissures discharging pus often present. Atrophic scar (often imperceptible) in the center. Occasionally exudative and crusted. Differentiation from warty lupus vulgaris difficult, perhaps unimportant. Lymphadenopathy uncommon.

Sites of Predilection

Affects sites prone to trauma: feet, hands, knees and ankles.

Course

Slow progression. Spontaneous healing unusual.

Scrofuloderma

Children or young adults. Skin involvement secondary to an underlying tubercular focus lymph node, bone or joint or testis.

Morphology

Combination of soft fluctuant nodules and chronic ulcers and sinuses with undermined edge and bluish hyperpigmentation. Serous discharge with thick crusting. Heals with irregular scarring. Surrounding skin may show features of lupus vulgaris.

Sites of Predilection

Neck, axillae, groins.

Metastatic Tuberculous Abscess (Tuberculous Gumma)

Uncommon. Children or young adults. Hematogenous spread from a primary focus.

Morphology

Ill-defined, firm, later softened and fluctuant subcutaneous swelling(s); may break down to form an ulcer with undermined edges. Signs of inflammation inconspicuous.

Sites of Predilection

Abdomen.

Tuberculides

Assumed cutaneous expression of hematogenous dissemination of tubercle bacilli from a systemic (often not demonstrable) focus in patients with heightened delayed hypersensitivity—strongly positive tuberculin skin test. Rare, even in populations with high prevalence of tuberculosis. Respond readily to antitubercular therapy; also resolve spontaneously. Classified as:

- *True tuberculides:* definitive tuberculous etiology. Includes lichen scrofulosorum and papulonecrotic tuberculide. And may be papulonecrotic tuberculide of glans/vulva.
- *Facultative tuberculides:* tuberculosis one of the several triggers. Includes erythema nodosum and erythema induratum.

True Tuberculides

Lichen scrofulosorum

Uncommon. Seen mainly in children. Appear as crops of asymptomatic grouped, small, flat topped, lichenoid, follicular, pale or skin colored papules with fine scales. Symmetrically on trunk, extremities. Involute over months, without residue.

Papular and papulonecrotic tuberculide

Appear as crops of bilaterally symmetrical papules and nodules; may necrose on top. Heal without residue. Or with scarring.

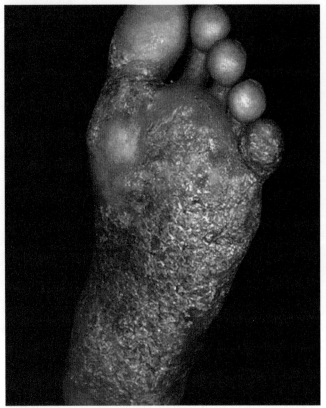

Tuberculosis verrucosa cutis: irregular hyperkeratotic indurated plaque with minimal scar.

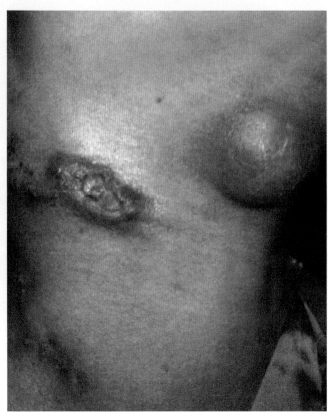

Scrofuloderma: combination of soft fluctuant nodules and chronic ulcers and sinuses with undermined edge and bluish hyperpigmentation. Lesions occur in relation to lymph nodes, joints, or bone or testis.

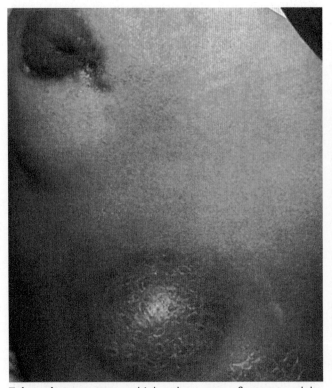

Tuberculous gumma: multiple subcutaneous fluctuant nodules will eventually rupture to form sinuses like in scrofuloderma.

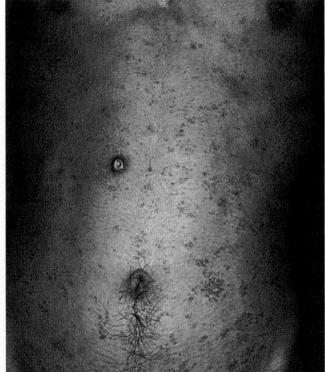

Lichen scrofulosorum: asymptomatic lichen nitidus-like scaly papules, symmetrically present on the trunk. Tuberculin test was strongly positive. Patient responded to ATT.

Papulonecrotic Tuberculide (of Glans)

Most reported from Africa, Asia subcontinent and Japan. Affects young to middle aged males (less frequently females). Cyclical episodes of papules which ulcerate in center. And self-heal to leave punched out and bridging or varioliform scars giving a 'worm-eaten appearance'. Glans/vulva involved.

Facultative Tuberculides

Erythema nodosum

Uncommon. Not all patients have associated tuberculosis; other causes such as sarcoidosis, streptococcal throat infections, drugs, Behcet's syndrome. Children and young adults affected, more often females. Painful and tender, non-ulcerating erythematous or purplish nodules. Each lesion self-limiting (2–6 weeks). Fresh lesions continue to appear. Resolve with hyperpigmentation. Bilateral and symmetrical, usually on the shins. Mild to moderate constitutional symptoms: fever, arthralgia.

Erythema Induratum (Bazin)

Uncommon. Affects young adult females. Painful, tender, dusky-red nodules which break down to form ulcers with bluish, irregular edges. Heal with scars. Erythrocyanotic lower extremities. Cold weather may precipitate lesions and warm weather improve the condition. Chronic and recurrent. Involves calves, often bilaterally. Many respond to adequate, prolonged antitubercular therapy.

INVESTIGATIONS

Always rule out tuberculosis of other organs by doing relevant investigations.

Tuberculin Test

Indicates immunity. Variable in lupus vulgaris, negative in tuberculous gumma and positive in scrofuloderma, tuberculosis verrucosa cutis. And strongly positive in tuberculides.

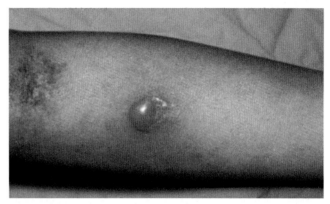

Tuberculin skin test (Mantoux test): strongly positive bullous reaction in a patient with lichen scrofulosorum; reflects good cell mediated immune response.

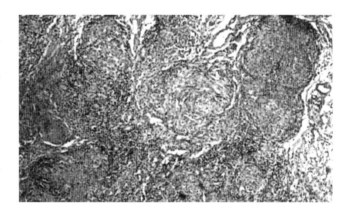

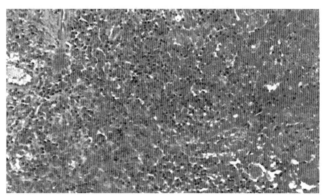

Lupus vulgaris: diffuse granulomatous infiltrate consisting of epithelioid cells, lymphocytes, plasma cells and giant cells; top (10x), bottom (40x).

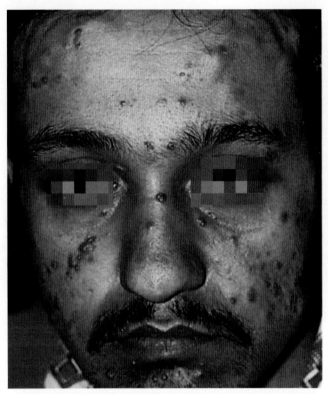

Papulonecrotic tuberculide: erythematous nodules surmounted with necrosis. Note symmetry. Patients tuberculin test was strongly positive and he responded to antituberculous treatment.

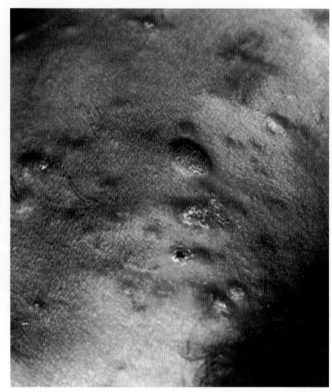

Papulonecrotic tuberculide: erythematous papules and nodules which over period of time developed necrosis.

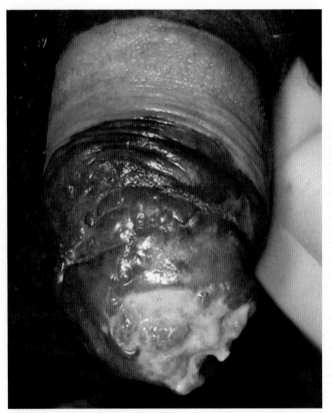

Papulonecrotic tuberculid of glans: Recurrent episodes of necrotic ulcer. Note healed punched out and bridging scars (worm eaten appearance).

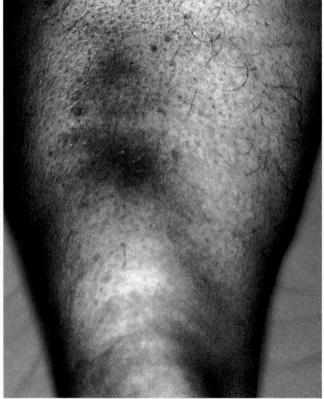

Erythema nodosum: painful, tender erythematous nodules on shin, which appear in crops. Resolve with hyperpigmentation in 2–6 weeks.

Histopathology

Cutaneous Tuberculosis and True Tuberculides

Basically tuberculoid granulomatous infiltrate. In lupus vulgaris and typical tuberculides conspicous. In scrofuloderma and gumma may be masked by necrosis and abscess formation. In TVC typical tubercles uncommon but epithelioid cells and giant cells seen. Tuberculoid granuloma also conspicous in lichen scrofulosorum and over whelmed by necrosis in papulonecrotic tuberculide.

Epidermal changes variable: acanthosis in lupus vulgaris, severe hyperkeratosis in warty tuberculosis or necrosis in scrofuloderma and the so-called tuberculides. *M. tuberculosis* demonstrable in scrofuloderma and tuberculous gumma; rarely in other forms.

Facultative Tuberculides

Erythema nodosum shows septal panniculitis with chronic perivascular infiltrate while erythema induratum shows tuberculoid granuloma with caseation necrosis.

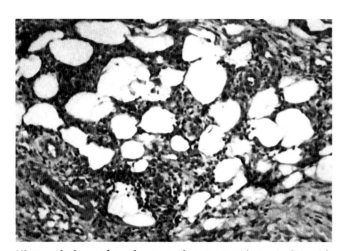

Histopathology of erythema nodosum: septal panniculitis with chronic perivascular infiltrate.

Identification of *Mycobacteria*

Direct Identification

By ordinary staining procedures not sensitive. Molecular techniques give better yield but not specific.

Culture

Not more sensitive.

Treatment

Systemic treatment with conventional antitubercular drugs. Essential to use 4 drugs (isoniazid, rifampicin, ethambutol and pyrazinamide) for initial intensive phase of 2 months; followed by 2 drugs (isoniazid, rifampicin) for 4 months, or longer. Drugs to be taken on empty stomach.

Treatment of cutaneous tuberculosis

	Duration	Drugs	Daily dose
Intensive phase	8 weeks	Isoniazid	5 mg/kg
		Rifampicin	10 mg/kg
		Ethambutol	15 mg/kg
		Pyrazinamide	30 mg/kg
Maintenance phase	16 weeks	Isoniazid	5 mg/kg
		Rifampicin	10 mg/kg

6

Diseases Caused by Arthropods and Parasites

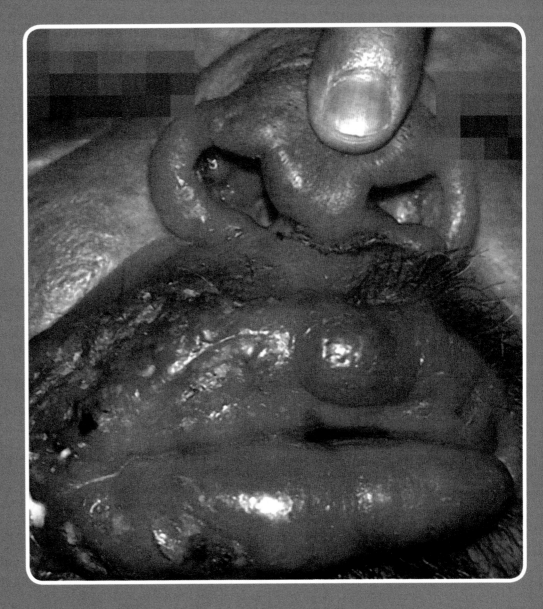

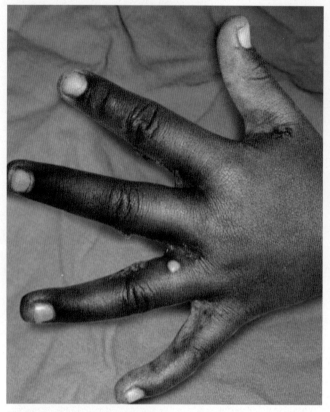

Scabies: characteristic involvement of web spaces of fingers. Secondary infection, a common complication.

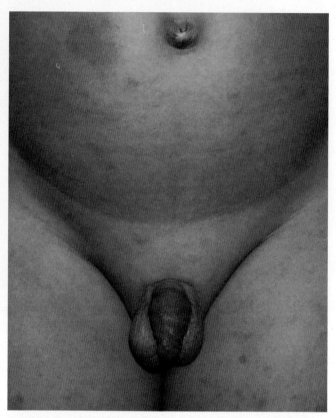

Scabies: papular and eczematous lesions in the belt area.

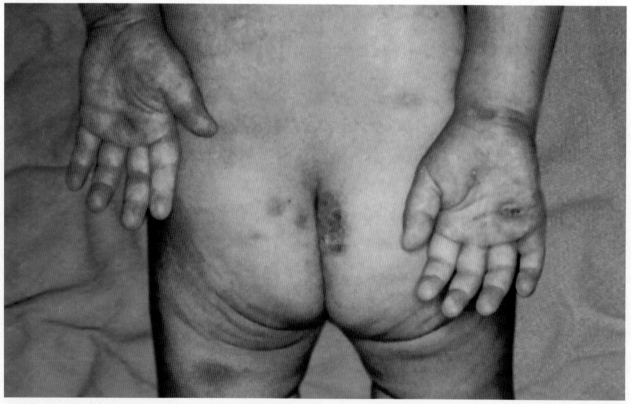

Scabies in an infant: palms (and soles) often involved.

Heterogeneous group of dermatoses caused by protozoa, worms or arthropods such as mites, lice, insects and fleas. Parasites living on skin, called ectoparasites, cause infestations; those living within the body, endoparasites, cause infections. May cause skin damage through mechanical injury, toxins and immune mediated mechanisms. Or act as vectors. Man may be the definitive or intermediate host. Most conditions, common in the tropics and wherever living conditions poor.

SCABIES

Etiology

Female of mite *Sarcoptes scabiei var. hominis*.

Epidemiology

An extremely common disease of the poor and underprivileged. Spreads by close personal contact; role of fomites uncertain, perhaps unimportant. Crowded living conditions and poor personal hygiene predispose. History of similar complaints in family or contacts often present. Also sexually transmitted.

Clinical Manifestations

Morphology

Intensely itchy (more pronounced at night), generalized papular eruption. Pathognomonic lesion a burrow, an irregularly linear skin colored ridge, produced by female mite tunneling through stratum corneum. Persistent nodules may develop on the male genitals (**nodular scabies**). Course of the disease variable—often a reflection of personal hygiene of patient.

Sites of Predilection

Burrows present in interdigital clefts of hands, flexors of wrists, elbows, anterior axillary folds, the 'belt' area and buttocks. And in children, additionally on the palms and soles. Male genitalia. And in females, the areolae of the breast. Head and neck conspicuously spared except in infants.

Complications

Excoriations, secondary pyococcal infection or eczematization common. Acute glomerulonephritis,

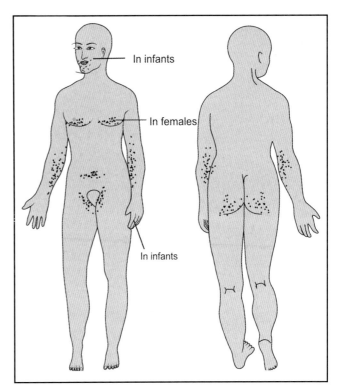

Sites of predilection: Scabies.

an occasional but serious complication of secondary streptococcal infection. Local applications of corticosteroids may make scabies unrecognizable (**scabies incognito**).

Norwegian Scabies

Rare. Caused by the same mite that causes ordinary scabies but in patients with compromised cell mediated immune status (e.g. AIDS). Or in mentally challenged. Manifests as hyperkeratotic and crusted lesions on the hands and feet. Keratotic, erythematous plaques on the trunk; occasionally generalized erythroderma. Itching minimal. Highly contagious condition, since there are numerous mites in the scales. May infect casual contacts to cause ordinary scabies.

Investigations

Diagnosis clinical.

Skin Scrapings

Sometimes skin scrapings done to demonstrate mite done by paring burrows from hands and wrists.

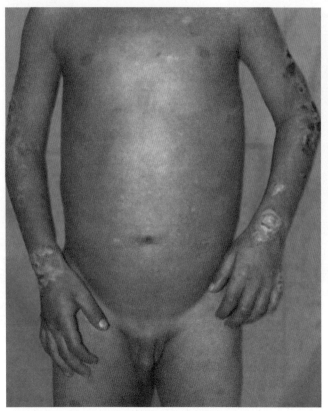

Scabies: infected and eczematous lesions.

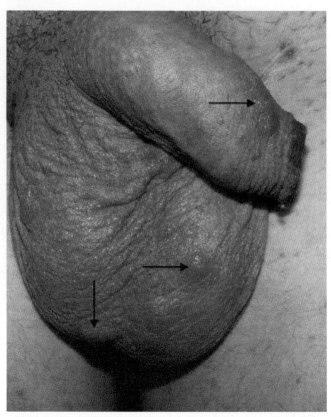

Scabies: note the serpiginous burrow on shaft of penis and the nodular lesions on scrotum.

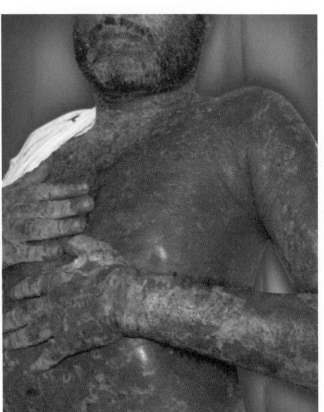

Norwegian scabies: presenting as exfoliative dermatitis.

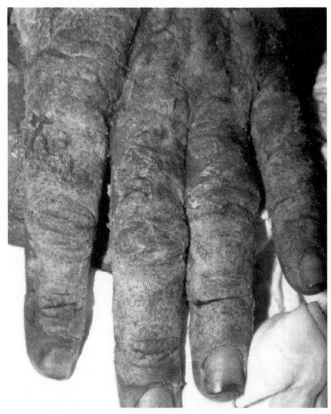

Norwegian scabies: hyperkeratotic lesions on the dorsa of the hands.

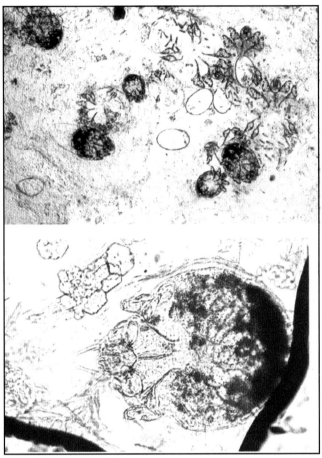

Skin scraping in Norwegian scabies: many acari seen in a scale (top); close-up view (bottom).

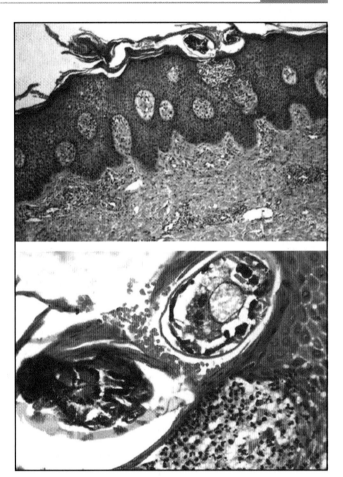

Histopathology of Norwegian scabies: acari in the stratum corneum, acanthosis and a perivascular infiltrate of lymphocytes, histiocytes and eosinophils (above); close-up view (below).

Biopsy

Shows acari in stratum corneum. And acanthosis and a perivascular infiltrate of lymphocytes and eosinophils.

Treatment

General Measures

All family members to be treated simultaneously. Itching (treated with antihistamines) persists for about 1–2 weeks, even after successful treatment; re-evaluate patient, if persists longer.

Specific Treatment

Antiscabitics, topical and systemic.

Topical treatment

Include permethrin, 5% cream, lindane (gamma benzene hexachloride, GBH), 1% lotion/cream and benzyl benzoate, 10–25% lotion/emulsion. Intralesional steroids used in nodular scabies.

Systemic treatment

Ivermectin (200 µg/kg), the only systemic agent. Used for Norwegian scabies and scabies epidemics in institutions (orphanages, old age homes).

PEDICULOSIS

Etiology

Pediculus humanus capitis (head louse). Or *Pediculus humanus corporis* (body louse). Or *Phthirus pubis* (pubic louse). *Pediculus humanus capitis* and *Pediculus humanus corporis* dorsoventrally flattened and oblong. Pubic louse (crab-louse) greater in width than length. Lice, obligate parasites. Blood-suckers literally. Cannot survive on inanimate objects.

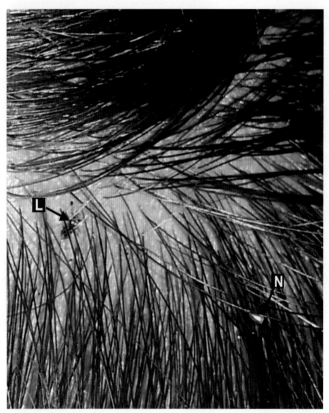

Pediculosis capitis: adult louse (L) appears as greyish white insects stuck to scalp or seen crawling. Generally more frequently nits (N) are seen as whitish oval particles attached to hair.

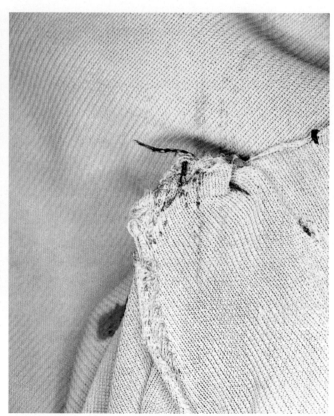

Pediculosis corporis: nits adherent to the seams of clothes.

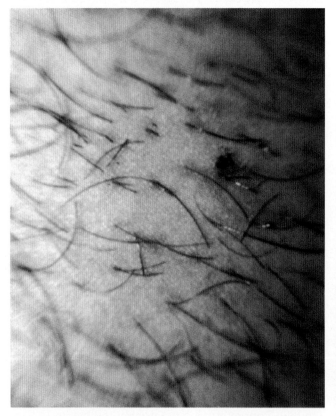

Pediculosis pubis: a louse and nits stuck to the hair.

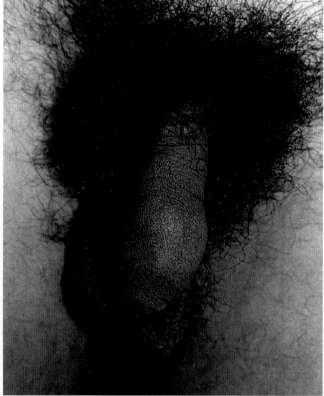

Pediculosis pubis: louse and nits attached to pubic hair.

Clinical Manifestations

Pediculosis Capitis

Common, particularly in girls and women. And men wearing long hair. Poor personal hygiene promotes infestation. Transmitted through combs, caps or hair brushes. Intensely itchy. Common sequence: scratching, exudation, secondary bacterial infection, infective eczema and cervical lymphadenopathy. Any bacterial infection in the occipital and postauricular areas, suspect pediculosis, so look for nits or lice. Nits (eggs of lice)-whitish, oval, firm particles easily detected near the root of the hair; cannot be flicked off the hair but can be slided along hair shaft. Adult lice: greyish insects, 3–4 mm long, stuck to the scalp or may be seen moving. Less frequently observed than nits.

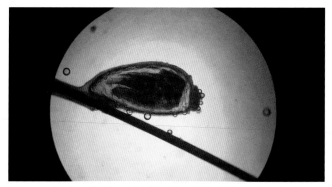

Nits attached to the hair shaft can be glided along the shaft with deep combing, but cannot be flicked off. Note the operculum (cap at the top of free end the nit) and the early louse inside the nit (saline mount, 10X).

Treatment

General Measures

Treat family and close contacts simultaneously. Remove nits with a fine-toothed comb. Treat combs and hair brushes in lysol or pediculocidal agents.

Specific Measures

Topical therapy

Topical permethrin, 1% applied for 10–15 minutes, treatment of choice. Repeat after 7 days to kill freshly hatched parasites. Alternates include GBH, 1% lotion. Malathion, 5% good for repeated infestation because of residual effect.

Systemic therapy

Ivermectin 250 μg/kg. Repeat after 7–10 days.

Pediculosis Corporis (Vagabond's Disease)

Rare. Seen in destitutes or mentally ill individuals with grossly neglected personal hygiene. Lice live on the seams of clothes but feed on blood. Vector of typhus, relapsing fever. Severely itchy condition. Small red macules turn to intensely pruritic papules with a central hemorrhagic punctum. Excoriations, pigmentation, bacterial infection, eczematization and crusting present on trunk and shoulders. Lice and nits demonstrable on seams of undergarments (rarely on body).

Treatment

General Measures

Improve patients hygiene. Treat contacts. High dose of antihistamines. And antibiotics if secondary infection.

Specific Measures

Treat clothes and bedding with DDT, 10% powder. Or GBH, 1%. Washing in hot water and hot ironing adequate to kill louse.

Pediculosis Pubis

Not uncommon. Sexually transmitted. Or occasionally through sharing bed or fomites. Intense itching. Louse stays stuck to the skin. Seen as dark brown specks in pubic region, axillae, eye lashes or body hair. Excoriations, secondary bacterial infection and eczematization common. Also bluish-grey macules (maculae cerulae) seen occasionally on the thighs or lower abdomen.

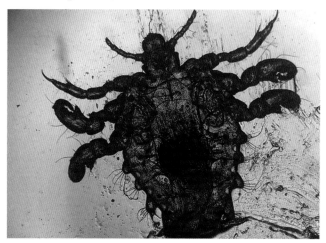

Pubic ('crab') louse: Note pincer like claws at free end of legs. (saline mount 10X)

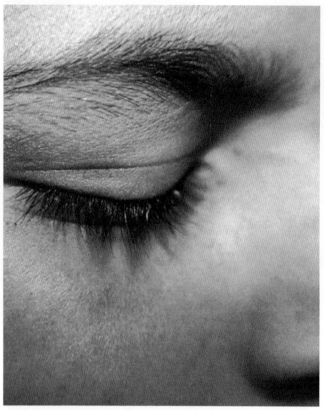

Pediculosis pubis: nits attached to the eyelashes.

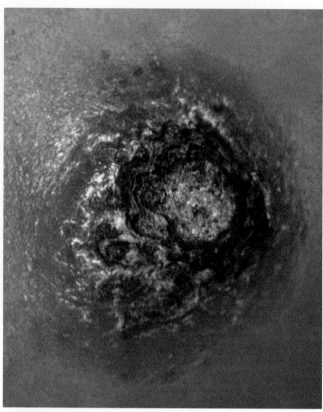

Acute cutaneous leishmaniasis: erythematous nodule showing ulceration.

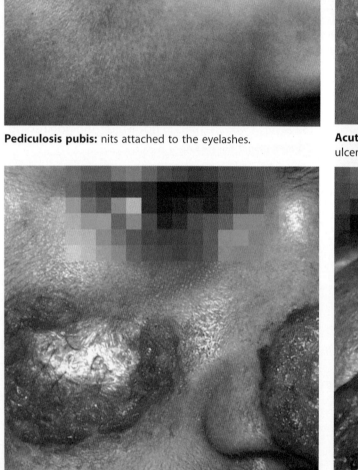

Chronic cutaneous leishmaniasis: with simultaneous progress and scarring.

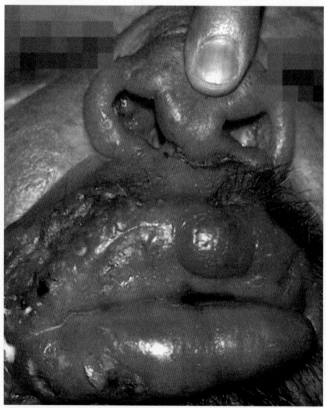

Mucocutaneous leishmaniasis: edematous nodules, some ulcerated on the lips and nose. Often leads to scarring and mutilation.

Treatment

General Measures

Treat sexual partners. Antihistamines and antibiotics.

Specific Measures

Treat with permethrin or GBH.

LEISHMANIASIS

Etiology

Caused by genus *Leishmania*. Different species cause varied presentation.

Causative agents of leishmaniasis	
Manifestation	*Agent*
Cutaneous leishmaniasis	*Leishmania tropica*
Mucocutaneous leishmaniasis	*L. major L. braziliensis*
Post kala-azar dermal leishmaniasis	*Leishmania donovani*

Vector for most is sand flies (*Phlebotomus species*), and reservoir, humans, dogs, rodents.

Pathogenesis

Clinical manifestations an interplay of virulence of the organism and cell mediated immunity (CMI) of the host. Spectral concept of leishmaniasis almost similar to that of leprosy.

Clinical Manifestations

Acute Cutaneous Leishmaniasis (Oriental Sore)

Common in the tropics. Children or adults. Variable incubation period-a few weeks to a year depending upon number of organisms and type (major or minor) of parasite. A solitary (or multiple) indolent edematous nodule or plaque with superficial ulceration and crusting. Or plaque surmounted by a crateriform ulcer. Associated satellite nodules; simultaneous progression and healing with scarring. Leishmanin skin test positive. Infection confers permanent immunity. Lesions on exposed sites (areas prone to be bitten by sandfly), like face, hands.

Chronic Cutaneous Leishmaniasis (Leishmaniasis Recidivans)

Uncommon. Reported from Iran and Afghanisthan. Reddish brown papules reappear in a healed lesion of leishmaniasis. Evolves into a plaque.

Disseminated Leishmaniasis

Uncommon. In patients with low CMI. Initial papulonodules, first spread locally. And then to distant cutaneous sites. No visceral involvement. Leishmanin test negative. Lesions rich in organisms.

Mucocutaneous Leishmaniasis

Common in Latin America. Due to *L. brasiliensis* incubation period shorter than for oriental sore. Primary lesion usually cutaneous papule or nodule with lymphangitis and lymphadenitis. Mucosal lesions usually simultaneous to, or a sequel to cutaneous lesions-erosive, ulcerative or grossly destructive. Nose, lips, soft palate and pharynx affected. Bones not involved. Course rapid progress, without healing.

Post Kala-azar Dermal Leishmaniasis (Dermal Leishmanoid)

A less common cutaneous aftermath of visceral leishmaniasis, generally after incomplete (sometimes even complete) treatment. Multiple, asymptomatic, hypopigmented macules on the trunk and extremities. And succulent nodules on the face; concentrated in the central part especially circumorally. Also malar erythema. Needs to be differentiated from lepromatous (and borderline) leprosy.

Investigations

Direct Microscopy

Samples obtained from lesion directly or through a slit skin smear. Stained with Giemsa. Wrights, or Leishman's stain. Shows amastigote LD bodies in and outside macrophages.

Culture

In NNN medium.

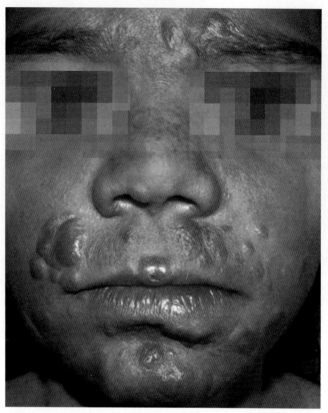

Post kala-azar dermal leishmaniasis: characteristic juicy papules and nodules in perioral distribution.

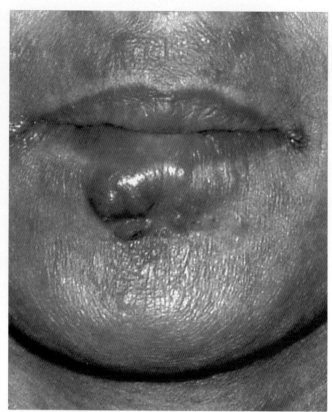

Post kala-azar dermal leishmaniasis: succulent centrofacial nodules.

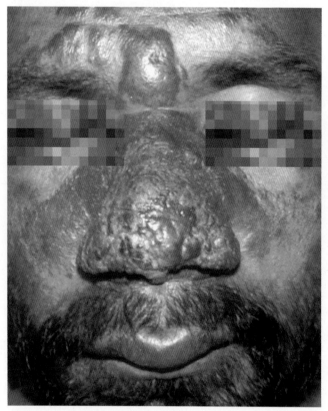

Post kala-azar dermal leishmaniasis: extensive facial involvement. Lesions predominantly centrofacial.

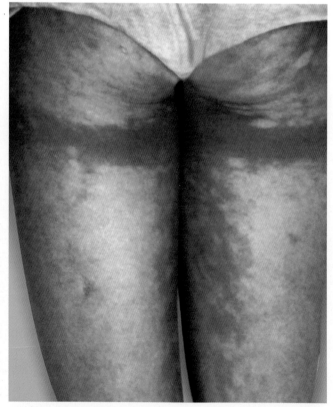

Post kala-azar dermal leishmaniasis: extensive hypopigmented macules.

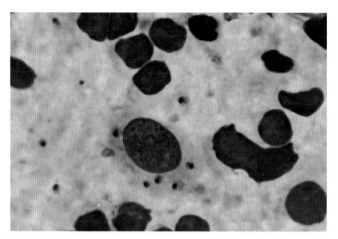

Tissue smear of post kala-azar dermal leishmaniasis: stained with Giemsa stain showing amastigote forms of leishmania (LD bodies) both within and outside macrophages.

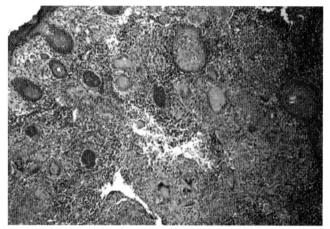

Histopathology of cutaneous leishmaniasis: dense mixed infiltrate of eosinophils, lymphocytes, plasma cells and macrophages filled with LD bodies.

Molecular Diagnosis

Kinetoplast minicircle DNA, highly sensitive and 100% specific.

Leishmanin Test

Montenegro test. Positive in most forms, except in initial phase of infection and in disseminated cutaneous leishmaniasis.

Serology

Elisa test to detect antibodies against various antigens of *Leishmania spp*, most notabily rr 39 and rk 16. Useful in visceral leishmaniasis and may be in PKDL.

Histopathology

Dense diffuse mixed infiltrate of histiocytes, lymphocytes, plasma cells (sometimes with intracytoplasmic eosinophilic Russel bodies), and eosinophils. Typically intracytoplasmic (in histiocytes) and extracellular dot-dash LD bodies diagnostic. Giemsa stained slides more sensitive. Chronic cutaneous leishmaniasis usually organism poor, with either diffuse or nodular non-caseating tuberculoid granuloma.

Treatment

Cutaneous Leishmaniasis

Intralesional pentavalent antimony, 15% paramomycin.

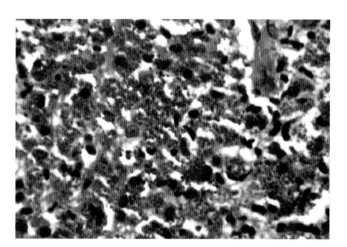

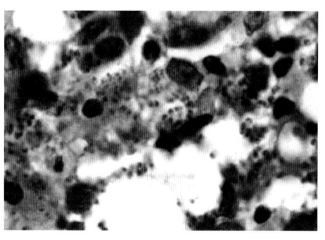

Histopathology of cutaneous leishmaniasis: Giemsa stained slide showing macrophages containing basophilic stained LD bodies; top (40x), bottom (100x).

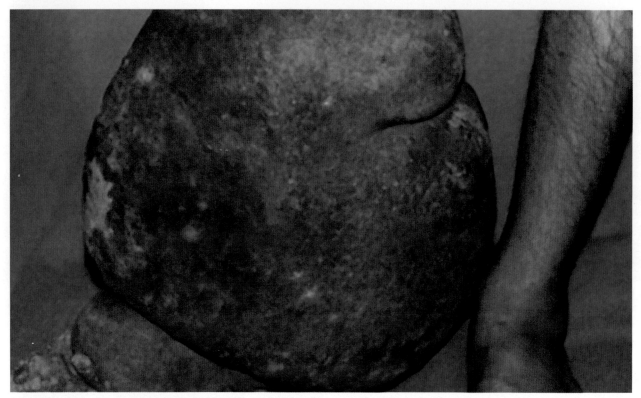

Filarial elephantiasis of the right leg and foot: lymphedema, hyperplasia of connective tissue with verrucosity of skin.

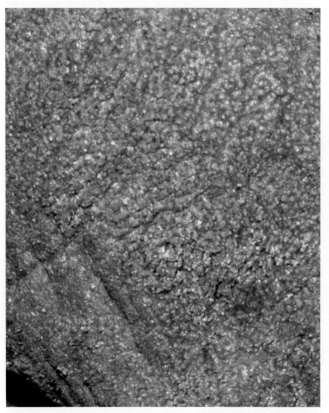

Lymphedema: close up of secondary changes—verrucosity and nodulation.

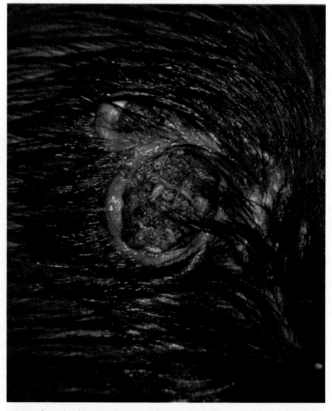

Wound myiasis: maggots in the wound.

Post Kala-azar Dermal Leishmaniasis

Pentavalent sodium antimony gluconate 10–20 mg/kg/day for 90–120 days, given parenterally. Ketoconazole, fluconazole, allopurinol, rifampicin given alone or in combination with antimony. If available miltefosine, 2.5 mg/kg/day orally for 28 days, is now first line of treatment.

FILARIASIS

Epidemiology

Endemic in parts of India, Asia and South America.

Etiology

Etiological Agents

Caused by *Wuchereria bancrofti* and *Brugia malayi*.

Vectors

Mosquitoes (*Culex*, *Mansonia*, *Aedes* and *Anopheles*), inject larvae into the skin.

Clinical Manifestations

Variable incubation period 3–12 months or more. Disease clinically indistinguishable irrespective of etiological agent. Presence of larvae (microfilariae) in circulation largely asymptomatic. Adult worms in the lymphatics cause symptoms.

Two stages recognized:

- **Early inflammatory phase:** Recurrent episodes of acute lymphangitis and lymphadenopathy, orchitis, funiculitis and fever.
- **Late obstructive phase:** Lymphedema, hyperplasia of the connective tissue and thickening of the skin and subcutaneous tissue with verrucous nodulation-elephantiasis.

Feet, legs or scrotum commonly affected.

Treatment

General Measures

Lower limb exercises. Foot end elevation. Hygiene and treatment of secondary bacterial infections.

Medical Treatment

Microfilariae respond to treatment with diethylcarbamazine in gradually increasing doses usually along with albendazole. DEC also used as mass drug administration (MDA) usually as fortified salt. Ivermectin also effective against microfilariae. Adult filariae not amenable to treatment.

Surgical Treatment

Elephantiasis needs surgical intervention—creation of lymphnode venous-shunt. Or/and removal of subcutaneous tissue.

CUTANEOUS MYIASIS

Infestation caused by the larvae (maggots) of flies (Diptera).

Clinical Manifestations

Can be:

- **Traumatic or wound myiasis:** which is common in patients with poor personal hygiene.
- **Obligatory myiasis:** which may manifest as furuncular form. Or as a creeping eruption.

INVESTIGATIONS

Usually clinical. Rarely histopathologically.

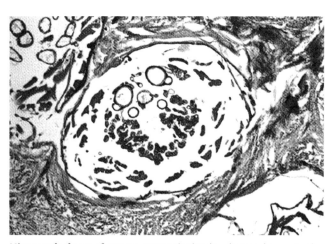

Histopathology of cutaneous myiasis: developing larvae in the dermis.

Treatment

Wound care paramount. Clean locally with chloroform, ether or other organic solvents or remove mechanically.

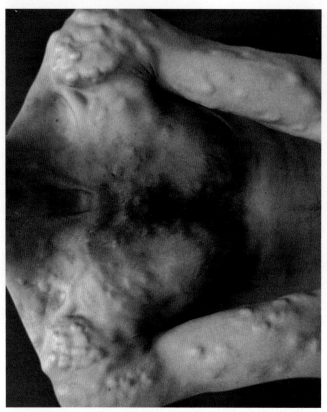

Cysticercosis of skin, extensive disseminated: multiple, round to oval, deep cysts.

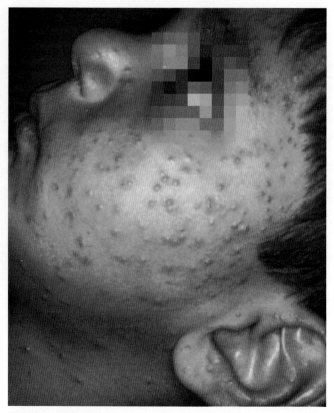

Papular urticaria: papular lesions on face and other exposed parts of body.

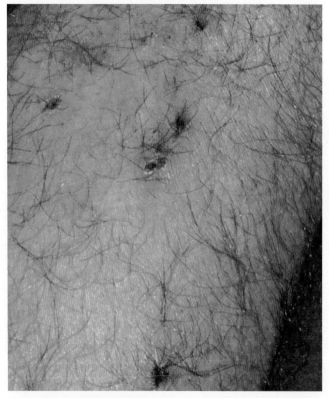

Insect bite hypersensitivity: excoriated papules on exposed sites. In an adult should arouse suspicion of an underlying lymphoreticular malignancy or HIV infection.

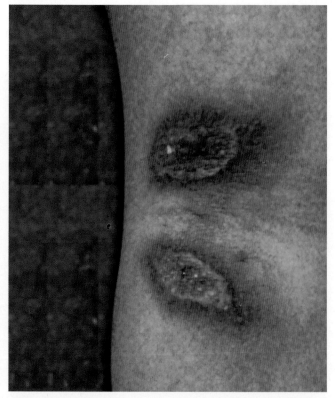

Pedrus dermatitis: due to chemicals from beetles; kissing lesions occur in flexural areas.

CYSTICERCOSIS

Uncommon. Results from ingestion of food or drink contaminated with the eggs of *Taenia solium*, subcutaneous, firm, asymptomatic 1–2 cm oblong nodules (larvae of taenia—*Cysticercus cellulosae*), vary in numbers. Brain, muscles and eyes may also be affected—may manifest as epilepsy or intracranial space occupying lesions.

Treatment

Surgical excision for skin lesions. Rule out neurocysticercosis.

INSECT BITES/REACTIONS

Etiology

Common, particularly in the tropics. Caused by hypersensitivity. Or injection squirting of 'toxic' substances.

Epidemiology

Children or adults. Seasonal.

Clinical Manifestations

Papular Urticaria

Common. Manifestation of hypersensitivity to insect bites. Children, 2–7 years. May manifest in immunocompromised adults (lymphoreticular malignancies, immunosuppression and HIV infection). Frequent in summers, remits in winter. Pruritic papules and weals or a 'combination-lesion' on an erythematous background. Individual lesions self-limiting. Excoriations and secondary bacterial infection frequent. Exposed sites.

Paederus Dermatitis

Outbreaks common at the end of rainy season. Acute erythematous vesicular reaction caused by beetle of genus Paederus (commonly *Paederus sabaeus*) due to a vesicant, paederin, released when the beetle is crushed. Kissing lesions common. Exposed sites-face, limbs.

Treatment

General Measures

Protection by physical barriers or insect repellents. Antihistamines. Secondary bacterial infections appropriately treated.

Specific Treatment

Acute lesions treated with topical corticosteroids.

DRACUNCULOSIS (GUINEA WORM INFESTATION)

Now eradicated. Caused by nematode-*Dracunculus medinensis*. Acquired by drinking water contaminated with parasitized cyclops (water fleas). The adult female dracunculus rests quietly in the subcutis, commonly of legs and feet. Emerges only on contact with water to discharge larvae. Blister or a superficial ulcer with the worm protruding. Prodrome of fever, urticaria, dyspnea. Cellulitis and abscess formation may complicate.

CUTANEOUS LARVA MIGRANS (CREEPING ERUPTION)

Etiology

Migratory skin lesions produced by movements within the skin of larvae of non-human hookworm (*Ancylostoma braziliense or A. caninum*). Normally harbored in the intestines of dogs and cats. Acquired on beaches or locations where soil contaminated with fecal matter.

Clinical Manifestations

Uncommon. Itchy, bizarre, tortuous, thread-like, pink or skin colored migratory ridge with tiny vesiculation. Variable course, largely self-limiting. Commonly seen on feet, hands, buttocks.

Treatment

Local application of 10% thiabendazole suspension 3–4 times a day for 7–10 days. Ivermectin 200 μg/kg, single dose, repeated after 7 days.

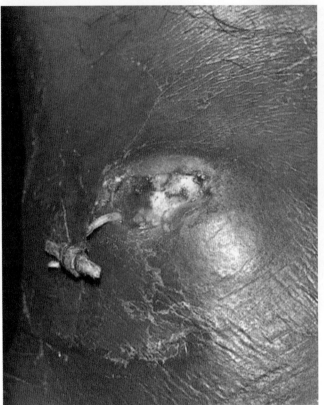

Dracunculosis: guinea worm protruding out of an ulcer.

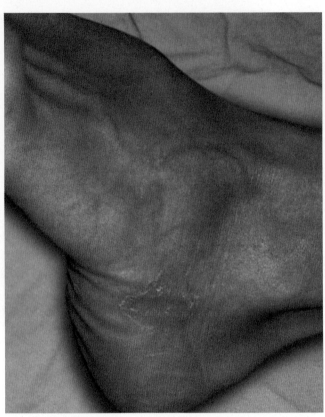

Creeping eruption: tortuous thread-like ridge.

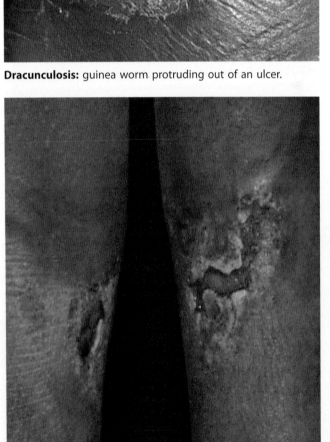

Onchocerciasis: lichenified and eroded dermatitis.

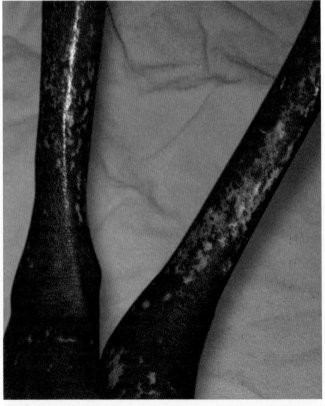

Onchocerciasis: late depigmented lesions on the shins-leopard skin.

ONCHOCERCIASIS

Etiology

Onchocerca volvulus.

Vectors

Members of *Simuliidae* family particularly *Simulium damnosum.*

Epidemiology

Common in Africa, Latin America and Yemen.

Clinical Manifestations

Pruritus. Localized acute (urticarial papules or pustules), chronic (excoriated papules or flat topped scars), or lichenified dermatitis accompanied by atrophy.

Late stage manifests as bilateral depigmentation, generally confined to pretibial skin (leopard skin). Visual impairment and blindness, a major complication.

Investigations

Diagnosis based on clinical features. And confirmed by demonstration of microfilariae in skin snips.

Treatment

Ivermectin, 100–200 µg/kg orally, single dose, causes pronounced reduction of microfilariae in the skin for 6–12 months. Repeat treatment. Alternatively use diethylcarbamazine. Suramin kills adult worms.

7

Dermatitis and Eczema

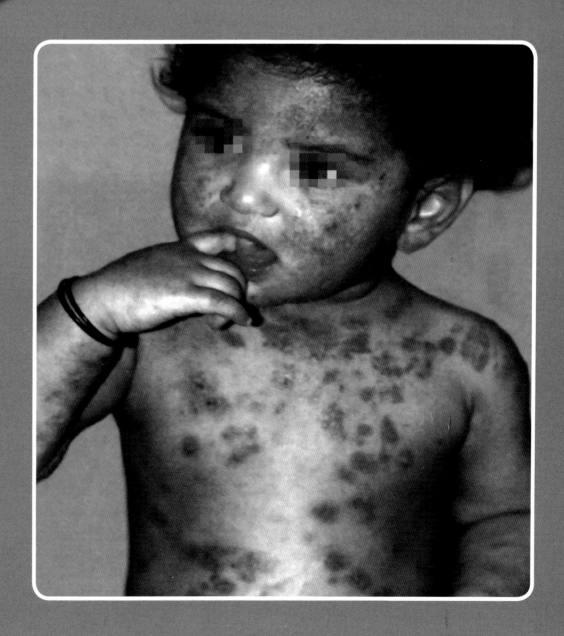

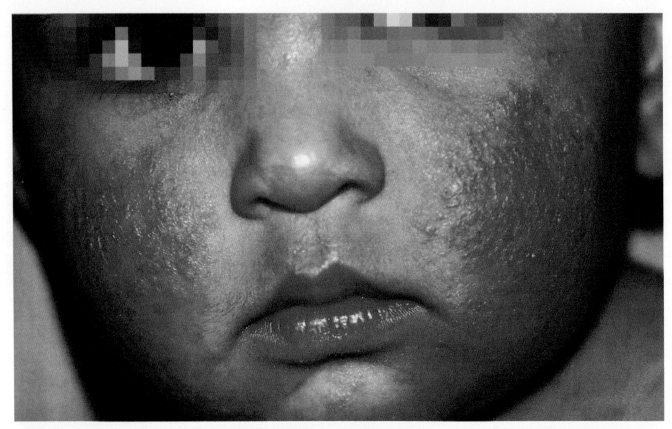

Atopic dermatitis, infantile phase: bilaterally symmetrical papulovesicular lesions on an erythematous background.

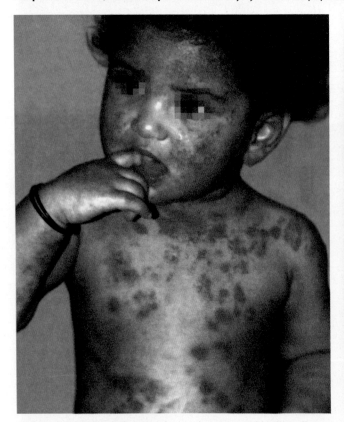

Atopic dermatitis, infantile phase: disseminated lesions all over the body.

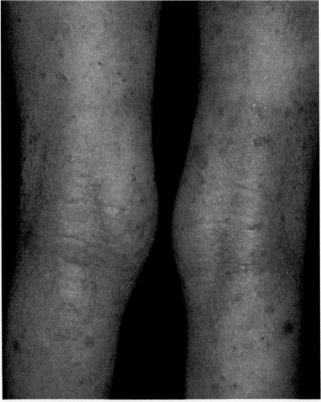

Atopic dermatitis, childhood phase: bilaterally symmetrical lichenified and excoriated lesions in the flexures of the knees.

INTRODUCTION

Dermatitis, a distinctive inflammatory response of the skin, secondary to a number of exogenous or endogenous factors. The terms dermatitis and eczema used synonymously and interchangeably. Genetic predisposition often important.

Classification

Several classifications proposed—some based on *etiology*—endogenous/exogenous. Others on *morphology/pattern* (nummular/seborrheic). Recent one combines both. Also as acute, subacute, chronic. *Acute phase*: characterized by erythema, edema, papulation, vesiculation, exudation, crusting. And *subacute or chronic phase*: characterized by scaling and lichenification.

Etiology

Reaction pattern to endogenous or exogenous stimuli. Genetic factors important in atopic while exogenous factors paramount in contact (irritant/allergic) dermatitis, diaper dermatitis. Also important to some extent in atopic dermatitis.

Histology

Epidermal intercellular edema (spongiosis) in acute eczema and acanthosis (hyperplasia of stratum malpighi), hyperkeratosis and parakeratosis (premature keratinization) in the subacute and chronic phase. Dermal inflammatory infiltrate, polymorphonuclear or lymphocytic, pronounced in acute eczema, less so in subacute or chronic eczema.

ATOPIC DERMATITIS (AD)

An itchy chronic remitting and relapsing inflammatory skin condition associated with other atopic disorders (asthma, hay fever) in patient or the family.

Etiology

Complex interplay between genetic factors (resulting in defective skin barrier), defective innate immunity and exaggerated immunological responses to allergens and microbes, by production of IgE.

Clinical Features

Common dermatosis. Three distinct or merging phases—**infantile**, **childhood** and **adult**. Itching, scratching, exudation and lichenification important features. More prone to acquiring viral and some bacterial infections. Dry, generally irritable skin that may not tolerate extremes of temperature or humidity such as dry cold, excessive sweating or contact with dust or wool. Patients anxious and sensitive.

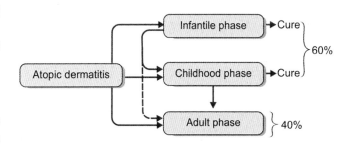

Infantile phase

Common. Often first born male infant. Onset at about 3rd month. Itching severe and paroxysmal. Bilaterally symmetrical, papulovesicular, exudative and crusted lesions. Cheeks predominantly involved. Later on extensors of extremities and trunk. Secondary bacterial infections common. Spontaneous remissions and relapses. May completely remit by about 2–3 years. Or may evolve into childhood phase.

Childhood phase

May evolve from the infantile phase or start *de novo*. Intensely pruritic papules. Sometimes lichenified and excoriated lesions. Symmetrically in the flexures of the elbows and knees. Also the wrists, ankles and sides of neck.

Adult phase

Less common. May evolve *per se*. Or from AD of infancy or childhood. Lichenified plaques, often in the flexures. Or as nummular dermatitis. Extensor aspects of the extremities occasionally involved. Itching a dominant complaint, thus patients more prone to develop lichen simplex chronicus.

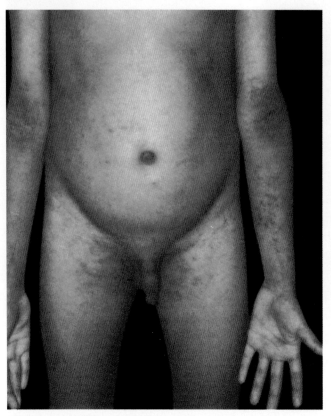

Atopic dermatitis, childhood phase: bilaterally symmetrical excoriated papules and lichenified lesions in the flexures.

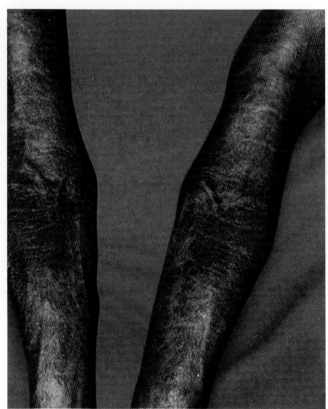

Atopic dermatitis, adult phase: lichenified lesions in the cubital fossae.

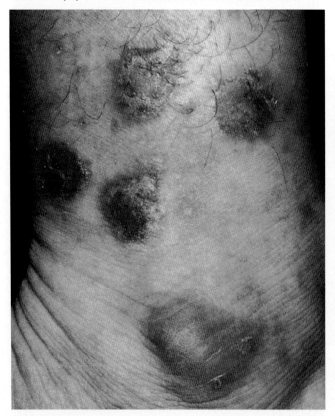

Nummular eczema: discoid (coin-like) exudative lesions with mild crusting.

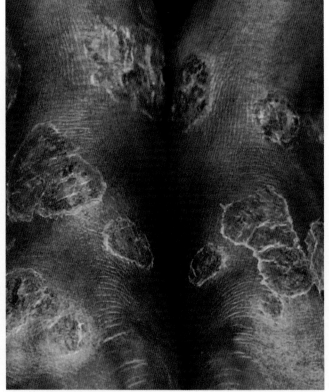

Dry discoid eczema: discoid plaques surmounted with scales.

Associations

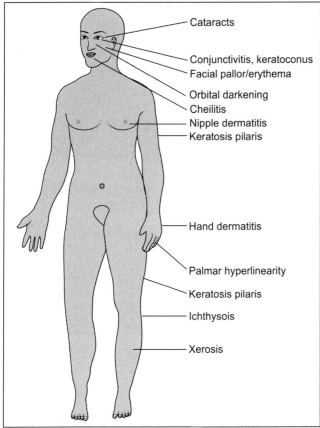

Associations of atopic dermatitis

Minor features
Cataracts (anterior subcapsular)
Cheilitis
Conjunctivitis, recurrent
Facial pallor/erythema
Food intolerance
Hand dermatitis: nonallergic, irritant
Ichthyosis
Elevated levels of IgE
Immediate (type I) skin test reactivity
Infections
Itching, when sweating
Keratoconus
Keratosis pilaris
Nipple dermatitis
Orbital darkening
Palmar hyperlinearity
Perifollicular accentuation
Pityriasis alba
White dermographism
Wool intolerance
Xerosis
* Arranged alphabetically

Treatment

General Measures

Scratching, the single most important factor, its avoidance the most desirable therapeutic measure. Though debatable, best controlled with antihistamines. Avoid dust, extremes of heat or dryness or direct contact with woolen fabrics—all of these being non-specific irritants. Role of diet controversial. Breast feeding probably protects. Routine childhood vaccinations not contraindicated. Skin continuosly treated with bland emollients-ointments, creams. Best used after hydration of skin. Best prophylactic measure too.

Specific Treatment

Topical therapy

Topical corticosteroids mainstay of therapy. Potency of steroid used based on disease severity, age of patient, site affected. Moderate-potency steroids used in acute state followed by mild to moderate steroids for maintenance. Combined with salicyclic acid in lichenified lesions and with antifungal agents in flexures. Topical immunomodulators (tacrolimus, 0.1 and 0.03% ointment and pimecrolimus 0.1% cream) found useful and steroid sparing. Wet wraps now considered important adjunctive treatment.

Systemic therapy

Short-term oral corticosteroids definitely useful in severe exacerbations. Recalcitrant cases may require oral cyclosporine, methotrexate, azathioprine and mycophenolate mofetil. Phototherapy, photochemotherapy, extracorporeal photopheresis and interferons other effective treatment measures, to be used in severe recalcitrant cases. Omalizumab a biological effective.

NUMMULAR ECZEMA

Etiology

A morphologic diagnosis. A number of unrelated factors such as atopy, infections, autosensitization (ide), physical trauma, particularly on a dry asteatotic skin may be responsible.

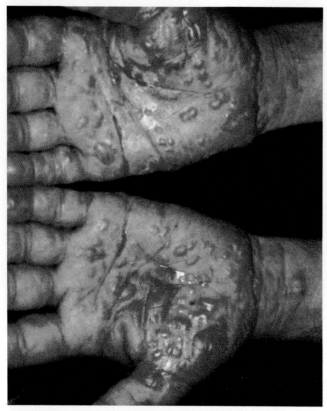

Pompholyx: deep seated bilaterally symmetrical vesicles on the palms.

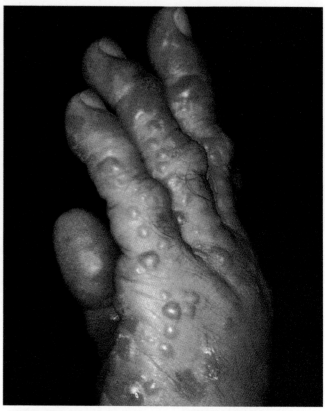

Pompholyx: vesicular lesions on the sides of the fingers.

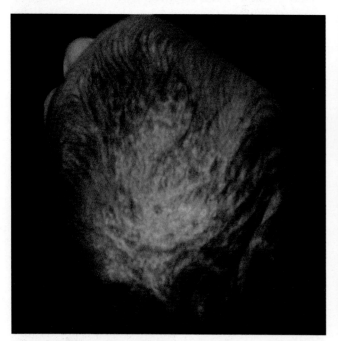

Seborrheic dermatitis, infantile: cradle cap.

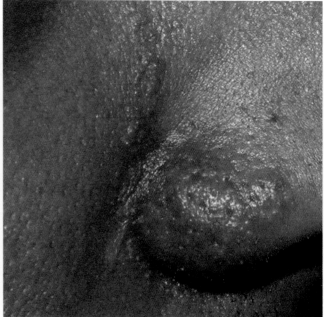

Seborrheic dermatitis: scaling nasolabrial fold.

Clinical Manifestations

Morphology

Erythematous, edematous discoid plaques of itchy, papulovesicular lesions which exude serous discharge and form crusts.

Sites of Predilection

Dorsa of the hands and extensor aspects of upper or lower extremities preferentially affected; bilateral but often asymmetrical.

Variants

Dry discoid dermatitis: A non-exudative variant of nummular eczema. Round or oval, dry, scaly plaques on extensors of extremities.

Course

Relapsing and remitting; relapses often abrupt in onset and frequent in winter.

Treatment

General Measures

Eliminate/treat predisposing factors. Moisturize skin.

Specific Treatment

Topical steroid (often combined with antibiotic cream). Antihistamines. Extensive lesions may warrant systemic steroids/immunosuppressives.

POMPHOLYX

Etiology

Multifactorial—atopic or other endogenous eczema. Or a dermatophytide (hematogenous dissemination of dermatophyte toxins from a focus of ringworm-generally tinea pedis).

Clinical Manifestations

More common in summers. Hyperhidrosis a common, association. Young adults of both sexes affected. Itchy or painful deep seated vesicular (sago-grain like) lesions on the palms, sides of the fingers and soles. Occasionally bullous or pustular lesions. Protracted relapsing course, each episode resolving in 2–3 weeks.

Treatment

General Measures

Saline compresses.

Specific Treatment

Potent topical steroids in moderate cases. Severe cases may need brief courses of systemic steroids. Relapsing cases pose a difficult therapeutic problem. Phototherapy or photochemotherapy may help.

SEBORRHEIC DERMATITIS

Etiology

Cause uncertain-possibly related to excessive growth of the commensal yeast, pityrosporum. Role of genetic factors debatable. Any relation to the quantity or composition of sebum uncertain. Individuals have a seborrheic diathesis. Dermatitis severe in patients with AIDS.

Epidemiology

Not uncommon. Two age peaks, in the first three months of life **infantile seborrheic dermatitis**. And second after fourth decade.

Clinical Manifestations

Morphology

Characteristic seborrheic look—oily skin with patulous, prominent follicular orifices. Scalp diffusely involved: ill-defined areas with greasy yellow scales on a dull red background (seborrhea capitis). Intertriginous areas: erythematous scaly lesions or exudative crusted and fissured lesions. Hairy areas—beard, trunk and pubic region show dull red, scaly plaques studded with follicular papules. Blepharitis and squamous otitis externa common association. Erythrodermic variant described as rarity.

Sites of Predilection

Characterized chiefly by its distribution. Scalp, retroauricular folds, eyebrows, nasolabial folds, beard area, interscapular and presternal regions, axillae, pubic region, groins, umbilicus and folds under pendulous breasts. Blepharitis: fine scaling of eyelid margin.

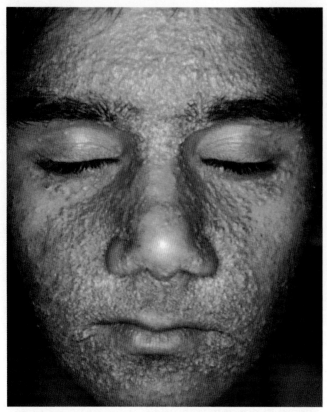

Seborrheic dermatitis: scaling and papulation on the face; nasolabial folds, eyebrows, upper lip and chin.

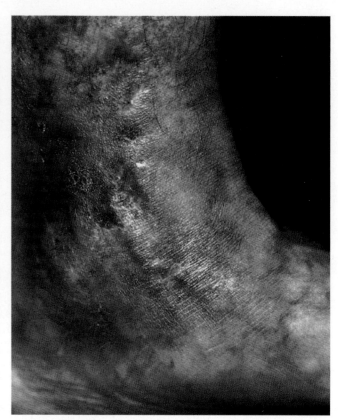

Stasis eczema: diffuse hyperpigmentation with depressed depigmented scar (atrophie blanche).

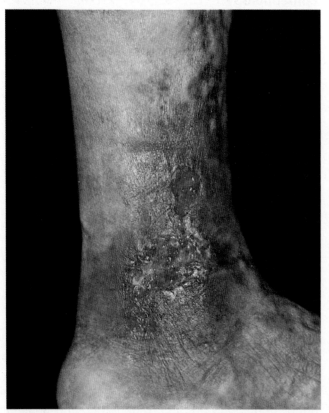

Stasis ulcer: ulcerative lesions surrounded by hyperpigmentation and erythema; tortuous dilated veins are seen.

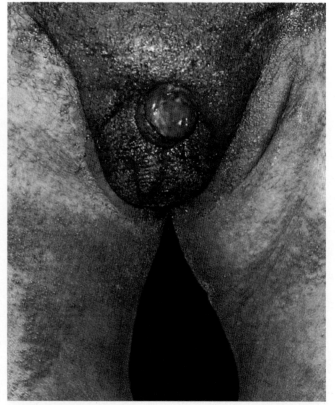

Irritant contact dermatitis: erythematous papulovesicles on the thighs due to application of cetrimide 20%.

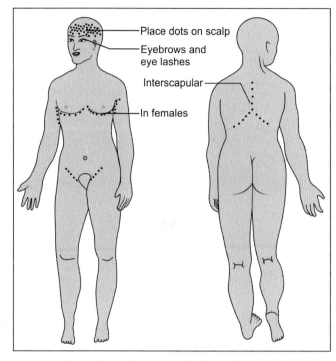

Sites of predilection: Seborrheic dermatitis.

- Place dots on scalp
- Eyebrows and eye lashes
- Interscapular
- In females

Course

Generally chronic with remissions and exacerbations. Patients predisposed to pyococcal infections.

Treatment

General Measures

Mild scaling of the scalp almost physiological. Ordinary shampooing alone adequate in mild cases. Application of hair oil best avoided.

Specific Therapy

Topical treatment

More severe scalp lesions treated with special medicated shampoos containing ketoconazole, fluconazole, selenium sulphide or zinc pyrithione, tar, salicylic acid. Shampoo best 'left on' for a few minutes before rinsing off. Repeated twice weekly or more frequently. Acute lesions at other sites treated with combination of topical steroids and antibiotics. Subacute stage, salicylic acid steroid combination helpful. Topical ketoconazole, 2% or butenafine, 1% cream give additional benefit.

Systemic treatment

For severe/extensive disease. Fluconazole, 150 mg weekly effective. Oral ketoconazole though effective best avoided because of its hepatotoxicity. For severe disease, narrow band UVB and PUVA therapy can be used.

STASIS ECZEMA

Epidemiology

Not uncommon. Middle aged individuals with compromised venous return. Related to long hours of continued standing.

Clinical Features

Slate-grey pigmentation. Later edema, acutely exudative and crusted lesions. Or scaly and lichenified areas; associated with obvious varicose veins or other evidence of venous stasis. Occasional ulceration that may heal with depigmented, atrophic scar (atrophie blanche). Medial aspects of ankles and lower legs involved. Autosensitization with generalized eczema not infrequent.

Treatment

General Measures

Relieve stasis. Keep feet elevated (at work also). Use pressure bandages/stockings.

Specific Therapy

Non-sensitizing, protective and bland local applications such as zinc oxide paste may help; compresses and non-fluorinated weak or moderate strength topical steroids in acute stages. Surgical or other intervention for correction of varicosities.

IRRITANT CONTACT DERMATITIS

Etiology

Non-immunologic dermatitis secondary to contact with an irritant substance in 'adequate' concentrations for a 'sufficient' length of time. Individuals with dry skin more prone. Single contact (usually accidental) with a strong irritant such as an acid, alkali, strong antiseptic. Or repeated contact (inadvertent, deliberate or occupational) with mild irritants such as detergents, cutting oils.

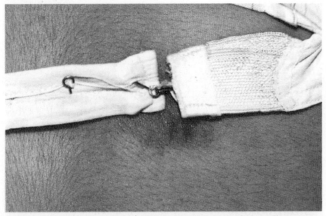

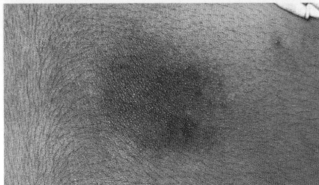

Allergic contact dermatitis: nickel in bra clips was causal.

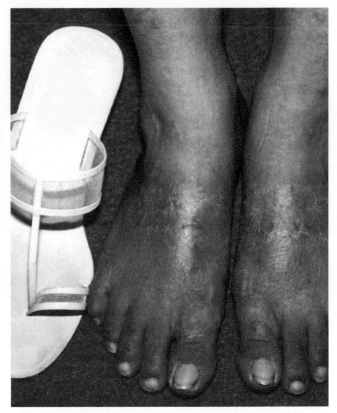

Allergic contact dermatitis, footwear: the skin in contact affected.

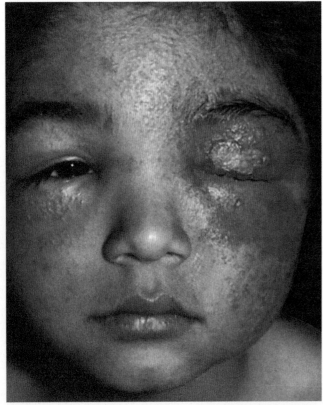

Allergic contact dermatitis: caused by a topical application following a minor injury; mild dissemination to the other side was due to accidental contact.

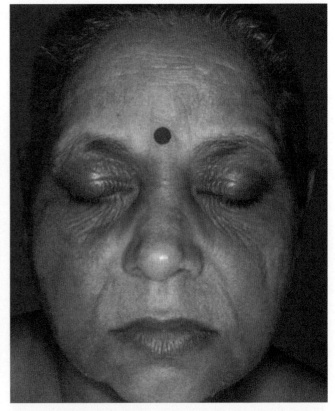

Airborne contact dermatitis: eyelids are conspicuously involved.

Clinical Manifestations

Common. Acute irritant dermatitis sharply limited to the area of contact. Similar in morphology to other acute eczemas—papules, vesicles or pustules, on an erythematous, edematous background. Heals with hyper/hypopigmentation. Strong irritants may cause necrosis or ulcers that heal with scars. Cumulative insult dermatitis due to repeated contact with weak irritants. Classic example **housewives' dermatitis**. Slow onset. Dryness and fissuring of the skin, followed by lichenification. Relapses on brief contact with mild irritants. Hands frequently affected.

ALLERGIC CONTACT DERMATITIS

A common dermatological problem, more frequent in the industrialized world.

Etiology

Type IV, delayed type hypersensitivity (DTH) response. Simple chemicals (haptens) become complete antigens on combining with a carrier, generally epidermal protein. Varying susceptibility of individuals. Racial and genetic factors, perhaps important. Sensitizing potential of substances variable. Nature of common contactants variable in different parts of the world. More frequent ones include nickel, cobalt, chromium, epoxy resins, antioxidants, textile dyes and finishes. *Plants*: such as *Parthenium hysterophorus* in India, poison ivy in the USA, *Primula obconica* in Europe and other members of the compositae family. *Medicaments*: such as nitrofurazone, neomycin, sulphonamides, penicillin, antihistamines, local anesthetics, lanolin, ethylene diamine and a host of 'home' remedies. *Cosmetics*: fragrances, paraphenylenediamine containing hair dyes, preservatives and eosin. The exposure to contactants would vary depending on sex, age, occupation, hobbies and living conditions. Damaged skin, occlusion, hyperhidrosis predispose. Immunocompromised states and debilitating conditions such as malignancies and lymphomas, interfere with the development of contact sensitivity.

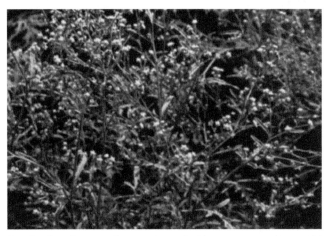

Parthenium hysterophorus: also called 'congress grass' is a wild compositae.

Clinical Manifestations

Morphology

Clinical features simulate those of acute, subacute or chronic dermatitis.

Sites of Predilection

Clue to suspecting the causal agent in allergic contact dermatitis. *Airborne contactants:* exposed sites face, particularly the eyelids, neck, hands and forearms. *Textile dermatitis*: axillae, flexures of elbows, thighs or other areas in intimate contact with clothing. *Shoe dermatitis*: areas in direct contact with the footwear-'V' shaped (with certain sandals), dorsa of toes or feet, depending on the shape of the shoe. *Occupational dermatitis*: hands and other exposed sites. *Metal dermatitis*: sites of contact with costume jewellery (ear lobules) watch straps on the wrist. Dermatitis due to local **medications** at the site of application for an injury or a surgical wound or on the hands in doctors, nurses and other paramedics. *Plant dermatitis*: sites of accidental or deliberate contact—hands, forearms. Or diffuse and generalized (airborne contact dermatitis-ABCD). *Hair dye dermatitis*—at the hair line.

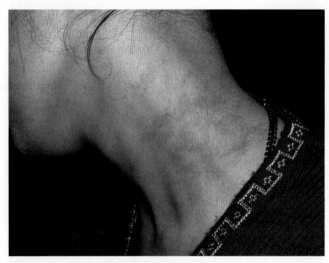

Allergic contact dermatitis: to perfumes.

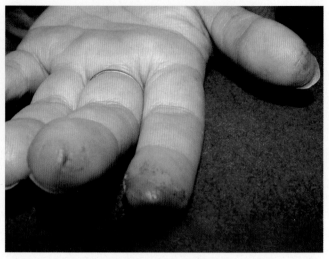

Allergic contact dermatitis: to vegetables.

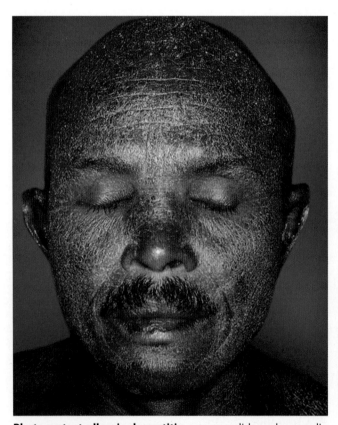

Photocontact allergic dermatitis: upper eyelids and upper lip are spared.

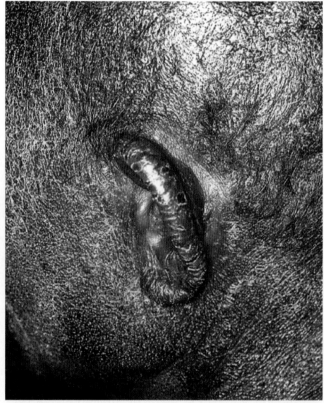

Photocontact dermatitis: retroauricular fold is conspicuously spared; helix of the ear is affected.

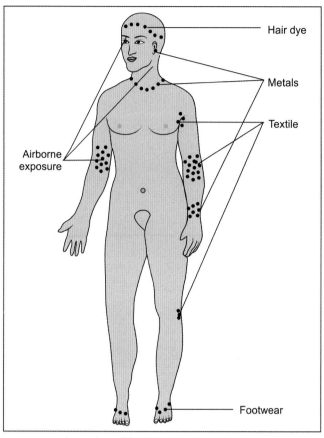

Sites of predilection: Contact dermatitis.

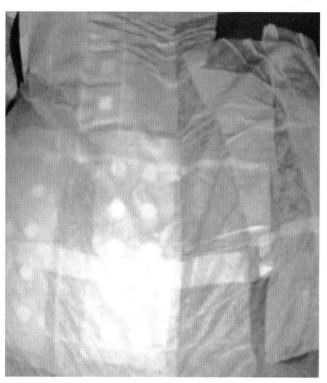

Patch test: involves application of antigen under occlusion for 48 hours and noting for reaction.

Investigations

Patch test diagnostic. Helps to identify trigger as also helps in determining substitutes.

PHOTOCONTACT ALLERGIC DERMATITIS

Etiology

Needs contactant and ultraviolet rays (UVA) for dermatitis to develop. Probably related to neoantigen formation. Several patients with parthenium dermatitis exhibit photoaggravation of a purely allergic dermatitis. Or develop the dermatitis only on exposure to light.

Clinical Manifestations

Morphology

Acute, subacute, chronic dermatitis.

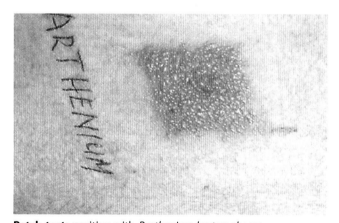

Patch test: positive with *Parthenium hysterophorus.*

Sites of Predilection

Photoexposed sites involved and photoprotected sites spared.

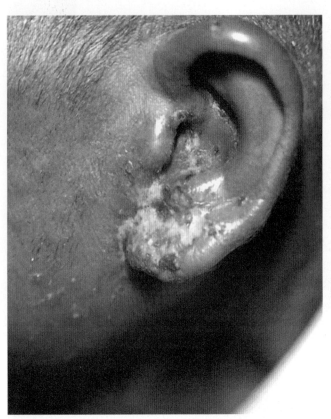

Infective eczema: eczematous reaction secondary to purulent discharge from the ear.

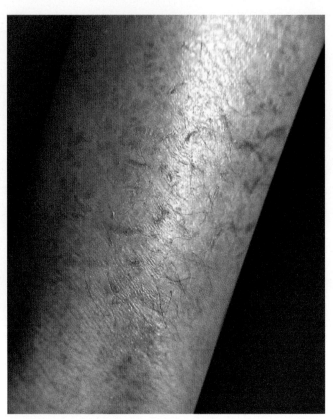

Asteatotic eczema: superficially fissured, dry lesions.

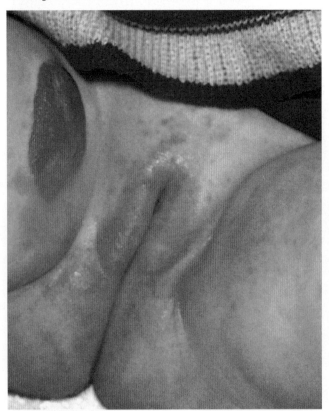

Napkin dermatitis: acutely inflamed diaper area; 'convex' surfaces affected, depth of fold spared.

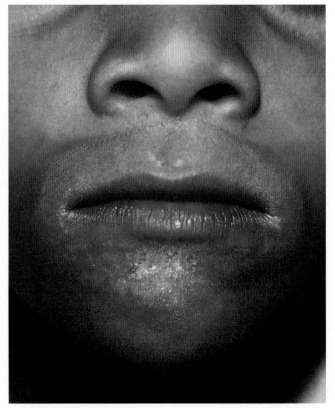

Lip-licking dermatitis: well-marginated dermatitis around the mouth.

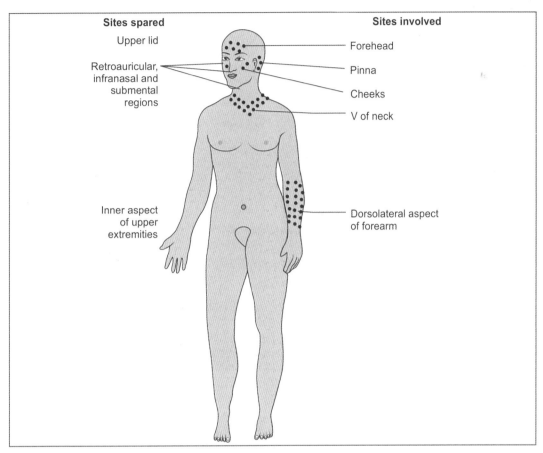

Sites of predilection: Photodermatitic.

Treatment

General Measures

Avoid contact. Often difficult to ascertain clinically (so use patch and photopatch tests to identify). Use substitutes instead. For photocontact dermatitis photoprotection paramount—avoid sun (light) exposure and use sunscreens.

Specific Therapy

Topical (systemic, in widespread disease) corticosteroids in acute phase. Airborne contact dermatitis due to parthenium may require systemic corticosteroids or other immunosuppressives like azathioprine.

INFECTIVE DERMATITIS (INFECTIOUS ECZEMATOID DERMATITIS)

Etiology

Acute eczematous reaction to contact with purulent discharge from a pyococcal lesion: a boil, a discharging ear, an infected wound, infected scabies or pediculosis.

Clinical Manifestations

Exuding, crusted, well or ill-defined plaques of vesiculopustular lesions. Discoid or bizarre shaped. Autoinoculation common. Often complicated by ide eruption.

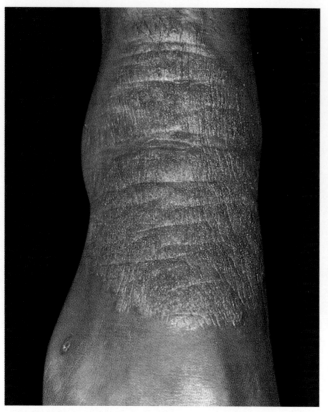

Lichen simplex chronicus: lichenified plaque showing hyperpigmentation, thickening and increased skin markings.

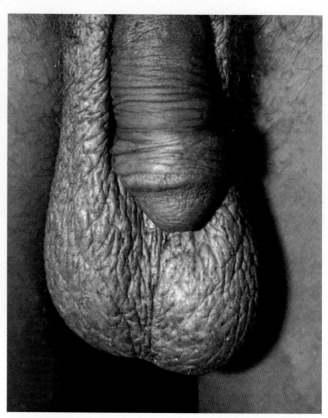

Lichen simplex chronicus: lichenified, excoriated scrotal skin.

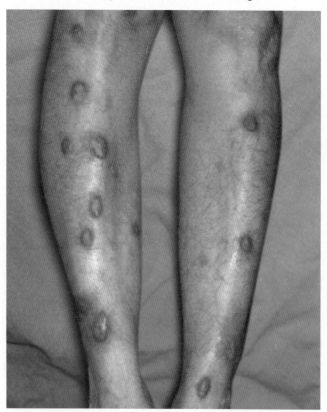

Prurigo nodularis: keratotic nodules surmounted by crusts.

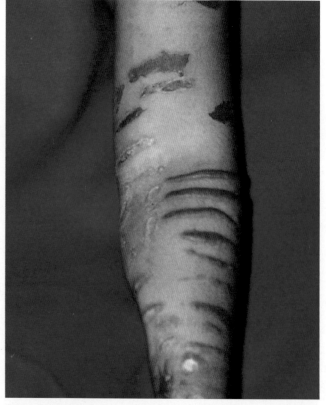

Dermatitis artefacta: superficial 'scalded' lesions and evenly spaced hypertrophic scars.

Treatment

Antibiotic or antibiotic-steroid combination creams for localized lesions. Patients with extensive lesions may, need systemic antibiotics.

ASTEATOTIC ECZEMA (ECZEMA CRAQUELÉ)

Elderly individuals with dry xerotic skin affected. Irregular or discoid patches of superficially fissured, dry, scaly and mildly crusted lesions on extensors of legs, dorsae of hands and trunk. Variable itching. Frequent baths, use of soap, detergents, dry and cold climates worsen.

Treatment

Use emollients-liberally, soon after shower. Avoid excessive use of soap. Mild steroids in acute cases.

NAPKIN DERMATITIS (DIAPER DERMATITIS)

Etiology

Use of occlusive diapers and lack of frequent changes predispose. Multifactorial etiology irritation with feces and urine or the presence of irritant detergents in the napkins.

Epidemiology

Common in the developed world. Less common in developing countries where infants frequently stay without occlusive napkins.

Clinical Manifestations

An irritant dermatitis of varying acuteness; diffuse glazed erythema with papules, vesicles or ulcerative and nodular lesions affecting the skin in contact with the soiled napkins. Depth of folds relatively spared. May persist unless properly managed.

Treatment

General Measures

Change soiled wet napkins promptly and rinse off detergents from cloth diapers. Avoid use of occlusive napkins. Keep diaper area clean, dry and free of irritating soaps; use thin film of talc. And avoid irritant antiseptics.

Specific Treatment

Treat acute dermatitis with topical non-fluorinated steroids such as hydrocortisone acetate preferably without occlusion.

LIP-LICKING DERMATITIS

Not uncommon; seen in children with a habit of licking their lips and around. Rule out atopic diathesis. Well defined, scaly lesions around the mouth.

Treatment

Avoid lip-licking. Use emollients.

LICHEN SIMPLEX CHRONICUS

Etiology

A common cutaneous response to scratching. More common in atopics and in orientals. May be primary. Or secondary to an itchy dermatosis. Pathogenetic mechanism: itch scratch-itch cycle.

Clinical Manifestations

Females affected more often. Circumscribed, lichenified plaques-thickened, pigmented plaques with pronounced skin markings. 'Mosaic' pattern; mild scaling. Occasional satellite lichenoid papules. *Common sites:* nape of the neck, ankles, lower legs, forearms, genitals. Secondary bacterial infection, a common complication.

Treatment

Avoid scratching. All efforts be directed towards breaking itch-scratch-itch cycle. Antipruritic measures include use of high potency corticosteroids like clobetasol propionate or betamethasone dipropionate often combined with salicylic acid (3%). Systemic antihistamines invariably needed. Prolonged use of potent steroids, however may cause skin atrophy and so best avoided.

PRURIGO NODULARIS

Not common. Often regarded as a nodular form of lichen simplex chronicus. Chronic persistent disease. Scratching is the cardinal feature.

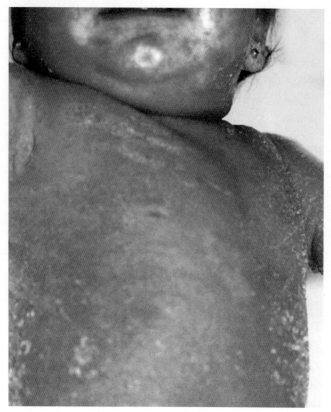

Erythroderma: due to psoriasis in a child.

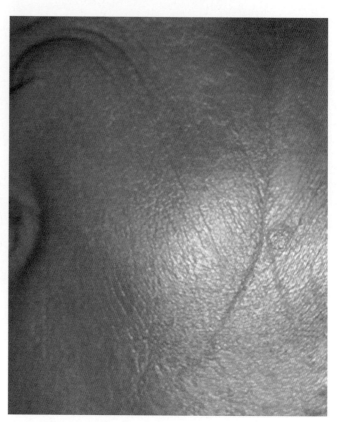

Erythroderma: sézary syndrome, in an elderly male.

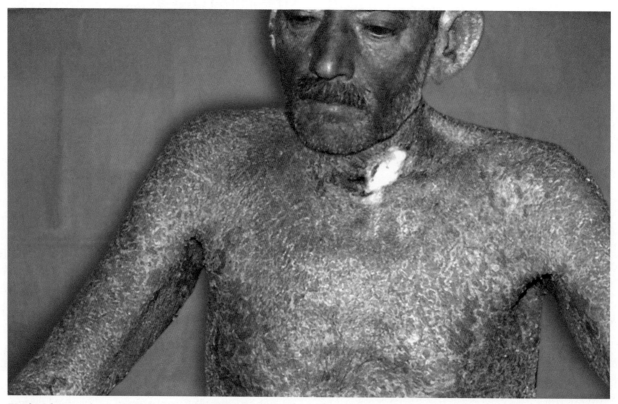

Erythroderma: drug-induced, due to phenytoin.

Intensely itchy, firm, pigmented, sometimes crusted keratotic warty papulonodules on the extensors of arms or legs; often bilaterally symmetrical. Itching paroxysmal and intense.

Treatment

Avoid scratching. Treat with potent topical steroids (initially under occlusion) or intralesional steroids. Always add antihistamines.

DERMATITIS ARTEFACTA (FACTITIAL DERMATITIS)

Uncommon. Severely disturbed, often hysterical women. Subconsciously self-inflicted injuries caused by physical, mechanical or chemical agents. Clinical lesions, not conforming to any disease pattern. Bizarre shaped, sized and destructive lesions, often appearing abruptly and repeatedly with varying periods of remission. Inaccessible areas of the body spared.

ERYTHRODERMA (EXFOLIATIVE DERMATITIS)

Etiology

Reaction pattern. End stage of several heterogeneous dermatosis.

Diseases associated with erythroderma

Psoriasis
Pityriasis rubra pilaris
Contact dermatitis including air borne and photo contact
Atopic dermatitis
Seborrheic dermatitis
Ichthyosis: keratinopathic ichthyosis; non-bullous ichthyosiform erythroderma
Drugs
Malignancies: cutaneous T-cell lymphomas, Sézary syndrome
Idiopathic.

Clinical Manifestations

Total or near total skin involvement with varying degree of erythema and scaling. Abrupt or insidious onset. Universal erythema—bright pink or dull red. Variable scaling—large, easily detachable or fine and branny. Skin warm, edematous and thickened. Nails and hair may be shed off. Palms and soles thickened, particularly in psoriasis and pityriasis rubra pilaris. *Lymphadenopathy:* generalized; sometimes specific, e.g. due to lymphomas but usually non-specific dermatopathic (lipomelanotic reticulosis). Thermoregulation poor, patient often feels cold. Loss of heat and water considerable.

Treatment

General Measures

Manage as for skin failure nutritional, electrolyte and fluid balance. Thermoregulation.

Specific Treatment

Topical therapy
Emollients and topical steroids.

Specific therapy
Treat underlying cause. If no cause discernable, antihistamines and immunosuppresives (steroids, methotrexate) mainstay.

8

Abnormal Vascular Responses

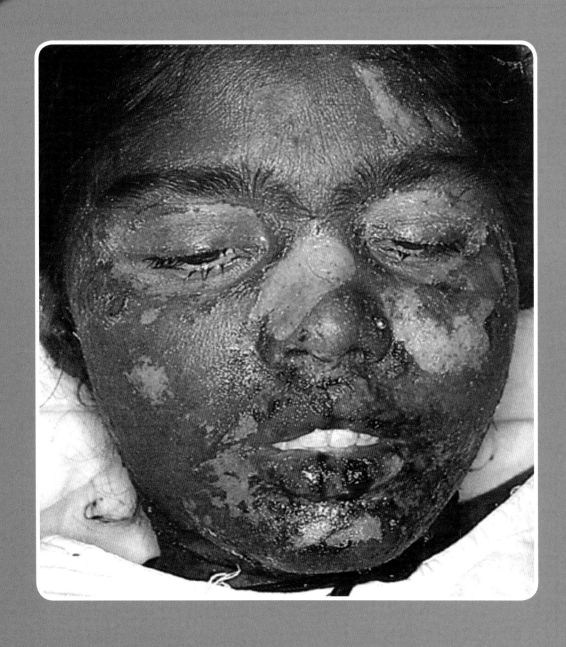

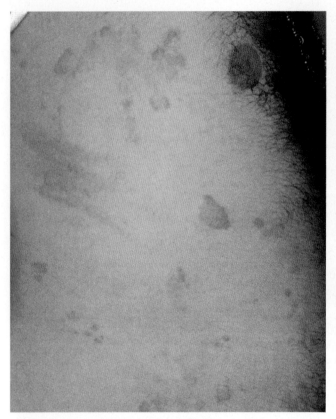

Urticaria: both irregular and linear wheals.

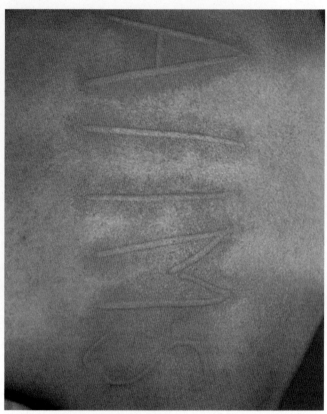

Dermographism: exaggerated triple response.

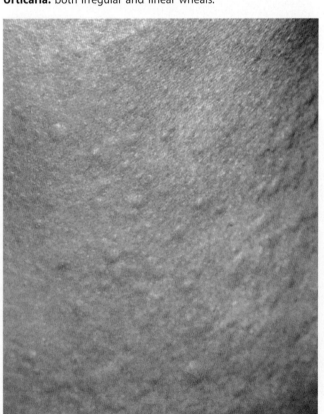

Cholinergic urticaria: small wheals which disappear in a few minutes.

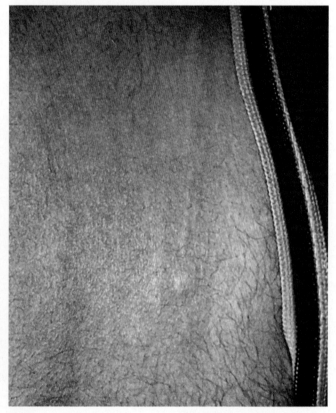

Pressure urticaria: wheal under tight undergarment.

Group of dermatoses in which blood vessel wall damage is the common denominator. Damage may be functional. Or structural. Injury may be physical. Or toxin- or immune-mediated. The spectrum of clinical manifestations varies from evanescent erythema to ischemic necrosis.

URTICARIA

A common vascular reaction characterized by production of wheals—itchy, evanescent, erythematous or pale, edematous swellings of the dermis. And subcutis (angioedema). Allergic or non-allergic in nature.

Etiology

Etiology of urticaria
Spontaneous
• Idiopathic
• Autoimmune
Ingestants
• Foods: like cheese, eggs, nuts, fish, mushrooms
• Food additives: yellow dye, tartrazine
• Preservatives: salicylates, benzoates
Inhalants: pollen, animal dander
Drugs: penicillins, salicylates, sulphonamides, sera
Infections: in teeth, tonsils, sinuses, gastrointestinal
Infestations: gut parasites
Contactants: foods, additives

Pathogenesis

Histamine and other mediators released from mast cells cause vasodilatation and escape of fluid in the dermis (and subcutis in angioedema). Either:

- **Allergic:** mostly type I, IgE mediated to variety of triggers. Less frequently type III, IgG mediated reaction.
- **Non-allergic:** varied etiology and pathogenesis.

Clinical Manifestations

Morphology

Morphology of lesions characteristic and similar in most urticarias except cholinergic urticaria and dermographism. Itchy evanescent (lasting few minutes to several hours, seldom >24 hours) edematous lesions. Episodes may recur daily or several times each day for days, weeks, or years. Variable sizes and shapes of wheals with or without an erythematous halo. Patients may have systemic symptoms (abdominal pain and flushing), if disease severe.

Angioedema: regarded as a deeper variant of urticaria; it involves the subcutaneous or submucosal tissue (rather than only the dermis). Urticaria and angioedema may coexist or occur independently. Large, deep seated, painful swellings; each may last >72 hours. Eyelids, lips, tongue, genitals, larynx, common sites for involvement. Laryngeal angioedema, a rare but serious complication.

Classification

- ***Spontaneous urticaria:*** which includes acute (which lasts < 6 weeks) and chronic (lasts > 6 weeks) urticaria. And includes autoimmune urticaria in which circulating auto-antibodies (detected by autologous serum skin test) present.
- ***Physical urticaria:*** which are triggered by physical stimuli. And are of different types.
  - *Dermographism:* an exaggeration of physiological triple response, so manifests as linear wheals on acute brisk stroking.
  - *Pressure urticaria:* results from constant pressure for long periods, e.g. under belts, straps or on the feet. May be immediate or delayed.
  - *Cholinergic urticaria:* small (1–2 mm) sized, evanescent lesions that last a few minutes to an hour or so. Precipitated by sweating, stress, heat and physical exertion.
  - *Cold urticaria:* lesions appear on exposure to cold wind or water; limited lesions or extensive. May cause histamine shock (and drowning while swimming in cold water).
  - *Solar urticaria:* young adults commonly affected. Occurs, on photo-exposed areas of the body within minutes of light exposure. Different wavelengths of light responsible. Exclude erythropoietic protoporphyria in patients with solar urticaria.
- ***Contact urticaria:*** occurs at sites of contact with substances like foods and food additives, furs, drugs.

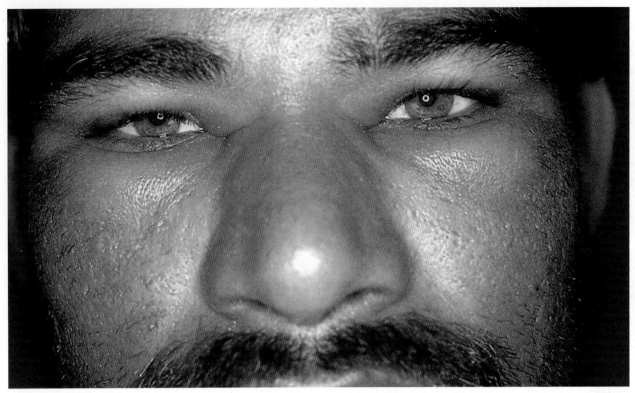

Angioedema: edematous swelling of the eyelids. Lesions last for >72 hours.

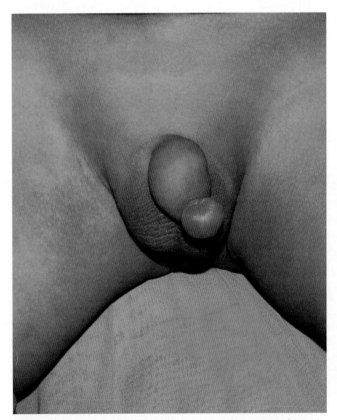

Angioedema: of penile skin leading to temporary paraphimosis.

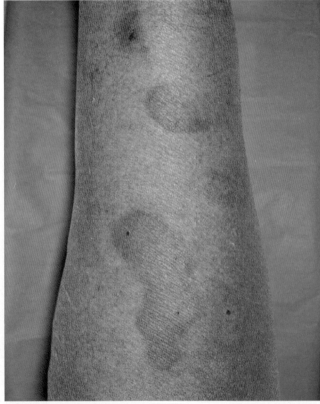

Erythema multiforme: target lesions with cyanotic center and erythematous halo.

Investigations

Often not required. Autologous serum skin test for autoimmune urticaria. Dermograder used for grading severity of dermographic urticaria. Cold stimulator for cold urticaria. Skin prick tests/serological tests for specific IgE of limited (? no) value.

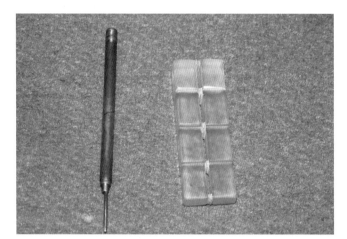

Dermograder: an instrument to grade urticaria.

Treatment

General Measures

Determining the cause (and then eliminating it) of chronic urticaria difficult. Clinical history may give a 'lead'; ideally followed by careful 'elimination' and 're-exposure' (challenge) to suspected causal agents. Diagnostic clues to etiology stem from pattern of occurrence, e.g. season, time of the day, relationship to food, sweating, physical activity, exposure to pressure, light, heat, cold. Food items containing dyes, preservatives and yeast and all drugs best avoided. Infective foci ought to be eliminated.

Specific Treatment

H1-receptor antihistamines mainstay of therapy. Antihistamines with low sedating and less anticholinergic effects which are long acting preferred. Average daily doses: chlorpheniramine maleate, 2–8 mg; promethazine, 25–100 mg; cyproheptadine, 4–12 mg; fexofenedine, 120–180 mg; cetrizine, 10–20 mg and levocetrizine, 5–10 mg. Some cases benefit from a combination of H_1 and H_2 antihistamines. Systemic corticosteroids should not be used routinely in acute urticaria. Unless severe, or associated with laryngeal angioedema.

Refractory cases: need cyclosporine, methotrexate, zafirlukast, monteleukast, zileuton, omalizumab.
Delayed pressure urticaria responds to NSAIDs, dapsone and sulfasalazine.
Angioedema: treat like urticaria.
Epinephrine and other emergency measures necessary in cases with laryngeal edema and cardiovascular collapse.

ERYTHEMA MULTIFORME

An acute reaction pattern affecting the skin and mucous membranes.

Epidemiology

Young adults of both sexes affected.

Etiology

Triggers

Triggers for erythema multiforme
Infections: frequent cause
• *Viral:* Herpes simplex virus (HSV, 1>2), varicella zoster virus, infectious mononucleosis, hepatitis B and C virus
• *Mycoplasma:* M. pneumoniae
Drugs: infrequent cause
Collagen vascular disease
Malignancies
Idiopathic

Pathogenesis

In HSV induced EM, fragmented DNA of virus demonstrated in keratinocytes. This probably induces immune mediated damage to blood vessels.

Clinical Manifestations

Morphology

Cutaneous lesion may be macular, papular, vesicular or bullous. The lesions may be monomorphous. Or polymorphous (multiforme), perhaps through

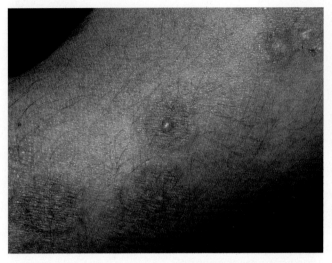

Erythema multiforme: typical target lesion with central bulla, dusky halo and marginal vesicles (herpetic iris of Bateman).

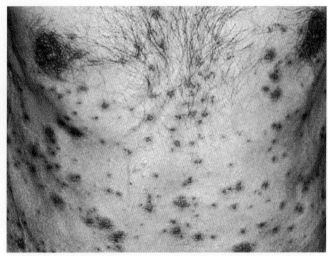

Erythema multiforme: iris (target) lesions on the trunk.

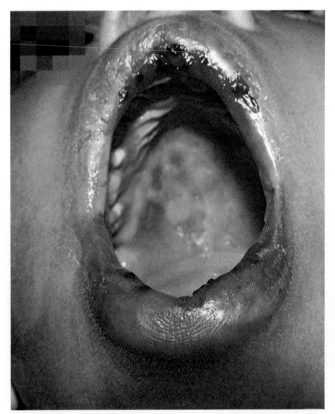

Erythema multiforme: mild oral lesions with hemorrhagic crusts on lips.

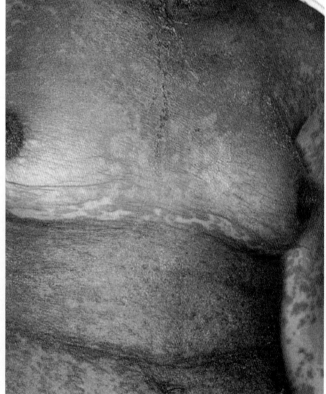

Toxic epidermal necrolysis: large areas of irregular dusky erythema developing flaccid bullae.

the process of evolution. Distinctive lesion is an 'iris' or 'target' plaque consisting of a cyanotic center and an erythematous halo; center sometime vesicular or bullous. Sometimes surrounded by rim of vesicles (**herpes iris of Bateman**). Vesiculo-bullous lesions seen in severe forms of erythema multiforme associated with severe constitutional symptoms (termed **EM major**). Mucosal lesions present in 70% patients. Mild, involving oral mucosa/eyes.

Course

Crops of lesions appear over several weeks. Individual lesions last about a week; heal with hyperpigmentation. Or occasionally depigmentation.

Sites of Predilection

Distribution of lesions commonly acral (palms and dorsae of the hands and feet), face. And on extensors of extremities, and less often the trunk.

Investigations

Diagnosis clinical. Sometimes biopsied.

Histopathology

Massive edema of upper dermis and perivascular infiltrate with individual keratinocyte necrosis.

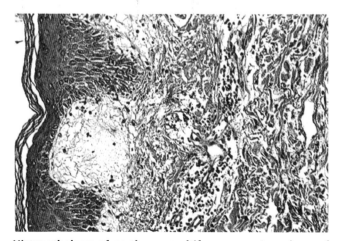

Histopathology of erythema multiforme: massive edema of upper dermis and perivascular lymphocytic infiltrate.

Identification of Trigger

Appropriate tests to identify the precipitating cause.

Treatment

General Measures

Eliminate/treat trigger. Reassure patient.

Specific Treatment

Mild forms, treat with systemic antihistamines. Severe cases may warrant oral steroids. Recurrent forms, acyclovir suppressive therapy.

EPIDERMAL NECROLYSIS

Manifests as two overlapping acute life threatening conditions Stevens-Johnson syndrome (SJS) and toxic epidermal necrolysis (TEN). Both rare categorized as:
- **SJS:** <10% body surface area (BSA) involvement.
- **SJS-TEN overlap:** 10–30 BSA involvement.
- **TEN:** >30% BSA involvement.

Etiology

Triggers for epidermal necrolysis
Drugs: most frequent (90%)
• *Anticonvulsants:* lamotrigine, carbamazepine, phenytoin, phenobarbitone
• *Antitubercular:* isoniazid, thiacetazone
• *NSAIDs:* oxicam derivatives, diclofenac
• *Others:* allopurinol, nevirapine.
• *Antibacterials:* sulphonamides, quinolones, aminopenicillins.
Others
• *Infections* like *Mycoplasma pneumoniae*
• *Collagen vascular diseases*: systemic lupus erythematosus.

Clinical Manifestations

Presence of mucocutaneous lesions typical.
- **Skin lesions:** Rapidly progressive large areas of irregular shaped dusky erythema, sometimes with atypical targetoid centers (scalded skin). Develop large, flaccid, clear or hemorrhagic bullae. Rupture to eventuate into large areas of denudation. Symmetrical distribution on face, upper trunk and proximal extremities. Severe constitutional symptoms. Serious, life threatening or fatal condition. Prognosticated using **SCORTEN**.

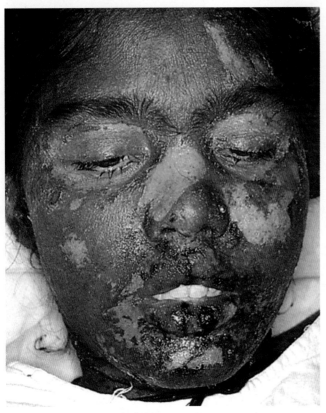

Toxic epidermal necrolysis: dark scalded-looking skin. Necrotic skin peels off in sheets leaving areas of denuded skin. Hemorrhagic crusts of lips.

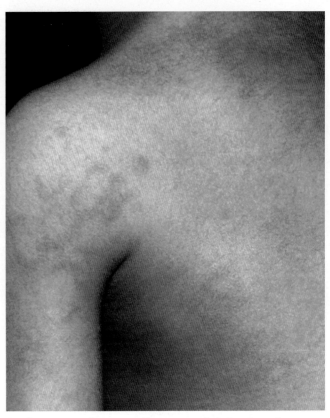

Erythema annulare centrifugum: well-defined erythematous scaly annular lesions.

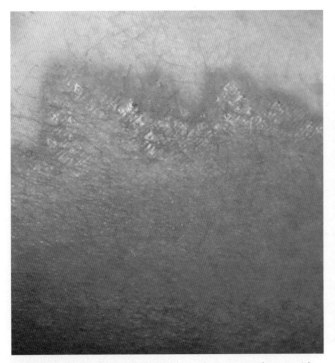

Erythema annulare centrifugum: erythematous plaque with a trailing edge of scales.

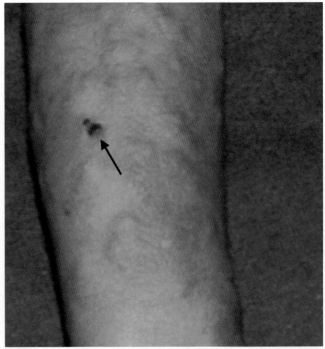

Erythema chronicum migrans: annular plaque with central tick bite.

- **Mucosal involvement:** Oral, ocular, nasal and genital; extensive oral ulceration and pseudomembrane formation, hemorrhagic crusts on lips. Purulent or catarrhal conjunctivitis, corneal ulceration. Severe balanitis, vulvovaginitis and urethritis.
- **Systemic involvement:** Frequent. Include respiratory and renal involvement.

Investigations

Diagnosis of EN clinical. Biopsy done mainly to circumvent legal issues. Evaluate for trigger. Regular monitoring of vitals, hematological and biochemical parameters imperative.

Biopsy

Early lesions show apoptic keratinocytes. Later lesions large areas of epidermal necrosis.

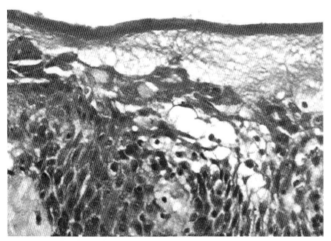

Histopathology of toxic epidermal necrolysis: necrotic keratinocytes (apoptosis).

Treatment

General Measures

Eliminate/treat (wherever feasible) precipitating factors such as drugs, infections. General management as for acute skin failure—maintain fluid and electrolyte balance, thermoregulation skin care with aseptic measures.

Specific Treatment

Mild forms, treat with systemic antihistamines and topical corticosteroids. Severe forms need aggressive treatment: moderately large or large doses of systemic corticosteroids—though use controversial. Intravenous immunoglobulin effective.

FIGURATE ERYTHEMAS AND CYCLOSPORINE (GYRATE ERYTHEMAS)

Uncommon.

Etiology

Varies with different annular erythemas.

Figurate erythema	Trigger
Erythema annulare centrifugum	Unknown mostly. Bacterial and fungal infection sometimes
Erythema gyratum repens	Cancer marker
Erythema chronicum migrans	Tick bite
Erythema marginatum rheumaticum	Rheumatic fever
Necrolytic migratory erythema	Glucagonoma marker

Clinical Manifestations

Reactive erythemas of varied configuration: annular, arcuate, serpiginous or irregular. Migratory character. Centrifugal spread with central clearing. Variable rate of progression (days-weeks). Each lesion lasts a few days; episodes recur for weeks, months, or years.

Erythema Annulare Centrifugum

A number of causal associations: tinea pedis, candidiasis, malignancies, drugs. Asymptomatic or mildly itchy. Annular or polycyclic lesions with peripheral extension and central clearing: palpable or flat. Trailing edge of scales characteristic. Discrete lesions distributed on the trunk, abdomen, or extremities.

Erythema Gyratum Repens

Rapidly moving waves of scaly erythematous lesions resembling grains of wood, commonly associated with malignancy, often of the breast or lung.

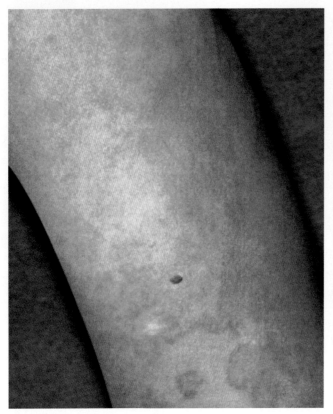

Erythema marginatum rheumaticum: indistinct erythematous lesions. Strong association with active rheumatic carditis.

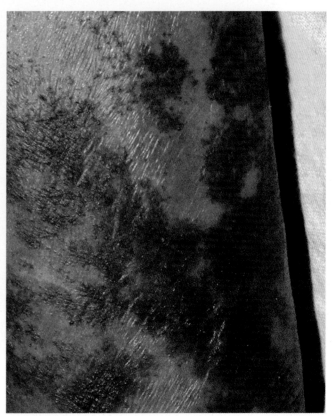

Necrolytic migratory erythema: polymorphous erythematous patches/plaques with erosions. Face, flexures and distal extremities. Due to underlying pancreatic glucagonoma.

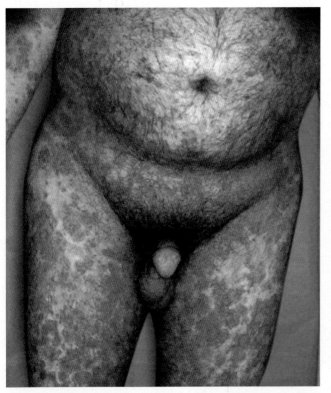

Drug eruption: bilateral erythematous papules, due to carbamazepine.

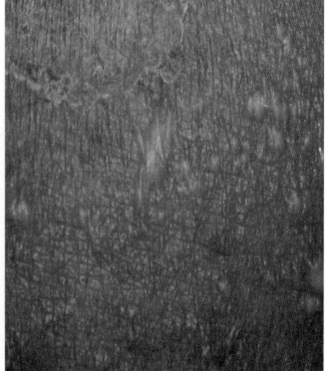

Acute generalized exanthematous pustulosis: small pustules on an erythematous background. Often starts on face or in flexural areas, rapidly becoming generalized.

Erythema Chronicum Migrans

Secondary to a tick bite or manifestation of Lyme's disease. Associated with Borrelia infection. Solitary macule or papule. Assumes large size by peripheral extension and central clearing.

Erythema Marginatum Rheumaticum

Rare. Children affected. Strong association with active rheumatic carditis. Asymptomatic, evanescent, almost fleeting, faintly red, barely palpable, discrete or polycyclic lesions. Easily missed on pigmented skin. Trunk, abdomen commonly involved.

Necrolytic Migratory Erythema

Due to underlying pancreatic glucagonoma. Polymorphous erythematous patches/plaques with erosions. Face, flexures and distal extremities.

Investigations

Histopathology

Variable often non-diagnostic. A sleeve of lymphocytes around the blood vessels in the upper and mid dermis usually seen. Variable changes in the epidermis: spongiosis and parakeratosis.

Other Investigations

To rule out underlying trigger.

Treatment

General Measures

Identify and attempt to remove the cause.

Specific Treatment

Symptomatic relief with topical steroids and systemic antihistamines or occasionally systemic corticosteroids. Antibiotics, e.g. penicillins, tetracyclines helpful in erythema chronicum migrans.

DRUG ERUPTIONS

Common. Undesirable cutaneous or mucocutaneous reactions to systemically prescribed drugs with or without associated other organ involvement.

Etiology

Virtually any drug may be responsible; the probability varies. Drugs that cause reactions with greater frequency are: phenytoin, barbiturates, sulphonamides, penicillins, phenothiazines, heavy metals, salicylates, phenylbutazone, thiazides, antimalarials. Presence of some genes predispose to development of drug hypersensitivity to specific drugs, e.g. presence of HLA B1502 allele predisposes to reactions to anticonvulsants while presence of HLA B5801 allele predisposes to development serious reactions to allopurinol.

Etiology of drug reactions

- *Exanthematous*: anticonvulsants, sulphonamides, penicillins.
- *Erythroderma*: sulphonamides, anticonvulsants.
- *Epidermal necrolysis*: anticonvulsants, antitubercular drugs, NSAIDs.
- *Acute generalized exanthematous pustulosis*: ampicillin, amoxicyllin.
- *Fixed drug eruption*: cotrimoxazole, tetracyclines NSAIDs.
- *Photosensitive drug eruptions*: tetracyclines, psoralens.

Pathogenesis

May be due to immune mediated or non-immune-mediated mechanisms.

Pathogenesis of drug reactions

- **Immunological**
  - IgE-mediated reactions
  - Cytotoxic reactions
  - Immune complex-mediated reactions
  - Cell-mediated hypersensitivity
- **Non-immunological**
  - *Predictable*
    - Side effects
    - Overdosage/cumulative toxicity
    - Delayed toxicity
    - Drug interactions
    - Exacerbation of pre-existing skin conditions
    - Teratogenicity/mutagenicity
  - *Unpredictable*
    - Idiosyncratic reactions
    - Intolerance

Clinical Manifestations

Usually sudden and abrupt onset, temporally related to drug intake. Severity variable—usually mild and self limiting. Sometimes severe and life

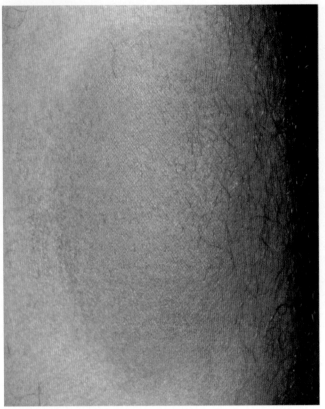

Fixed drug eruption: circular lesions; bluish center with peripheral erythematous halo.

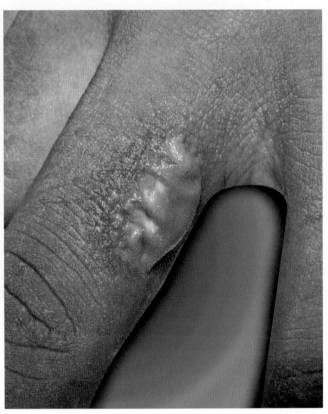

Bullous fixed drug eruption: bulla surrounded by erythematous halo.

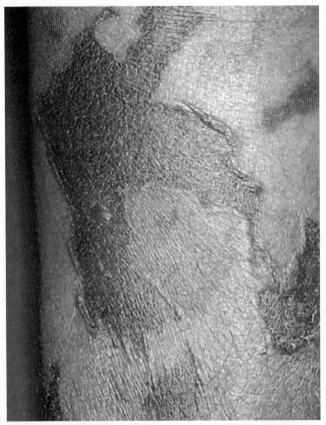

Cutaneous vasculitis: superficial ulcers and large hemorrhagic bullae.

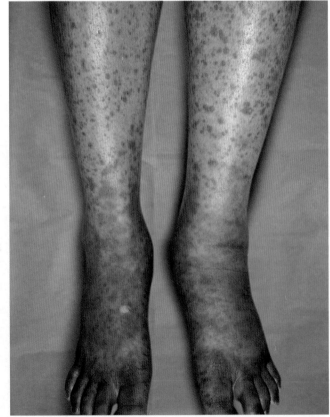

Henoch-Schönlein purpura: bilaterally symmetrical palpable purpuric lesions.

threatening (SJS/TEN, EM major, anaphylaxis). May mimic any morphologic pattern—exanthematous, erythodermic, epidermal necrolysis, acute generalized exanthematous pustulosis, fixed drug eruption, photosensitive. Different morphologic patterns in different patients with the same drug. Course variable; often prompt remission upon withdrawal and relapse on readministration.

Exanthematous Eruptions

Commonest drug eruption. Itchy symmetrical papulosquamous lesions on the trunk which spread centrifugally. Rash begins within 1–2 weeks of starting the therapy and subsides (with desquamation) 1–2 weeks after stopping. Drug rash with eosinophilia and systemic symptoms syndrome (DRESS), a severe variant.

Acute Generalized Exanthematous Pustulosis

Small pustules develop rapidly on an erythematous background. Often starts on face or in flexural areas, rapidly becoming generalized. May be associated with fever and malaise.

Fixed Drug Eruptions (FDE)

Single, a few, rarely multiple lesions. Distinctive morphology: circular or oval, erythematous macules or plaques with a bluish, sometimes vesiculated middle and an erythematous halo. Mucocutaneous junctions particularly affected. Site(s) once affected always gets reactivated on readministration of the drug; fresh lesions may appear at other sites. No constitutional symptoms. Self limiting course; heal with characteristic bluish-black pigmentation.

Treatment

General Measures

Prompt withdrawal of the drug essential. Patients with SJS-TEN need excellent nursing and supportive care (*vide supra*).

Specific Treatment

Mild rash: soothing topical applications like zinc calamine lotion, or cold cream adequate. *Moderate or severe:* systemic antihistamines and corticosteroids. SJS-TEN need urgent

attention and sometimes large doses of systemic corticosteroids. In FDE, if necessary, challenge under supervision may be justified.

CUTANEOUS VASCULITIS

A reaction pattern with a spectrum of manifestations varying from erythema to frank necrosis of the skin. Common denominator, a histological vasculitis. Acute or recurrent and chronic. Progression and prognosis depend on the primary cause and associated organ involvement.

Etiology

Reaction pattern to variety of triggers.

Triggers causing vasculitis

- **Infections**
  - Bacterial: Streptococcal
  - Viral: hepatitis B, C
  - Mycobacterial
- **Connective tissue disorders:** systemic lupus erythematosus, rheumatoid arthritis, antiphospholipid antibody syndromes
- **Malignancies**
- **Drugs**

Pathogenesis

Usually immune complex mediated.

Clinical Manifestations

Vasculitis can manifest both in skin. And in internal organs. Cutaneous manifestations depend on size of vessel involved (venular involvement as palpable purpura, arterial as ulcers). And type of infiltrate (neutrophils as papules, granulomatous as nodules). Internal organ involvement depends on pattern of involvement. Several patterns recognized.

Henoch-Schönlein Purpura

A common small vessel (venular) vasculitis. Obscure etiology: streptococcal infection or drugs incriminated. Children of either sex affected. Onset often abrupt. Triad of palpable purpura, arthritis and gastrointestinal involvement. Crops of urticarial, edematous papular and purpuric lesions. On ankles, lower legs. Polyarthritis: knee, elbow, ankle or small joints of the hands, painful, tender and swollen. Abdominal pain, vomiting, melena

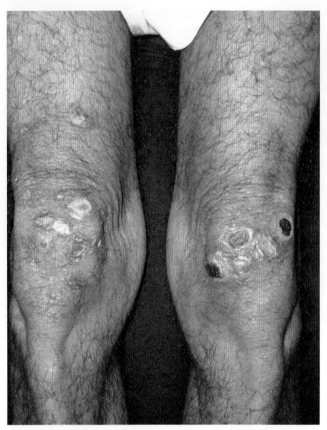

Erythema elevatum diutinum: symmetric erythematous papules on knees.

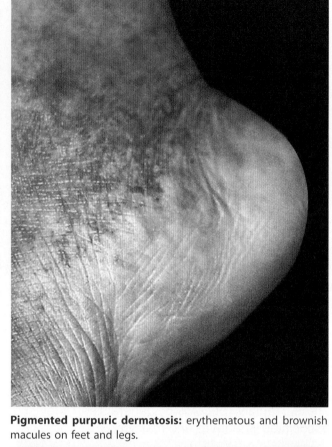

Pigmented purpuric dermatosis: erythematous and brownish macules on feet and legs.

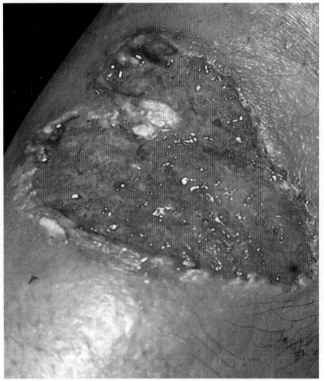

Pyoderma gangrenosum: large ulcer with bluish edematous necrotic edge.

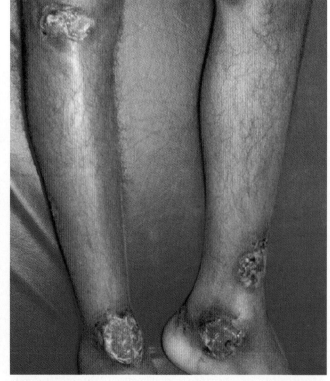

Pyoderma gangrenosum: multiple lesions on both lower limbs.

9

Papulo-Squamous Disorders

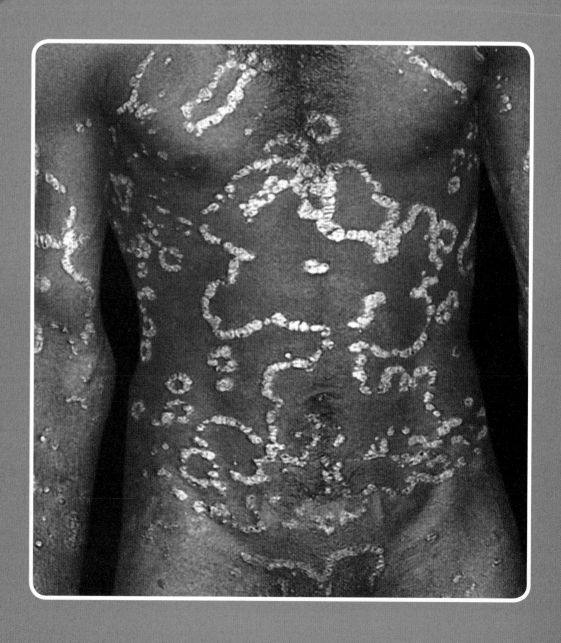

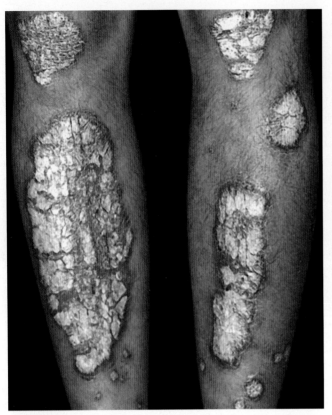

Psoriasis: red scaly plaques involving the extensors of the legs and knees.

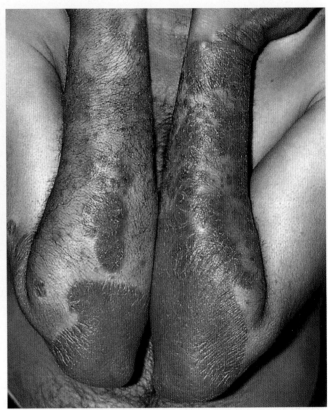

Plaque psoriasis: involving the extensor surfaces of the elbows and forearms.

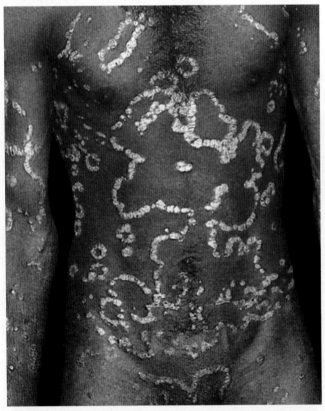

Psoriasis: bizarre geographical patterned lesions. Annular lesions conspicuous.

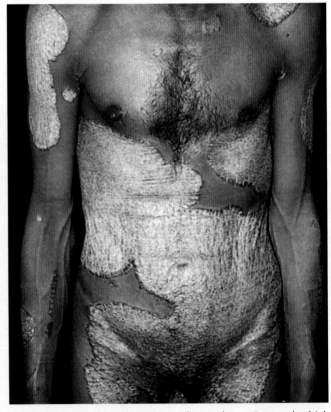

Psoriasis: large plaques covering almost the entire trunk; thick scales.

Heterogeneous group of dermatoses characterized by erythematous papules or plaques surmounted with scales. Color of lesions varies from faint pink (pityriasis rosea) to dull red (psoriasis) to purple or violaceous (lichen planus). Scales vary from minimal (lichen planus) to abundant (psoriasis), easily removable (chronic plaque psoriasis) to adherent (rupioid psoriasis).

PSORIASIS

Epidemiology

Extremely common dermatosis with worldwide distribution. Plaque psoriasis has bimodal age distribution, early (2nd decade) onset, with more severe course and more frequent arthropathy. And late (5th decade) onset with milder course.

Etiology

Genetic predisposition: autosomal dominant inheritance with incomplete penetrance. Multifactorial. Strong association with HLAB13, HLA-Bw17 and HLA-Cw6. *Environmental factors* contribute: trauma, infections, emotional stress, climatic changes may precipitate relapses. Sunlight usually protects. Patients with AIDS present with severe psoriasis.

Pathogenesis

Basic pathogenetic mechanism ill-understood. Earlier thought to be a disorder of aberrant keratinization with secondary inflammation. Now recognized as primarily an inflammatory disorder induced and sustained by T-cell mediated immune response (complex cascade of humoral and cellular immunomechanisms) which leads to accelerated growth of epidermal and vascular cells. Chief cutaneous manifestations result from hyperplasia of the epidermis—epidermopoiesis more rapid. And transit time of epidermal cells diminished with immature nucleated epidermal cells present in the stratum corneum (parakeratosis).

Clinical Manifestations

Morphology

Classical psoriasis characterized by asymptomatic (or itchy), well-defined erythematous, scaly papules and plaques of varying sizes and configurations (discoid, gyrate, annular). Sometimes lesions uniformly 1–3 cm only (so called **small plaque psoriasis**). Lesions covered with varying amount of loosely attached silvery white scales overlying an adherent translucent membranous scale. Removal of the latter reveals punctate bleeding spots (from the elongated capillary loops in dermal papillae) —the characteristic **Auspitz sign**. Sometimes lesions hyperkeratotic—rupioid (cone shaped), ostraceous (oyster shaped) or elephantine (grossly hyperkeratotic). **Ring of Woronoff**, occasionally seen as a hypopigmented halo around the plaques. Lesions often elicited at sites of trauma (**Koebner's isomorphic phenomenon**).

Sites of Predilection

Distributed generally on extensors of the body— knees, elbows, lower lumbosacral region. As also umbilicus and intergluteal cleft. Palms and soles, scalp (frequently) and genitals also involved. Facial involvement a late and infrequent feature. Less commonly a flexural distribution (**inverse psoriasis**). And rarely a photodistribution.

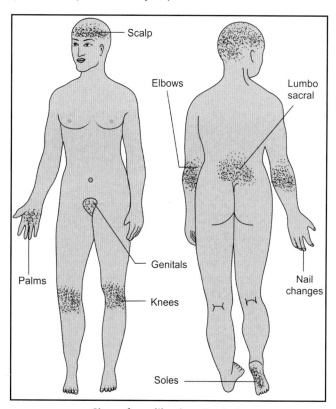

Sites of predilection: Psoriasis.

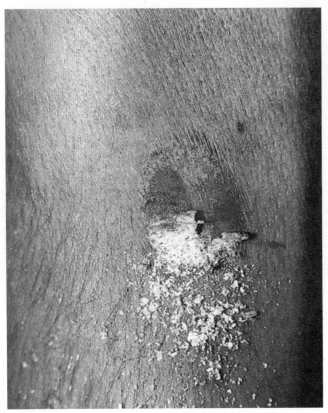

Psoriasis: auspitz sign showing bleeding points.

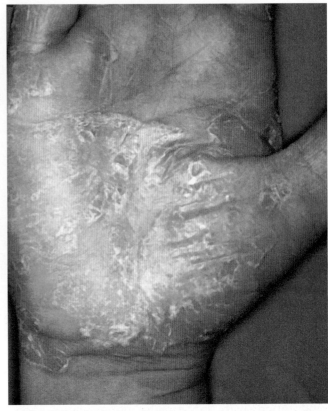

Palmar psoriasis: well-defined scaly, erythematous plaques on the palms.

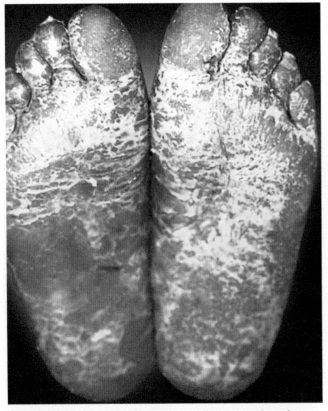

Plantar psoriasis: scaly erythematous plaques on the soles.

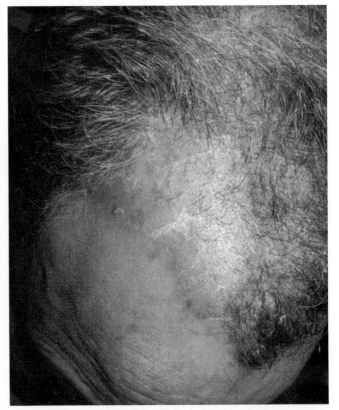

Psoriasis of scalp: rather diffuse, but well marginated involvement, spilling beyond scalp margin.

Variants

Palmoplantar psoriasis

Varied manifestations. Well-defined, erythematous, plaques with thick scales. Or hyperkeratotic, fissured, erythematous, ill-defined plaques on the heels or other parts of the soles (usually sparing insteps) and palms. Often bilaterally symmetrical.

Psoriasis of scalp

Common. Well marginated, erythematous, scaly, discrete or confluent plaques. Often spillage beyond hair margin. When associated with seborrheic dermatitis, labelled as **sebopsoriasis**.

Flexural psoriasis

Inverse distribution. Confined to the flexures—axillary, gluteal, inframammary or retroauricular folds. Scaling less pronounced due to moistness, but otherwise still well-defined and erythematous. Candidal superinfection frequent.

Genital psoriasis

Male genitals more frequently affected. Well marginated erythematous lesions. Scaling minimal in uncircumcised.

Guttate psoriasis

Adolescents and young males. Generally follows streptococcal pharyngitis. Crops of small, erythematous papules/plaques with minimal scaling. Trunk and proximal parts of extremities affected.

Erythrodermic psoriasis

May follow chronic or unstable psoriasis. Or start *de novo*–particularly in children. Irritant topical therapy or phototherapy may precipitate. Characteristically bright red erythema with extensive moderate–severe scaling. Almost the entire cutaneous surface involved. No islands of normal skin (c.f. pityriasis rubra pilaris). Associated nail and scalp involvement. Thermoregulation poor–patient feels cold. *Course:* complete clearing or reversion to plaque psoriasis. Serious with occasionally fatal outcome.

Pustular psoriasis

Localized

Generally on palmoplantar lesions with or often without associated psoriasis elsewhere on the body. Superficial sterile pustules on an erythematous background.

Generalized (von Zumbusch) pustular psoriasis

Rare. Serious, could be fatal. Spontaneous onset particularly in children. Or precipitated by withdrawal of systemic steroids, presence of a systemic infection, or application of an irritant. Affects previously diseased or unaffected skin. Generalized/extensive superficial sterile pustules on sheets of erythema. Confluence of pustules leads to lakes of pus. Paronychial involvement typical. Severe constitutional symptoms—fever, arthralgia. And leucocytosis, hypoalbuminemia, hypocalcemia.

Impetigo herpetiformis

Rare. Perhaps a variant of pustular psoriasis seen in late pregnancy. Pustulation on an erythematous background. Associated toxemia. Serious, may be fatal. High fetal and perinatal mortality. Tendency to recur with subsequent pregnancies.

Associations

Psoriasis of nails

Common. Due to involvement of nail matrix or nail bed, often both. Associated psoriatic lesions elsewhere. Occasionally isolated manifestation. All nails may be affected, finger nails more often. Common presentation: pitting of nail plates, subungual hyperkeratosis, onycholysis, dystrophy and yellowish or greenish discoloration. Classical psoriatic distal interphalangeal arthritis often associated with nail involvement.

Psoriatic arthropathy

Less common association. Both sexes affected, females more often. May precede, accompany or follow appearance of skin lesions. Nail involvement

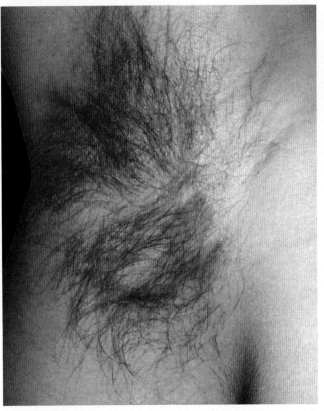

Flexural psoriasis: well-marginated erythematous lesions with minimal scaling.

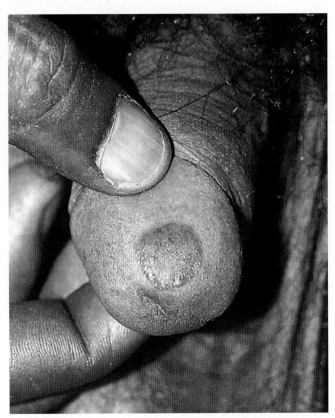

Penile psoriasis: well-circumscribed, mildly scaly lesion.

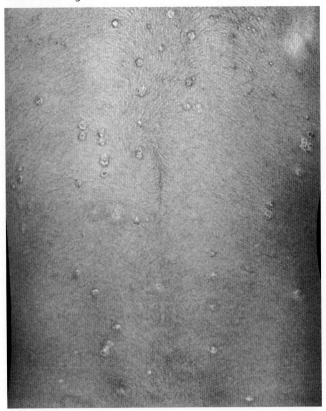

Guttate psoriasis: scaly, erythematous small papules.

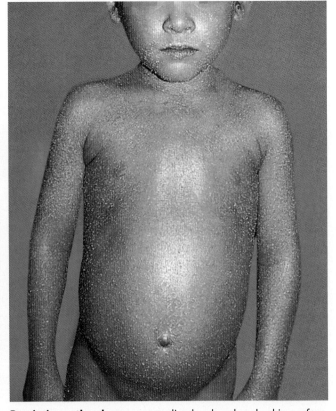

Psoriatic erythroderma: generalized red and scaly skin surface.

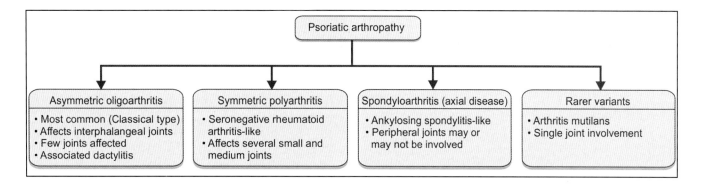

frequent. Several patterns recognized: asymmetric distal interphalangeal joints involvement; symmetrical seronegative rheumatoid arthritis like; ankylosing spondylitis-like arthritis mutilans; oligoarthritis.

Metabolic syndrome

Recent reports suggest association of psoriasis with metabolic syndrome.

Course

Course unpredictable and variable–spontaneous remissions and relapses a characteristic feature. Most patients worse in winter, some in summer. Patients with ill-defined erythematous and warm lesions indicate an unstable form; could progress on to **erythroderma**.

Investigations

None generally required. In doubtful cases biopsy required.

Histopathology

Biopsy characterized by parakeratosis and orthokeratosis, loss of granular cell layer, uniform, club shaped elongation of rete ridges and suprapapillary thinning of epidermis. Neutrophilic collections in parakeratotic stratum corneum form subcorneal pustule (**Munro's micro-abscess**) in psoriasis and a spongiform pustule (**spongiform pustule of Kogoj**) in stratum spinosum in pustular psoriasis. Papillary blood vessels dilated, elongated and tortuous. Perivascular mononuclear infiltrate in dermis.

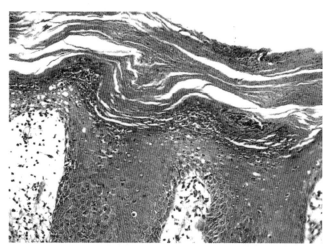

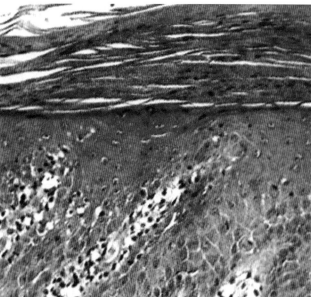

Histopathology of psoriasis: parakeratotic hyperkeratosis, pronounced and uniform acanthosis and suprapapillary thinning of the epidermis; top (x10), bottom (x40).

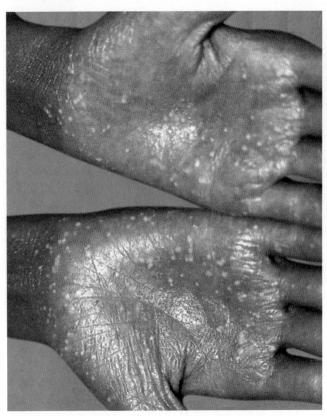

Pustular psoriasis, localized: superficial discrete pustules on the palms.

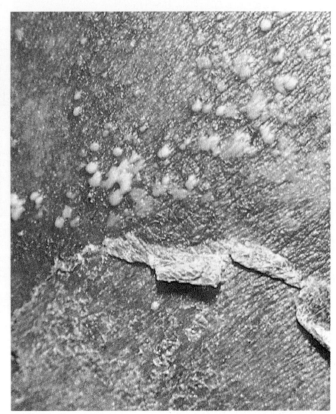

Pustular psoriasis, generalized: superficial discrete and confluent pustules on a generalized 'fiery' background.

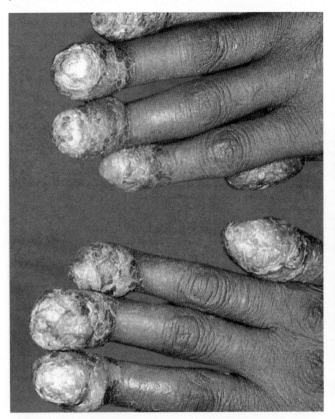

Pustular psoriasis: nail and paronychial involvement.

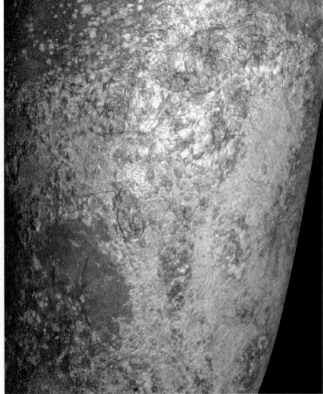

Impetigo herpetiformis: superficial pustules at the periphery of an erythematous lesion. Pustular psoriasis of pregnancy.

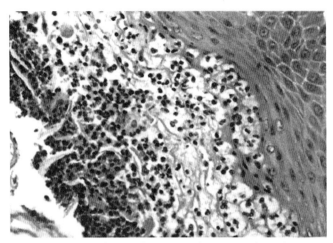

Histopathology of pustular psoriasis: intraepidermal neutrophilic pustule (spongiform pustule of Kogoj).

Treatment

Aimed at bringing about remission. And maintaining it, but relapses occur despite therapy. Various topical, systemic or photo-therapeutic modalities available. Rationale mostly ill understood.

General Measures

Counselling patient regarding chronicity, relapses paramount. Avoidance of smoking, alcohol intake.

Specific Treatment

Topical therapy, the preferred modality of treatment. Used exclusively for localized disease. And as adjuvant to systemic therapy which is necessary mostly for extensive disease (>10% body surface area), pustular, erythrodermic and arthritic psoriasis. Also for debilitating localized disease (palmoplantar psoriasis).

Topical therapy

Several agents available. *Crude coal tar*, 3–10% or solution of liquor carbonis detergens applied once or twice a day. Exposure to sunlight or UVB of additional value. Combining with salicylic acid (2–5%) helps in removing scales especially in thick lesions. As also on palms and soles. *Anthralin* used as conventional therapy (0.05–0.1% applied overnight) or as short contact therapy (2% applied for ½–2 hours); removed with any oil. *Calcipotriol*, a synthetic analogue of vitamin D, used as 0.005% ointment. Total application not

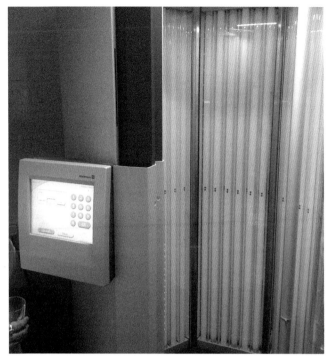

Phototherapy/photochemotherapy units: consists of vertically mounted UV tubes which emit either UVA or UVB (311 nm).

to exceed 100 gm/week of ointment, as increases calcium absorption and cause hypercalcemia or hypercalcuria. May also cause local irritation.

Phototherapy and photochemotherapy

Phototherapy involves exposure on alternate days to incremental doses of ultraviolet B (narrow band, 311 nm, given using UVB chambers) after application of emollient (to reduce scattering of light). Clearance generally in 6–8 weeks. *Photochemotherapy* involves intake on alternate days of oral 8-methoxypsoralen, 0.6 mg/kg, 2–3 hours before exposure to gradually increasing doses of sunlight (PUVA sol) or UVA delivered using UVA chambers (PUVA). Initial dose of light and increments depend on skin type. Response in psoriasis better with photochemotherapy than phototherapy (probably related to greater penetration of UVA).

Systemic therapy

Methotrexate, perhaps the most frequently used medication. Used for extensive plaque psoriasis. And pustular, erythrodermic and arthritic psoriasis. Also for debilitating palmoplantar psoriasis. Dose

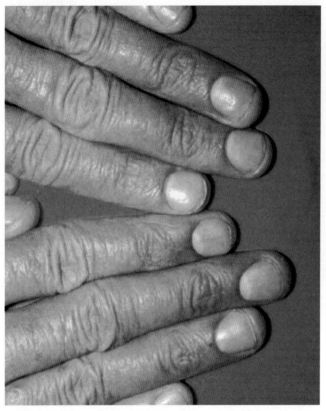

Psoriasis nails: conspicuous pitting of the nail plates with mild-subungual hyperkeratosis.

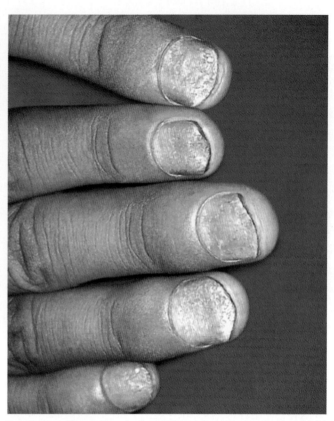

Psoriasis nails: uniformly dystrophic nails with proximal nail fold involvement.

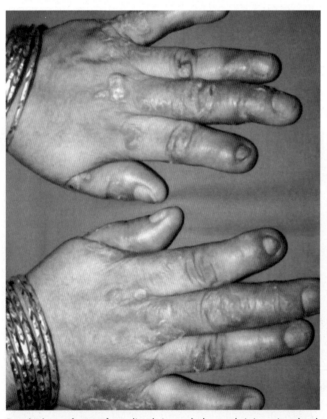

Psoriatic arthropathy: distal interphalangeal joints involved. Note nail changes, a common association.

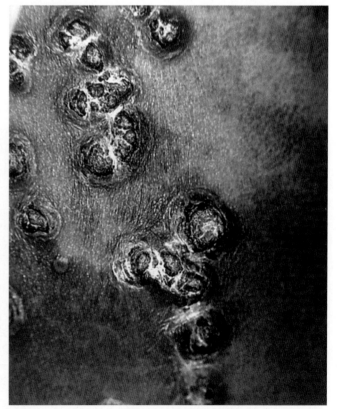

Rupioid psoriasis: heaped up scales on large papules.

0.2–0.3 mg/kg given weekly or less frequently as a single dose. Avoid concomitant use of aspirin, tetracyclines or other protein binding agents. Monitor for hepatotoxicity and bone-marrow toxicity, which are reduced by supplementing with folic acid, 5 mg weekly. *Acitretin*, 0.25–0.75 mg/kg, to be taken with food. Very effective in pustular psoriasis. Less so in plaque psoriasis, but the drug of choice in immunecompromised individuals. Dryness of skin and cheilitis universal. Potentially hepatotoxic, hyperlipidemic and teratogenic. Contraindicated in child-bearing females. So prolonged contraception (long half life) mandatory. *Cyclosporine* 3–5 mg/kg/day useful in recalcitrant cases. And in extensive and pustular psoriasis. Cost and side effects (hypertension, nephrotoxicity) preclude routine use. Other drugs used include *mycophenolate mofetil* and *leflunomide*. Corticosteroids, perhaps the most frequently **misused** systemic therapy in psoriasis. Advisable, to avoid as withdrawal may precipitate attacks of pustular or erythrodermic psoriasis. Only indication probably pustular psoriasis in pregnancy. Advancement in knowledge in pathophysiology of psoriasis, has shifted focus of treatment towards control of inflammatory cascade. Biologicals target specific steps in the immunoinflammatory mechanisms. Include etanercept, infliximab and adalimumab which block activity of TNF α, an important cytokine involved in psoriasis, alefacept which is a T-cell blocker and ustekinumab which targets interleukin-12 and IL-23.

REITER'S SYNDROME

Now known as reactive arthritis.

Epidemiology

Two forms recognized; epidemic (post dysenteric, also labeled enteric acquired reactive arthritis, EARA) and endemic (venereal, also labeled sexually acquired reactive arthritis, SARA). Disease of young adult males.

Etiology

Reactive phenomenon to a host of infections. Some sexually acquired (*Chlamydia trachomatis, Ureaplasma urealyticum* and probably *Mycoplasma genitalium*). Others enteric (*Campylobacter, Salmonella, Yersinia* and *Shigella*).

Pathogenesis

Pathogenesis complex. Genetically orchestrated immune response to an antigen, probably infectious, focused on skin and joints. HLA-B27 positivity in 50–90% cases.

Clinical Manifestations

Syndrome characterized by triad of **arthritis** (non-suppurative, asymmetric seronegative predominantly of lower extremities), **urethritis** and **inflammatory eye disease**. **Mucocutaneous findings** include rupioid/pustular psoriasis, circinate balanitis and keratoderma blenorrhagicum. Chronic relapsing course in 60% cases.

Treatment

Rest, physiotherapy, NSAIDs and antibiotics (e.g. doxycycline to treat *C. trachomatis*) during acute phase. Methotrexate (0.2 mg/kg/week), azathioprine (1.5–2.5 mg/kg/d), sulfasalazine, acitretin and cyclosporine for severe, recalcitrant skin and joint involvement. Systemic steroids in debilitating disease. Recent reports of gratifying response to infliximab.

LICHEN PLANUS

Epidemiology

Common dermatosis particularly in some parts of the world such as India. Any age, mostly young adults of both sexes, affected.

Etiology

Obscure etiology, uncertain pathogenesis. Probably a reaction pattern precipitated by a variety of unrelated and mostly unknown, factors. Drugs (thiazides, chlordiazepoxide, gold, chloroquine), contact with paraphenylenediamine and exposure to light responsible in some cases.

Clinical Manifestations

Morphology

Intensely pruritic, violaceous, flat-topped, polygonal, well-demarcated papules of variable size, marked by criss-cross whitish streaks (**Wickham's striae**). Scaling minimal. Lesions discrete, confluent or

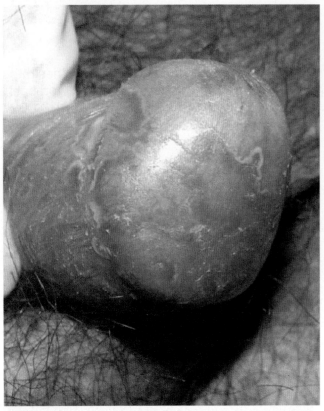

Reiter's disease: characteristic circinate balanitis. Moist erythematous plaque with polycyclic margin.

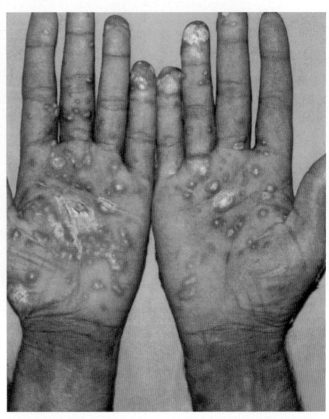

Reiter's disease: pathognomonic, keratoderma blenorrhagicum.

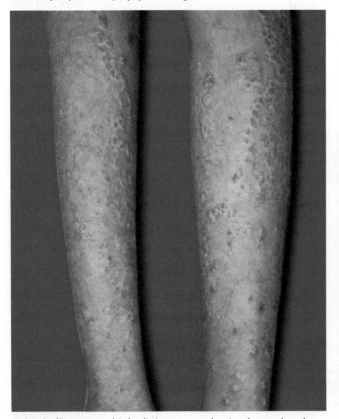

Reiter's disease: multiple discrete to coalescing heaped-up keratotic papules.

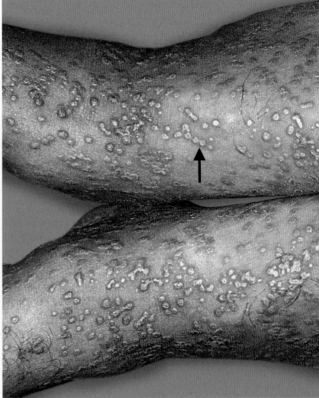

Lichen planus: pink and purplish papules. Note Koebner's phenomenon.

grouped. **Koebner's isomorphic phenomenon** indicates active disease.

Variants

Hypertrophic LP
Verrucous hyperkeratotic papules and nodules with central depigmentation. On shins.

Lichen planopilaris
Hair follicles involved; scalp often affected, with cicatricial alopecia. Other parts: violaceous keratotic follicular papules; heal with follicular atrophy.

Palmoplantar LP
Yellowish, keratotic papules; occasionally ulcerated plaques.

Annular LP
Annular (clear, sometimes atrophic center with a ring of papular lesions). Usually on face and glans.

Rarer variants
Vesicular and *bullous* lesions occasionally seen. *Actinic LP* on photoexposed parts; typically annular lesions with hypopigmented halo.

Associations

Oral LP
Nearly 0.6–2% of population affected. May occur in absence of skin lesions. Asymptomatic in a third but usually symptomatic (pain and burning sensation). Clinical types include reticular (most common) and plaque variants. And erosive (which has an infrequent premalignant potential). Runs chronic remitting and relapsing course.

Genital LP
Annular or flat, violaceous papules or plaques on the glans or shaft of penis. Vulvar lesions often erosive.

LP of nails
Less frequently affected but may present without any skin or mucosal lesions. Thinning of nail plate frequent. In severe cases, complete loss of nail plate (**onychomadesis**). Or extension of proximal nail fold to nail bed—splitting and destroying nail plate (**pterygium unguis**).

Sites of Predilection
Predilection for extremities (flexors of wrists and shins) and lower back. Follicular lesions on scalp and thighs, hypertrophic LP on shins and actinic LP on photoexposed sites.

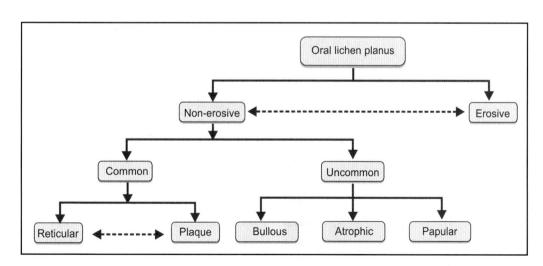

Oral lichen planus: Classification.

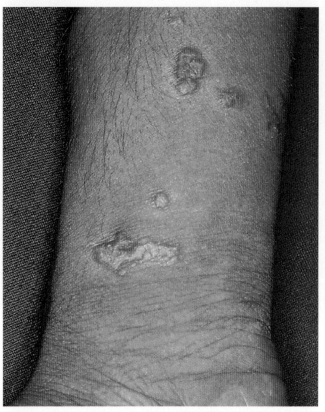

Lichen planus: typical lesions distributed on the wrist and forearm.

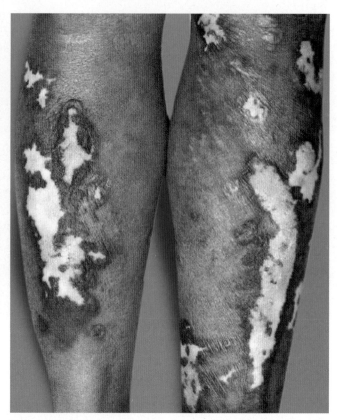

Lichen planus hypertrophicus: hypertrophic plaques with central depigmentation.

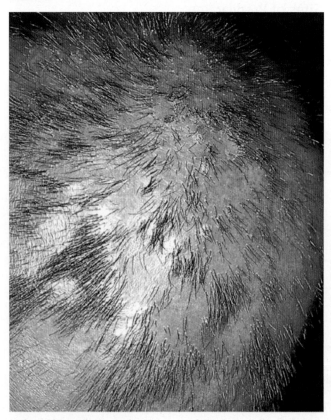

Lichen planopilaris, scalp: slate-grey follicular papules with cicatricial alopecia.

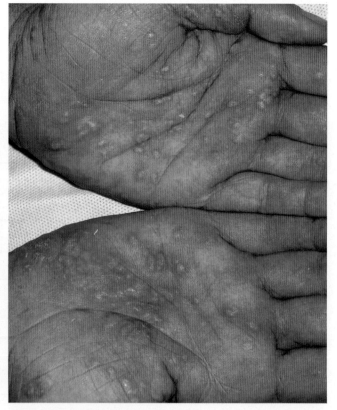

Lichen planus of palms: yellow brown keratotic papules and plaques, many showing pitting.

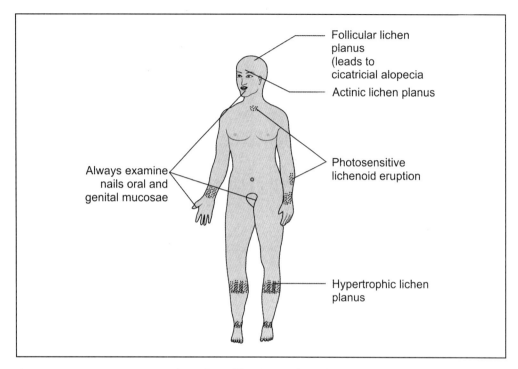

Sites of predilection: Lichen planus.

Course

LP runs a self-limiting course lasting several months. Relapses uncommon. Hypertrophic lesions last for several years. Occasional malignant change in buccal or hypertrophic lesions.

Investigations

None required. Biopsy done occasionally in doubtful cases.

Biopsy

Compact hyperkeratosis, irregular hypergranulosis and acanthosis (pronounced in hypertrophic variety) with saw-tooth appearance of rete ridges (c.f. club shaped in psoriasis). Liquefactive degeneration of basal cell layer (with formation of Max Joseph's space) and band of lymphocytes and histiocytes apposing the epidermis pathognomonic. Cytoid or colloid bodies at the dermoepidermal interface. Melanin incontinence in upper dermis. Perifollicular infiltrate in lichen planopilaris. Subepidermal split in bullous LP.

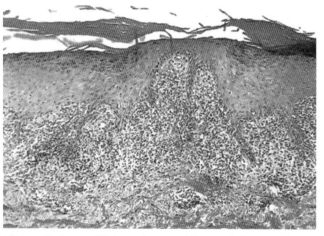

Histopathology of lichen planus: obliterated dermoepidermal interface with vacuolar degeneration of basal cells and a dense band of lymphohistiocytic infiltrate in upper dermis.

Treatment

General Measures

Remove suspected precipitating agent such as drugs, hair dyes. Protect from sunlight in actinic form. Antihistamines as antipruritics.

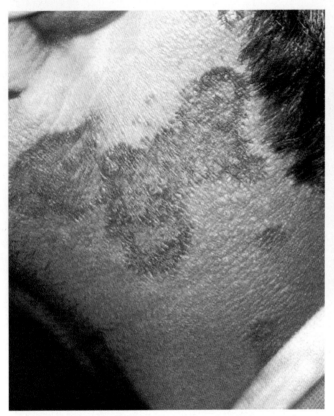

Lichen planus actinicus: small and large violaceous papules assuming annular configuration on the side of the neck.

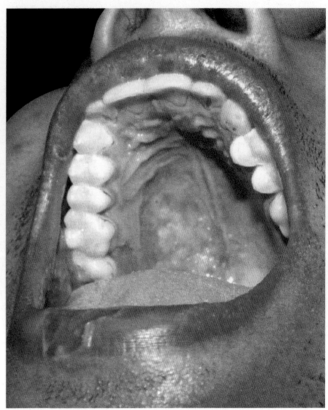

Mucosal lichen planus: of the palate and lips.

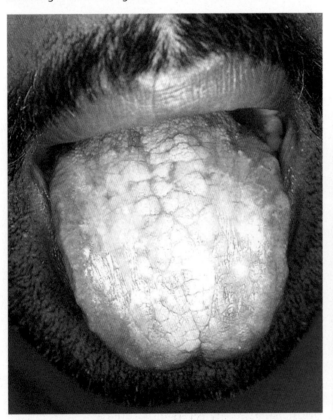

Mucosal lichen planus: whitish plaque on the tongue.

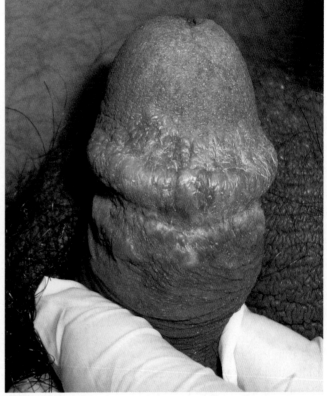

Genital lichen planus: violaceous papules and plaques over the glans penis and coronal sulcus.

Specific Treatment

Topical therapy

Topical corticosteroids (cream base ordinarily and in ointment base in hypertrophic lesions) mainstay in localized lesions. Formulations in orabase paste for oral lesions. Also topical tacrolimus or pimecrolimus.

Systemic therapy

Systemic corticosteroids in widespread progressive lesions. Extensive lesions also respond to photo/photochemotherapy, retinoids (acitretin), immunosuppressives (azathioprine, methotrexate, cyclosporine) and dapsone.

LICHEN PLANUS PIGMENTOSUS

Probably a macular variant of lichen planus.

Epidemiology

Common in India. Also described from Latin America, Japan and Europe variously as **erythema dyschromicum perstans** and **pigmented cosmetic dermatitis**. Young adults affected.

Etiology

Probably represents a lichenoid reaction pattern to an unknown agent though cosmetics including fragrances, hair dyes and mustard oil incriminated.

Clinical Manifestations

Asymptomatic or mildly itchy. Small or by confluence, large, irregular or oval macules of slate-grey to blue-black color. Starts from preauricular region with gradual spread to face, upper extremities, trunk and abdomen. Associated with other, particularly follicular, lichen planus. Mucosal involvement infrequent. Progressive course.

Investigations

None usually required, though biopsy ofen performed.

Biopsy

Histopathology variable. Active lesions show features of LP. Late lesions, focal incontinence of pigment with mild to moderate lymphohistiocytic infiltrate. And melanophages.

Treatment

Resistant to therapy. Repeated (8–10) courses of vitamin A in daily doses of 100,000 units for 2–3 weeks in a month may help. Recent reports of systemic retinoids being helpful.

LICHEN NITIDUS

Perhaps a micropapular form of lichen planus.

Clinical Manifestations

Actinic and non-actinic variants. *Actinic form (micropapular lichen planus)*: present more often in women, on the light-exposed parts of the forearms, chest, upper back; face sometimes affected. May be associated with ordinary lichen planus. Actinic variant may relapse on exposure to sunlight.

Non-actinic variant: on the male genitals or elsewhere. Asymptomatic or itchy, flat topped or dome-shaped, pale or skin colored papules. Self limiting.

Investigations

Diagnosis usually clinical. Confirmation histopathological.

Biopsy

Histopathology shows an atrophic, flattened epidermis with patchy degeneration of basal cell layer with lymphohistiocytic infiltrate. Epithelioid cell granuloma encircled by elongated rete ridges typical—'**ball in claw**' a typical appearance. Occasionally histology indistinguishable from lichen planus.

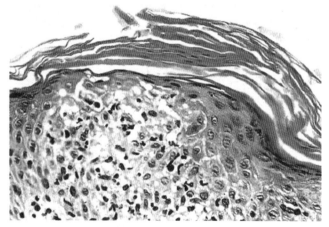

Lichen nitidus: focal collection of lymphocytes and histiocytes with atrophy of overlying epidermis; note elongated rete ridges at the edges giving 'ball in claw' appearance.

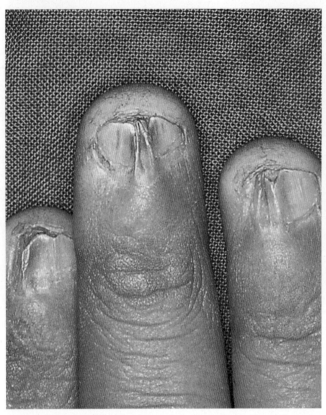

Lichen planus, nails: note dystrophy of several nails with pterygium unguis. Nail plates thin.

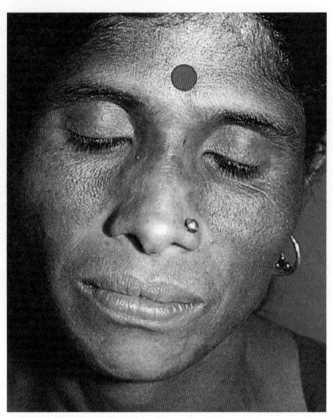

Lichen planus pigmentosus: diffuse bluish-grey pigmentation in a photosensitive distribution.

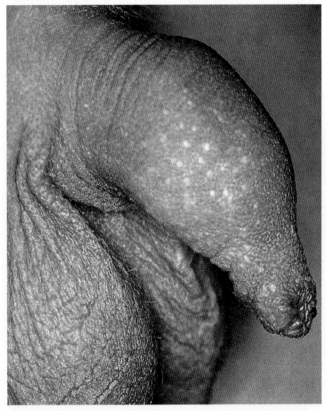

Lichen nitidus: small grouped shiny papules on shaft of penis.

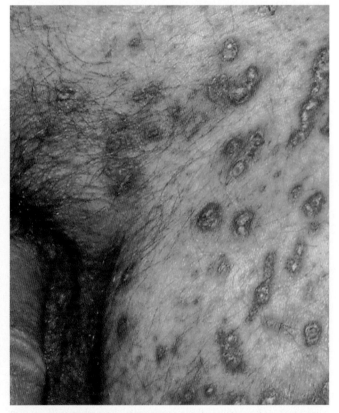

Keratosis lichenoides chronica: violaceous hyperkeratotic papules in linear configuration.

Treatment

Self resolving condition. Topical steroids. And photoprotection for actinic variant.

KERATOSIS LICHENOIDES CHRONICA (NEKAM'S DISEASE)

Rare. Chronic and progressive usually affecting individuals aged 20–40 years. Presents as violaceous and hyperkeratotic papules in linear, reticular or plaque form. Located on the trunk and limbs. Oral/genital lesions occasional.

PITYRIASIS ROSEA

Epidemiology

Common.

Etiology

Unknown, possibly a viral etiology (HHV-7).

Clinical Manifestations

Morphology

Clinically distinctive papulosquamous rash with primary lesion, the **herald patch**, a hypopigmented or erythematous, oval plaque with a peripheral collarette of fine scales. Similar but smaller lesions appear over the next few days. Mildly pruritic or asymptomatic. Minimal constitutional symptoms. Lymphadenopathy frequent. Heal spontaneously in 6–10 weeks with or without some hypopigmentation. Second attack is unusual.

Sites of Predilection

Chiefly on trunk along lines of cleavage and proximal portions of the upper and lower extremities. Occasionally distal parts of extremities and face involved (**inversus variety**).

Treatment

Reassurance—about self-limiting nature. Bland applications such as calamine lotion or emollients. Occasionally topical steroids. Systemic antihistamines to relieve itching.

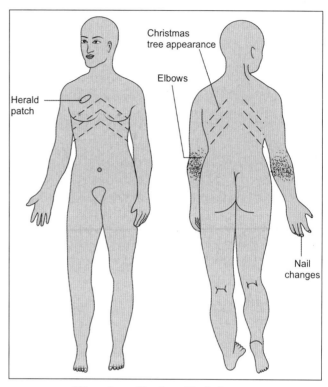

Sites of predilection: Pityriasis rosea.

PITYRIASIS RUBRA PILARIS

Epidemiology

Rare.

Etiology

Etiology obscure. Genetic influence perhaps operative in some forms.

Clinical Manifestations

Several variants—*juvenile (classical/atypical/circumscribed) and adult (classical/atypical) onset. And HIV-associated.* Onset abrupt or gradual. As an erythroderma or a seborrheic picture affecting scalp and face. Gradual development of asymptomatic erythematous, acuminate follicular papules on the dorsae of proximal phalanges, knees, elbows and later elsewhere. May become confluent to form salmon colored plaques with fine branny or frankly psoriasiform scales. Erythroderma shows characteristic skip areas—islands of normal skin. Palmoplantar keratoderma is diffuse and pale yellow in color, the so-called keratotic

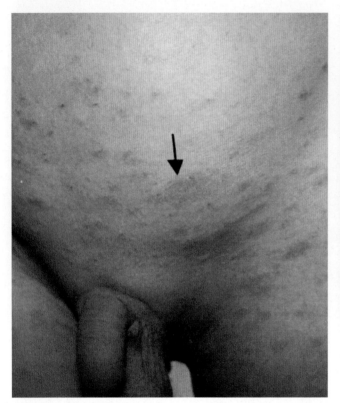

Pityriasis rosea: multiple, red scaly plaques on the trunk. Note herald patch in the suprapubic area.

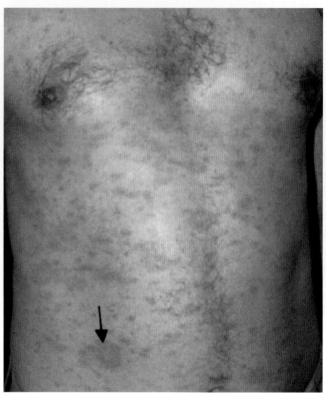

Pityriasis rosea: multiple erythematous plaques with collarette of scales on the trunk. Note herald patch in the right iliac fossa.

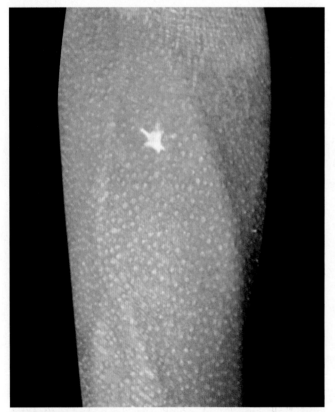

Pityriasis rubra pilaris: keratotic follicular papules.

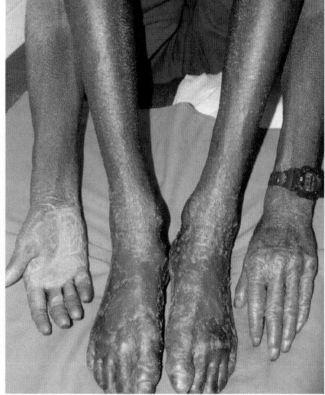

Pityriasis rubra pilaris: keratoderma with yellow to orange hue, hyperkeratotic lesions on the knuckles with follicular papules on the dorsa of proximal phalanges.

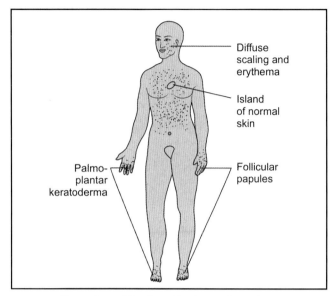

Sites of predilection: Pityriasis rubra pilaris.

Diffuse scaling and erythema

Island of normal skin

Follicular papules

Palmo-plantar keratoderma

sandal (**keratodermic/PRP sandals**). Mucous membrane involvement rare. Nail involvement not characteristic. Protracted course; occasional spontaneous resolution. Relapses unusual.

Investigations

None usually required. Biopsy sometimes done especially in erythroderma to confirm the diagnosis.

Biopsy

Histopathology shows alternating orthokeratosis and parakeratosis in both vertical and horizontal directions (checker board pattern). Keratotic plugs in the hair follicles with focal parakeratosis in the follicular shoulder with perifollicular lymphocytic infiltrate in the dermis.

Treatment

General Measures

Emollients.

Specific Treatment

Combination of topical and systemic therapy.

Topical treatment

Use moderately potent corticosteroids or tretinoin or a combination of the two.

Systemic treatment

Oral retinoids (acitretin, 0.5–1 mg/kg/day) or methotrexate. Response less satisfactory than in psoriasis.

10

Autoimmune Vesiculobullous Dermatoses

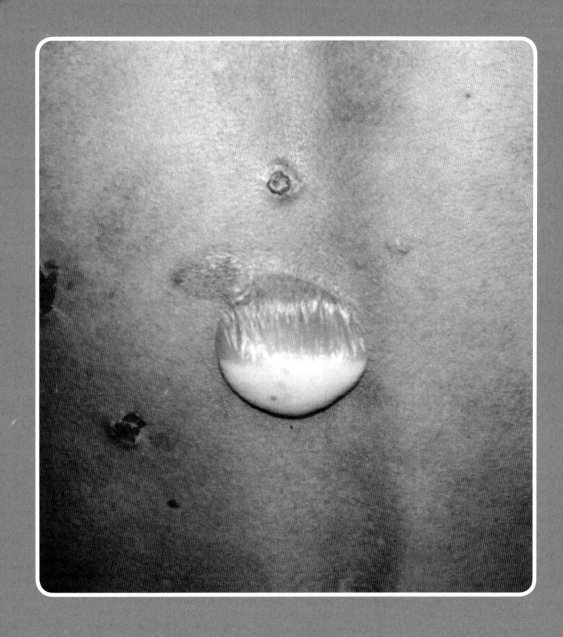

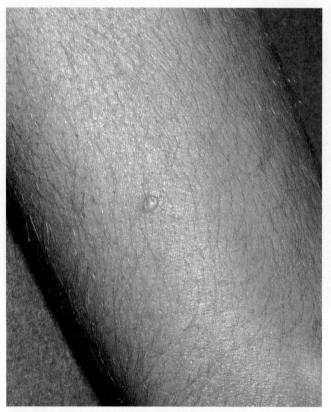

Pemphigus vulgaris: early lesion small vesicle on normal skin.

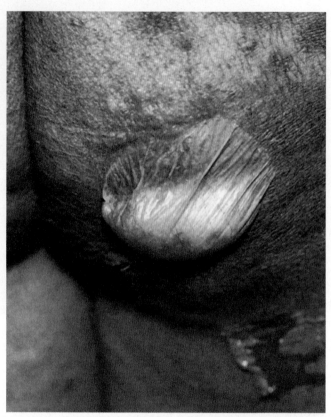

Pemphigus vulgaris: large flaccid turbid-fluid filled bulla.

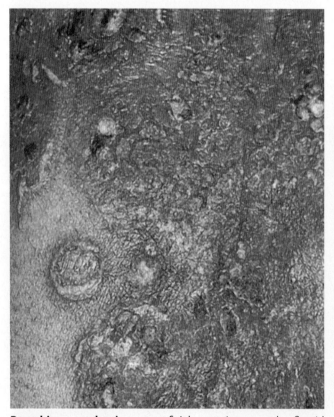

Pemphigus vulgaris: superficial erosions and flaccid vesiculopustules.

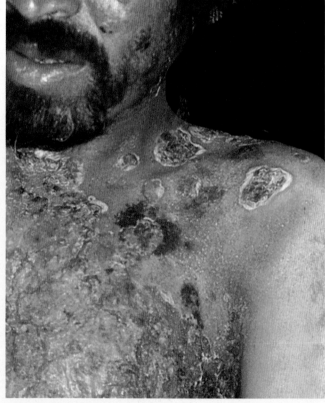

Pemphigus vulgaris: extensive lesions.

A group of dermatoses of autoimmune etiology characterized by appearance of vesiculobullous lesions with or without mucosal involvement. Induced by antibodies against antigens present in epidermis (pemphigus group). Or in dermoepidermal junction (the subepidermal immunobullous disorders). The pathogenitically important antibodies deposited in a fish net pattern against intercellular substance in epidermis (in pemphigus). Or in a uniform linear pattern in basement membrane zone (in pemphigoid and linear IgA dermatoses). Or in granular pattern in dermal papillae (in dermatitis herpetiformis). Morbidity and mortality, systemic manifestations and associations variable. Diagnosis confirmed by direct immunofluorescence (DIF) on skin biopsy. Or by demonstration of circulating antibodies by indirect immunofluorescence (IIF) or by ELISA.

Antigenic targets in autoimmune bullous disorders	
Disease	*Target antigens*
Pemphigus vulgaris and variants	Desmoglein 3 and 1
Pemphigus foliaceus and variants	Desmoglein 1
IgA pemphigus	
• SCPD* type	Desmocollin 1
• IEN** type	Desmoglein 1 and 3
Paraneoplastic pemphigus	Desmoplakin 1 and 2, Envoplakin, Periplakin, Desmoglein 3
Bullous pemphigoid	BP*** 180, BP*** 230
Herpes gestationis	BP*** 180, BP*** 230
Cicatricial pemphigoid	BP*** 180, laminin 5
Linear IGA disease	BP*** 180, collagen (type VII)
Dermatitis herpetiformis	Unknown

* Subcorneal pustular dermatosis
** Intraepidermal neutrophilic
*** Bullous pemphigoid

PEMPHIGUS

The most common of the vesiculobullous dermatoses.

Epidemiology

Not uncommon in India and South East Asia. Rare in the West. Middle aged, occasionally young adults and rarely children, of both sexes affected.

Classification

Several types recognized:
• Pemphigus vulgaris
• Pemphigus vegetans
• Pemphigus foliaceus
• Pemphigus erythematosus
• Paraneoplastic pemphigus.

Etiology

Autoimmune etiology. Occasionally drug induced or paraneoplastic in nature.

Pathogenesis

IgG antibodies directed, in pemphigus vulgaris, against desmoglein 3 and 1 (desmosomal cadherins involved in epidermal adhesion). And in pemphigus foliaceus against desmoglein 1. Bind to and cause loss of cohesion of epidermal cells (**acantholysis**). Intraepidermal blisters characterized by presence of acantholysis and **acantholytic cells** (rounded epidermal cells with large dense nuclei). Epidermal split at different levels in different types—subcorneal in pemphigus foliaceus and pemphigus erythematosus, suprabasal in pemphigus vulgaris and pemphigus vegetans.

Clinical Manifestations

All variants characterized by presence of superficial, flaccid bullae which are absent/transient (pemphigus foliaceus and pemphigus erythematosus) to relatively more persistent (pemphigus vulgaris and pemphigus vegetans).

Pemphigus Vulgaris

Most common and most serious type. Adults affected. Insidious onset of mucosal and/or cutaneous lesions. *Mucosal lesions:* generally buccal but other mucosae also involved. Bullae

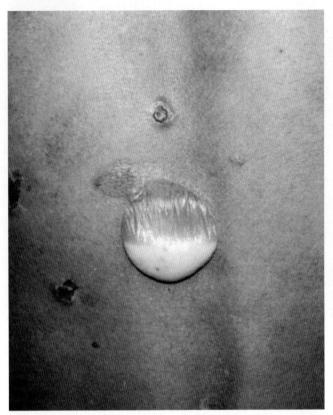

Pear sign: positive in pemphigus vulgaris, collection of fluid in the lower part of the bulla.

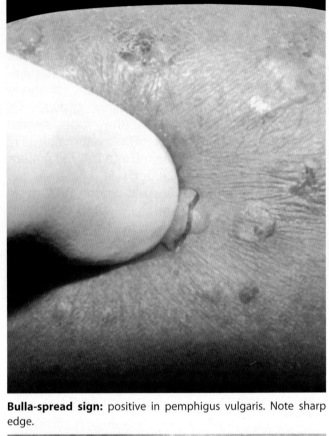

Bulla-spread sign: positive in pemphigus vulgaris. Note sharp edge.

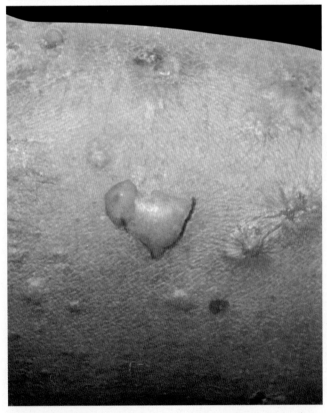

Bulla-spread sign: positive in pemphigus vulgaris. Note sharp edge of extended bulla and easily ruptured bulla.

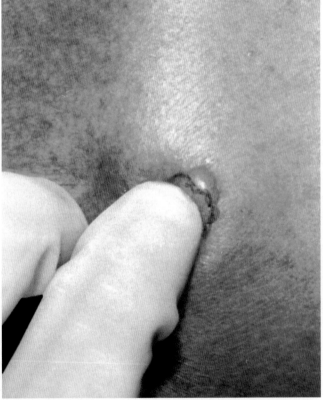

Bulla-spread sign: sometimes positive in bullous pemphigoid, but note rounded edge.

rare. Manifests as painful, superficial erosions; often (in 50%) precede appearance of cutaneous lesions. *Cutaneous lesions*: superficial and flaccid vesicles and bullae; rupture easily, leaving large denuded areas; extend peripherally. Occasional bleeding. Clinically normal epidermis peeled off by gentle tangential pressure **(Nikolsky's sign)**. Healing slow, with hyperpigmentation. Pressure areas and sites of friction more prone. Flexural lesions prone to becoming hypertrophic and vegetative. Paronychial lesions typical. Little toxemia. Remissions mostly induced by systemic corticosteroids or other immunosuppressives. Relapses common. Mortality, though still moderate, has come down considerably.

Pemphigus Vegetans

An uncommon variant of pemphigus vulgaris. Hypertrophic vegetative lesions with superficial fissuring with or without obvious vesiculation. In axillae, groins, perineum, perianal areas and lips. Mucosal lesions infrequent. Prognostically better than pemphigus vulgaris.

Pemphigus Foliaceus

Less common, less serious than pemphigus vulgaris. Elderly individuals or children. Scale-crusts, sometimes with, but more often without, superficial vesiculation. Gradual spread, from face, scalp, upper trunk (seborrhoeic distribution) to becoming generalized. May simulate exfoliative dermatitis. Mucosal lesions infrequent.

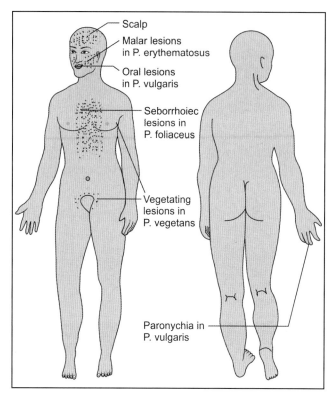

Sites of predilection: Pemphigus.

Mechanical signs in bullous disorders			
Sign	*Description*	*Interpretation of positive sign*	*Clinical diagnosis*
Nikolsky's sign	Peeling-off of clinically normal skin (due to acantholysis)	Intraepidermal bulla and disease active	• Pemphigus • Staphylococcal scalded skin syndrome
Pseudo-Nikolsky's sign	Peeling-off of skin (due to apoptotic necrosis)	Intraepidermal bulla	• Toxic epidermal necrolysis • Stevens-Johnson syndrome • Erythema multiforme
Pear sign	Collection of fluid in lower part of blister due to gravity	Intraepidermal flaccid bulla	• Pemphigus
Bulla-spread sign (Asboe-Hansen sign)	Extension of blister in direction opposite to side of pressure		• Edge sharp: Pemphigus • Edge rounded: Bullous pemphigoid
Sheklakov sign	Pin-point bleeding spots on peeling-off of the remnant of blister (analogous to Auspitz sign)	Subepidermal bulla	• Bullous pemphigoid • Epidermolysis bullosa acquisita

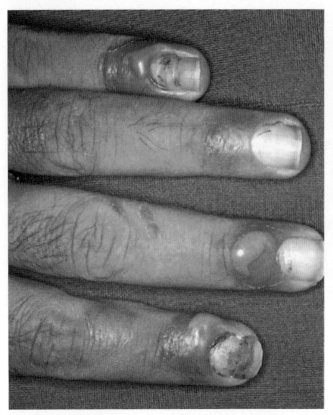

Pemphigus vulgaris: paronychia, a typical involvement.

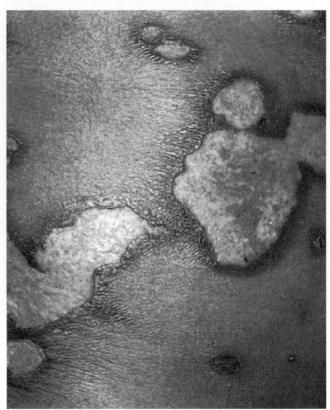

Pemphigus vulgaris: healing lesions.

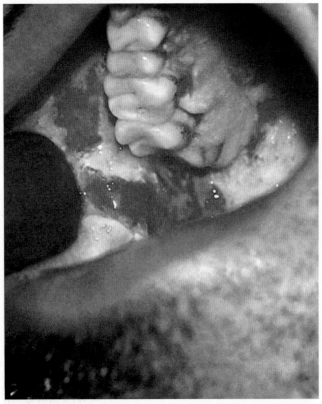

Pemphigus vulgaris: buccal mucosal lesions showing ragged margin.

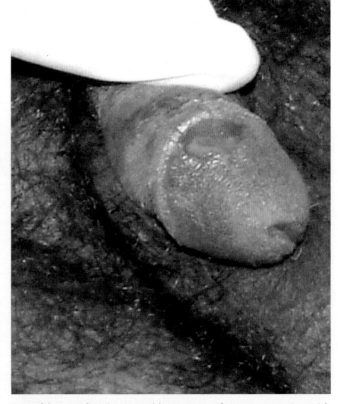

Pemphigus vulgaris: genital lesions manifesting as erosion with irregular margins.

Pemphigus Erythematosus (Senear-Usher Syndrome)

Uncommon variant of pemphigus foliaceus; Erythema and scale-crusts in malar area (butterfly distribution). And scaly lesions also on the scalp and elsewhere.

IgA Pemphigus (Intraepidermal Neutrophilic IgA Dermatosis)

Recently described variant of pemphigus. Involvement of mucous membranes rare. Two types recognized:

- *Subcorneal pustular dermatosis (SCPD) type*: Superficial (subcorneal) pustules with predilection for intertriginous areas (like classic SCPD).
- *Intraepidermal neutrophilic (IEN) type*: Flaccid blisters and pustules in annular or sunflower like configuration, with central erythema and peripheral vesiculation. Erode to form crusts.

Paraneoplastic Pemphigus (Paraneoplastic Autoimmune Multiorgan Syndrome)

Malignancy associated autoimmune phenomenon with circulating antibodies against components of desmosomes and hemidesmosomes. *Malignancies associated*: non-Hodgkin's lymphoma, chronic lymphocytic lymphoma, Castelman's disease, thymoma, sarcoma, Waldenstrom's macroglobulinemia, lung cancer. At presentation, malignancy not detectable in one-third of patients. Severe painful mucosal erosions and polymorphic skin lesions-erythema multiforme-like, pemphigoid-like, pemphigus-like, graft-vs-host disease-like, lichen planus pemphigoides-like. Trunk and extremities, particularly acral parts including palms and soles and paronychia. Response to therapy poor, unless malignancy removed.

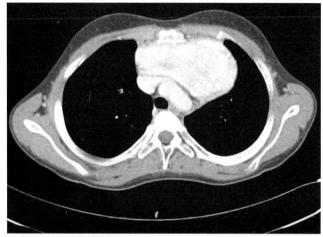

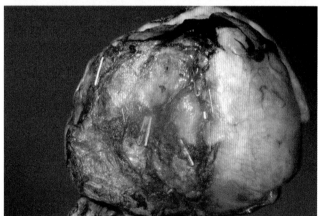

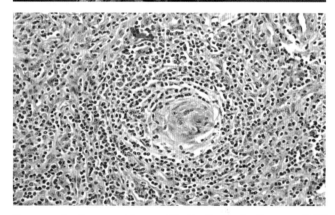

Paraneoplastic pemphigus with Castleman's disease: CECT chest showing a large, highly vascular tumor with its attachments to anterior chest wall. Surgical excision showed large-sized highly vascular mass with bosselated surface. Histopathology of tumor showed well-formed lymphoid follicles rich in plasma cells and central blood vessels seen at follicular center with concentrically arranged lymphoid tissue and plasma cells in interfollicular areas, suggestive of Castleman's disease.

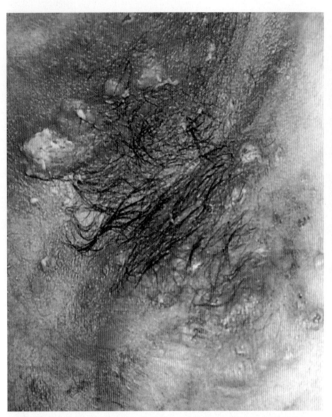

Pemphigus vegetans: exuberant vegetative and fissured lesions in flexures.

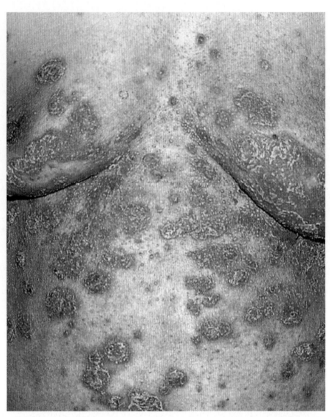

Pemphigus foliaceus: scale-crusts in seborrheic distribution.

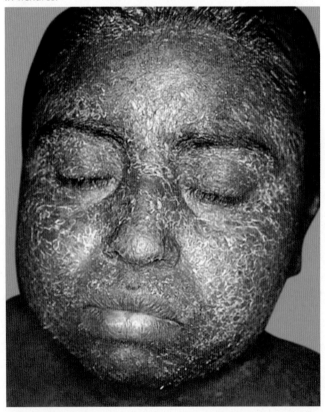

Pemphigus foliaceus: scale-crusts all over the face (similar lesions also present on the body).

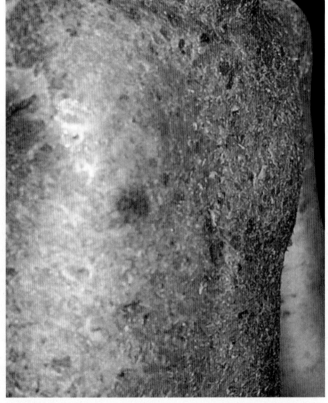

Pemphigus foliaceus: scale-crusts over trunk. Removal of scale-crust reveals minimally moist skin or an erosion.

Course

Depends on the type of pemphigus. And individual variation. Relapses generally frequent. Some patients maintain remission without steroids and adjuvants after a couple of years of therapy. Varying mortality: due to the disease (paraneoplastic pemphigus >> pemphigus vulgaris >> pemphigus foliaceus). Or sepsis or complications of therapy.

Investigations

Diagnosis needs to be confirmed cytopathologically (**Tzanck smear**), histopathologically. And with immunofluorescence.

Cytopathology

Tzanck smear done by scrapping floor of the bulla. And staining with Giemsa/Leishman stain. Shows acantholytic cells, which are large keratinocytes with big rounded nuclei and cytoplasm condensed peripherally.

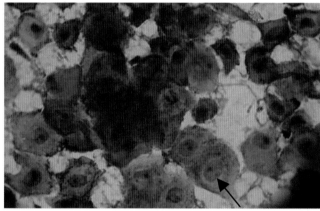

Tzanck smear stained with Giemsa stain: shows acantholytic cells which are large keratinocytes with big rounded nuclei and a perinuclear halo.

Histopathology

Biopsy taken from edge of the bulla shows acantholytic intraepidermal split containing acantholytic cells (rounded epidermal cells with large rounded nuclei) and eosinophils. *Location of split*: suprabasal in pemphigus vulgaris (and vegetans) and subcorneal in the foliaceus (and erythematosus). *Vegetans variant:* also shows acanthosis, hyperkeratosis and large intra-epidermal eosinophilic abscesses. *IgA pemphigus*: neutrophilic collections either in lower epidermis or in entire epidermis with sparse acantholysis.

Paraneoplastic pemphigus: intraepidermal acantholysis, keratinocyte necrosis and vacuolar interface dermatitis.

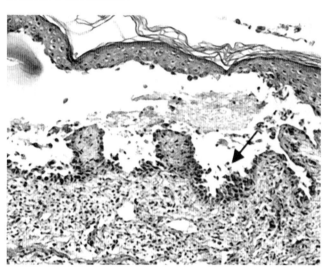

Histopathology of pemphigus vulgaris: suprabasal intraepidermal split with acantholysis.

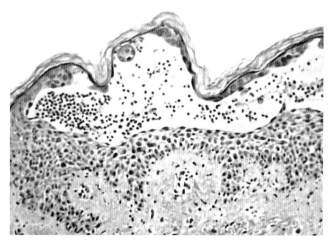

Histopathology of pemphigus foliaceus: subcorneal split containing acantholytic cells and eosinophils.

Immunofluorescence

Direct immunofluorescence

In pemphigus vulgaris, vegetans, foliaceus, erythematosus: IgG autoantibodies along keratinocyte cell membrane giving a fish net appearance. *IgA pemphigus*: IgA antibodies distributed in upper epidermis. *Paraneoplastic pemphigus*: IgG and complement in intercellular spaces. As well as granular/linear deposit of complement along basement membrane zone (BMZ).

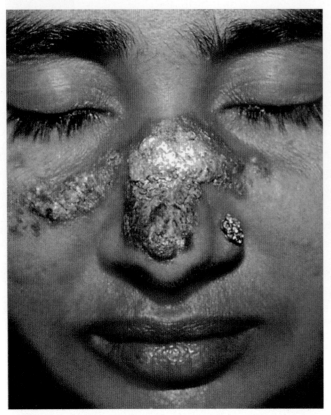

Pemphigus erythematosus: scale-crusts with underlying erythema in butterfly distribution.

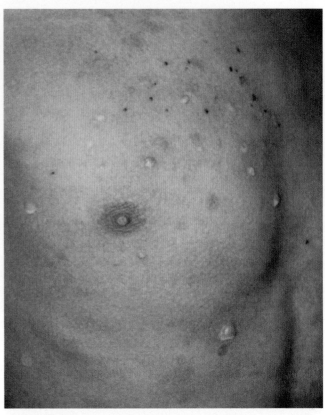

IgA pemphigus: subcorneal pustular type with hypopyon.

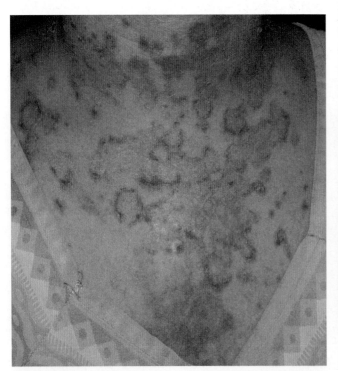

IgA pemphigus: intraepidermal neutrophic variant. Flaccid blisters in annular configuration. Note central erythema and peripheral vesiculation and erosions.

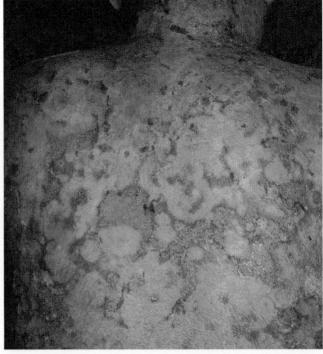

IgA pemphigus: IEN variant flaccid blisters in an annular configuration.

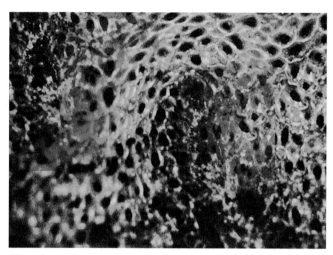

Direct immunofluorescence of pemphigus: fish-net like deposit of IgG in epidermis.

Indirect immunofluorescence

In pemphigus vulgaris/ vegetans/ foliaceus/ erythematosus: circulating IgG autoantibodies always present. Titers reflect disease activity. *In IgA pemphigus:* circulating IgA autoantibodies in 50% of patients. Titers of IgA pemphigus autoantibodies much lower than titers of IgG autoantibodies in IgG-mediated pemphigus. *Paraneoplastic pemphigus:* pattern similar to pemphigus. In addition, circulating antibodies to rat bladder transitional epithelium. In all variants, antibodies also detectable by ELISA.

Treatment

General Measures

Depends on extent of involvement. For extensive lesions, care for electrolyte/fluids. Also prevention/treatment of skin/mucosal infections—bacterial and candidal.

Specific Treatment

Topical therapy

Care of wound important-use topical antibiotic-steroid combinations. Epidermal growth factor probably hastens healing.

Systemic therapy

Aim is to bring about remission rapidly and maintain it. Systemic corticosteroids, mainstay of treatment. Large doses (60–80 mg/day of prednisolone equivalent) given daily orally. Or as oral (betamethasone) or parenteral (dexamethasone), 100 mg pulse, given monthly or fortnightly. Pulse therapy perhaps brings about remission more rapidly. Use of adjuvants (azathioprine, 50–100 mg/ day, cyclophosphamide, 50–100 mg/ day and methotrexate, 7.5–15 mg/week) steroid sparing; also help maintain remission. Daily oral steroids, though required to maintain remissions in some patients. Biologicals, in form of rituximab, the new drug.

PEMPHIGOID (BULLOUS PEMPHIGOID, BP)

Etiology

Autoantibodies (usually IgG, sometimes IgE, occasionally both) against 2 BP antigens: BPAG1 (BP230 antigen) and BPAG2 (BP180 antigen) in BMZ probably directly (and/ or indirectly) responsible for pathogenesis.

Pathogenesis

BP IgG antibodies capable of inducing dermal–epidermal separation in presence of complement and leukocytes.

Epidemiology

Uncommon in the East, relatively common in the West. Elderly individuals.

Clinical Manifestations

Morphology

Large, tense at times, hemorrhagic, bullae on an erythematous or urticarial background. Bulla do not rupture but roof settles. So cutaneous lesions heal faster than in pemphigus. Healing with minimal scarring with hyperpigmentation and milia formation. Mucosal lesions infrequent.

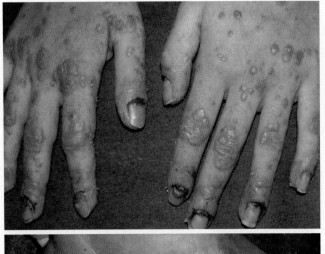

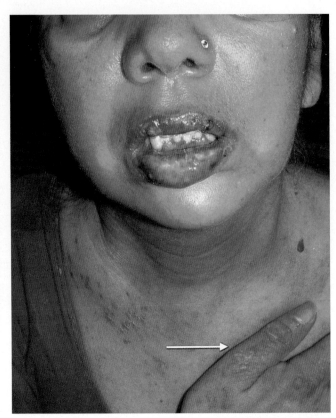

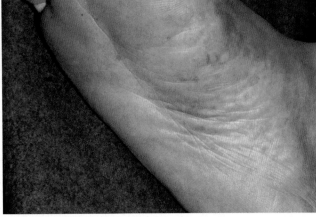

Paraneoplastic pemphigus: indolent oral lesions with lichenoid plaques in acral areas.

Paraneoplastic pemphigus: lichenoid lesions in the acral parts, and erythema multiforme like lesions on soles. Patients also had indolent mucositis.

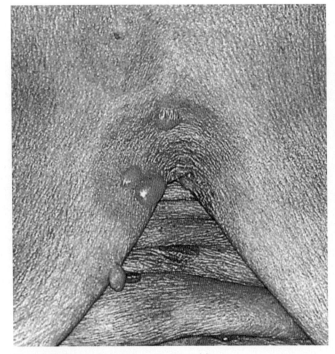

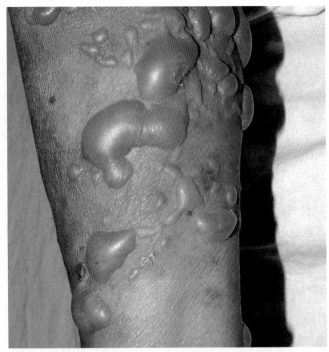

Pemphigoid: early bullae on urticarial base.

Bullous pemphigoid: large tense bullae on urticarial base.

Sites of Predilection

Lower limbs, abdomen, trunk.

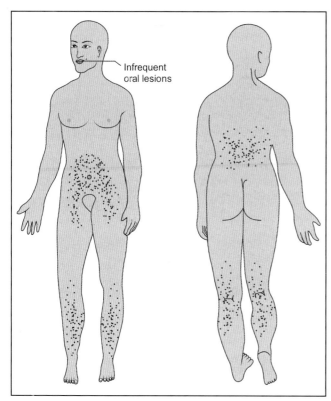

Infrequent
oral lesions

Sites of predilection: Bullous pemphigoid.

Course

Little toxemia. Spontaneous or (more often) therapeutic remission. Relapses less frequent than in pemphigus. Prognosis generally good, unless associated with malignancy.

Associations

Occasional association with systemic malignancies, particularly lymphomas (? just age related).

Investigations

Histopathology

Subepidermal bulla with eosinophils.

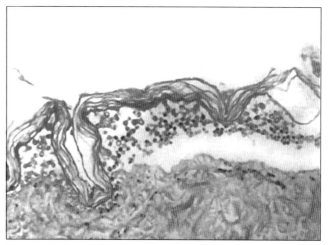

Histopathology of bullous pemphigoid: subepidermal bulla with eosinophils.

Immunofluorescence

Direct immunofluorescence

Linear deposit of IgG (less frequently IgE) and complement C3 at BMZ.

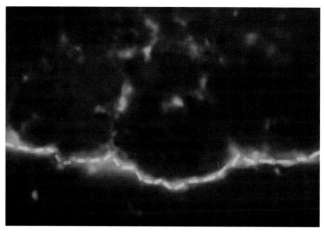

Direct immunofluorescence of bullous pemphigoid: linear deposit of IgG and C3 along the basement membrane.

Indirect immunofluorescence

About 70% (higher, if salt split skin used as substrate) of patients have circulating IgG (more frequently) and IgE (less frequent, but associated with more severe disease) autoantibodies that bind to BMZ

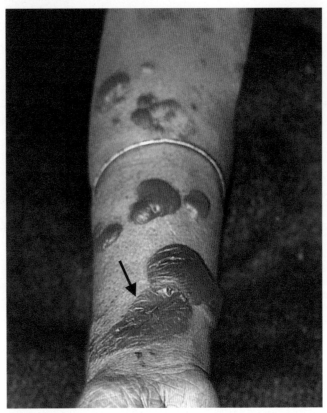

Pemphigoid: large, tense, clear and hemorrhagic blisters on the forearms. Bullae do not rupture, but roof settles as fluid is reabsorbed.

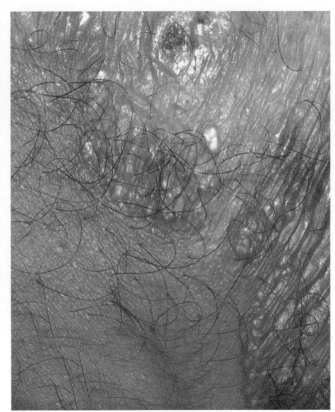

Pemphigoid: bullae heal with hyperpigmentation and milia formation.

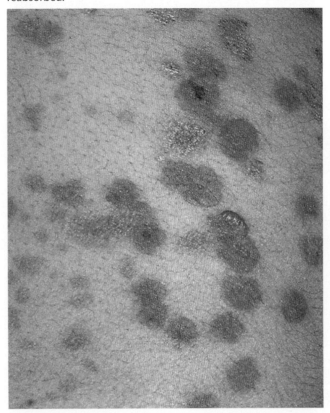

Herpes gestationis: erythematous plaques with clear vesicles at the edges. Some lesions targetoid.

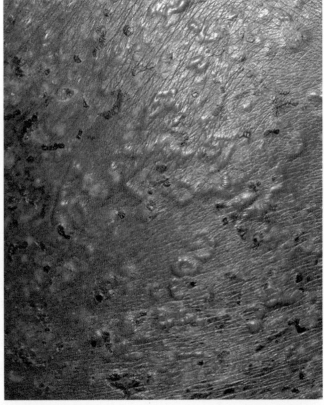

Herpes gestationis: clear vesicles on trunk. Many blisters arranged in arcuate/annular pattern. Patient prematurely delivered a small for date baby.

of normal human skin or monkey esophagus. Also detected by ELISA.

Treatment

General Measures

Patient usually well maintained.

Specific Treatment

Topical therapy

If few lesions, managed with potent corticosteroids topically.

Systemic therapy

If extensive, dapsone, 200 mg/ day, first line drug. Add 30–40 mg prednisolone equivalent, if control inadequate. Finally, wean off corticosteroids and maintain on small dose of dapsone. Combination of tetracyclines and high dose of niacinamide, also safe and effective.

HERPES GESTATIONIS (PEMPHIGOID GESTATIONIS, PG)

Epidemiology

Rare. More frequent in populations with higher prevalence of HLA-DR3 and -DR4.

Etiology and Pathogenesis

Occurs during pregnancy. Or in those on oral contraceptives. All (nearly) patients have IgG antibodies (to BP180), deposited at BMZ which induces deposition of C3 also along BMZ.

Clinical Manifestations

Morphology

Tense vesicles arranged in an annular/arcuate fashion on an erythematous or urticarial background. Erythema multiforme like targetoid lesions also present.

Sites of Predilection

Abdomen, lower trunk, lower extremities, palms and soles.

Course

Generally self limiting; remits at parturition. Occasionally continues post partum. Recurs in subsequent pregnancies.

Complications

No increased maternal morbidity or mortality. Increased risk of premature and small-for gestational-age babies.

Investigations

Histopathology

Subepidermal bulla with eosinophils.

Immunofluorescence

Direct immunofluorescence

Linear deposit of C3 and sometimes IgG demonstrable at BMZ.

Indirect immunofluorescence

Occasionally detects circulating IgG deposition. Increased sensitivity using complement-added IIF. Also detected by ELISA.

Treatment

Moderate doses (40–60 mg) of prednisolone with or without dapsone.

BENIGN MUCOSAL PEMPHIGOID (CICATRICIAL PEMPHIGOID, CP)

Etiology

Autoantibodies (usually IgG, sometimes IgA, occasionally both) against antigens (mostly BPAG2, sometimes laminin332, and several others) in epidermal BMZ probably directly (and/or indirectly) responsible for pathogenesis of CP.

Epidemiology

Rare. Elderly individuals.

Clinical Manifestations

Predominantly mucosal lesions, heal with scarring, adhesions and contractures. Eyes and mouth

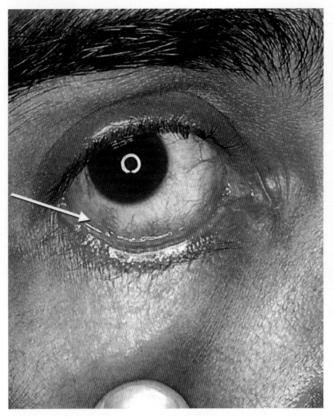

Benign mucosal pemphigoid: ocular involvement with chronic conjunctivities and adhesions.

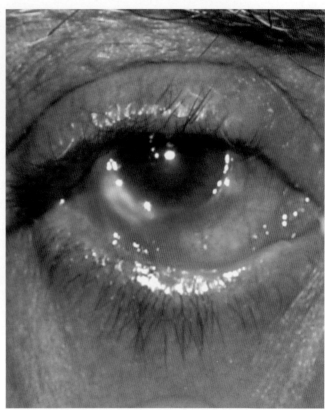

Benign mucosal pemphigoid: symblepheron.

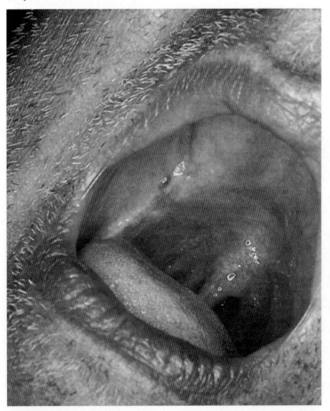

Benign mucosal pemphigoid: palatal lesions. Begin as transient vesicles which rupture to form chronic erosions.

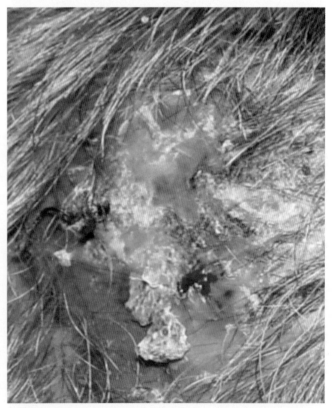

Benign mucosal pemphigoid: skin lesions, often tend to occurs at the same site on scalp leading to cicatricial alopecia.

commonly affected. Skin lesions less common (30%) and localized to scalp, head and neck. Progressive course interspersed with remissions. Complicated by symblepheron, loss of vision. And laryngeal stenosis. And cicatricial alopecia.

Investigations

Histopathology

Subepidermal bulla. Dermal infiltrate of lymphocytes and plasma cells, later replaced by fibroblasts.

Immunofluorescence

Direct immunofluorescence

IgG and C3 at BMZ. More frequently demonstrable in mucosal lesions.

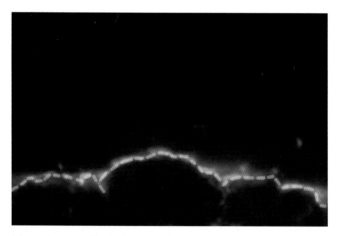

Direct immunofluorescence of cicatricial pemphigoid: linear deposit of IgG and C3 along the basement membrane in mucosal lesions.

Indirect immunofluorescence

Low levels of circulating usually IgG (less frequently IgA).

Treatment

Systemic corticosteroids with an adjuvant usually azathioprine. Aggressive treatment initiated early to prevent scarring. Occasionally topical or intra-lesional corticosteroid therapy.

CHRONIC BULLOUS DERMATOSIS OF CHILDHOOD (CBDC)

Epidemiology

Rather common. Young children; both sexes.

Etiology

IgA mediated disease.

Clinical Manifestations

Morphology

Acute onset. Asymptomatic or itchy. Clear, tense bullae often grouped to give a **cluster of jewels appearance**. New lesions sometimes appear around the periphery of previous lesions with a collarette of blisters, giving the so called **string of pearl appearance**. Mucous membrane involvement occasional.

Sites of Predilection

Face, trunk, perigenital area and extremities.

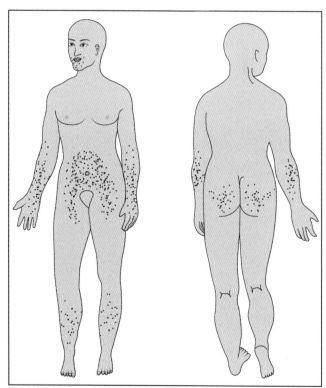

Sites of predilection: Chronic bullous dermatosis of childhood (CBDC).

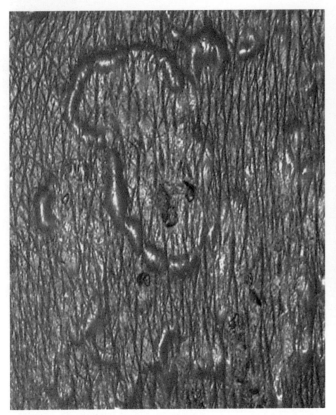

Chronic bullous dermatosis of childhood: typical string of pearl appearance of tense bullae.

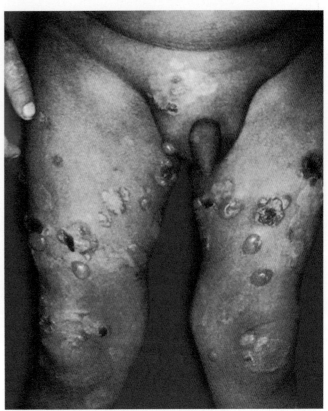

Chronic bullous dermatosis of childhood: tense bullae in perigenital region.

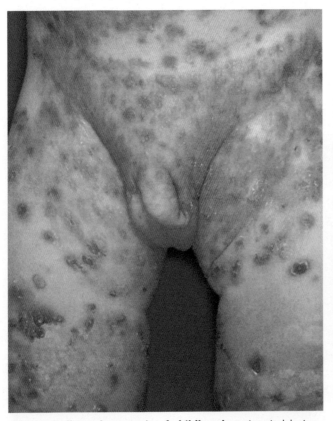

Chronic bullous dermatosis of childhood: perigenital lesions very characteristics.

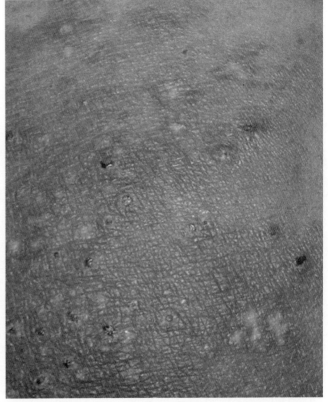

Linear IgA bullous dermatosis: itchy grouped small papulovesicles on urticarial background. Most vesicles have been excoriated.

Variants

Linear IgA bullous dermatosis

Rare variant seen after fourth decade of life. May be triggered by drugs (vancomycin), inflammatory bowel disease or associated with malignancy (lymphoid). Clinical presentation like CBDC/BP/ dermatitis herpetiformis. Drug induced may mimic toxic epidermal necrolysis.

Course

CBDC: relapsing and remitting, with eventual resolution. LABD: variable with both spontaneous remissions and long-standing disease.

Investigations

Histopathology

Subepidermal bulla, with collections of neutrophils along dermoepidermal junction often accumulating at the papillary tips.

Immunofluorescence

Direct immunofluorescence

Linear IgA deposits in BMZ.

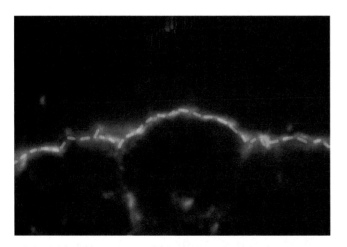

Direct immunofluorescence of CBDC/LABD: linear deposit of IgA along the basement membrane in perilesional skin.

Indirect immunofluorescence

Majority of patients with LABD have low-titers of circulating IgA antibodies against the epidermal side of the split skin substrate.

Treatment

Dapsone and sulphapyridine effective. Some patients need systemic corticosteroids.

DERMATITIS HERPETIFORMIS (DH)

Etiology

Genes encoding the DQ2 present in almost all patients of DH. As also in gluten sensitive enteropathy (GSE). Aberrant processing/response (due to genetic predisposition) to gluten, a protein in wheat, barley, and rye, critical to pathogenesis.

Pathogenesis

Epidermal transglutaminase (TGases) the dominant autoantigen. Circulating IgA antibodies directed against TGases also observed. IgA-TGases immune complexes formed locally within papillary dermis, lead to neutrophil chemotaxis (with formation of neutrophilic abscesses), proteolytic cleavage at BMZ and subepidermal blister formation.

Epidemiology

Uncommon. Young adult males.

Clinical Manifestations

Morphology

Intensely pruritic, bilaterally symmetrical, grouped, small vesicles or papules on an urticarial background. May form annular plaques with vesicular edge. Heal with hyperpigmentation. Grouped excoriations sometimes the only manifestation. Mucosal lesions not seen.

Sites of Predilection

Shoulders, elbows, back, buttocks, trunk and extensor aspects of extremities.

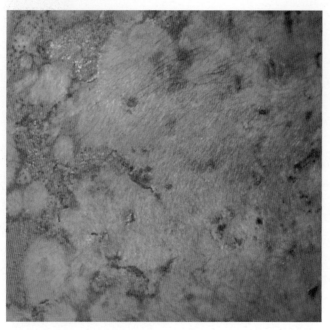

Linear IgA bullous dermatosis: drug induced LABD mimicking toxic epidermal necrolysis.

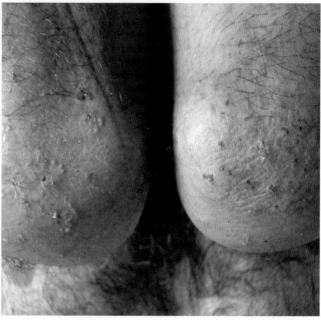

Dermatitis herpetiformis: grouped excoriations and intervening vesicles over both elbows.

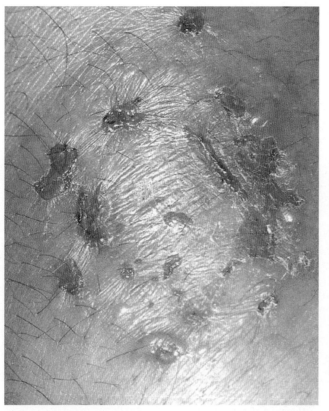

Dermatitis herpetiformis: grouped vesiculation on an erythematous background. Many vesicles have been excoriated.

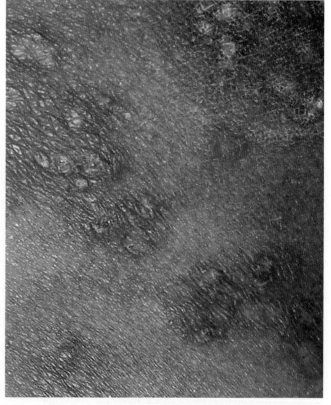

Dermatitis herpetiformis: grouped excoriation often the only manifestations.

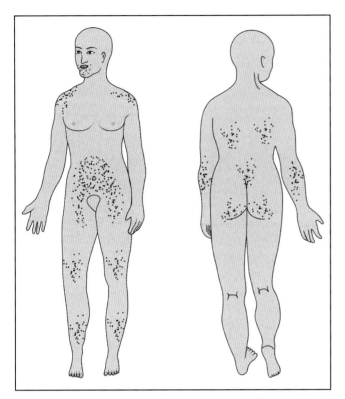

Sites of predilection: Dermatitis herpetiformis.

Course

Relapsing and remitting course.

Association

Associated GSE invariable; mostly asymptomatic.

Investigations

Histopathology

Small, subepidermal bulla with large number of neutrophils in a fibrinous exudate. Small dermo-epidermal split in the peribullous location with papillary apical neutrophilic abscesses.

Immunofluorescence

Direct immunofluorescence

Granular deposits of IgA at apices of dermal papillae in peribullous location.

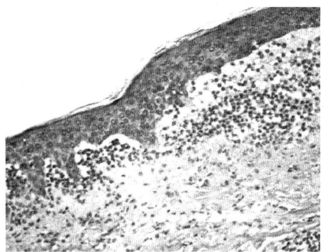

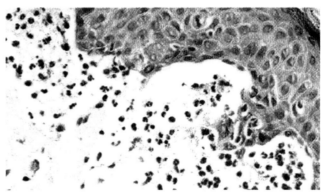

Histopathology of dermatitis herpetiformis: subepidermal split with papillary apical abscesses containing large number of neutrophils. Top (10x). Bottom (40x).

Indirect immunofluorescence

Antireticulin IgA and IgG antibodies sometimes detected.

Treatment

Gluten free (wheat-free) diet helps both skin pathology and enteropathy. But slow in action. Dapsone, almost specific. Daily adult dose, 100–200 mg; dramatic remission in a couple of days. Maintain remission with diet control and small dose of dapsone (25–50 mg/day). Sulphapyridine, 2 g/day, a more toxic alternative.

11

Metabolic and Nutritional Dermatoses

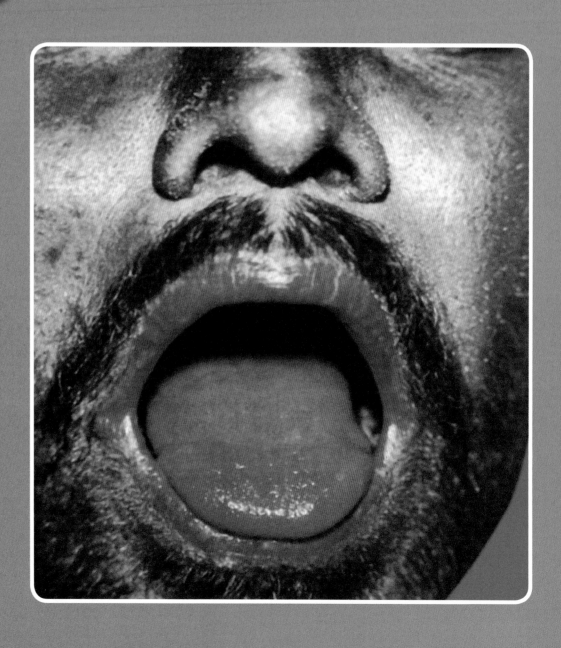

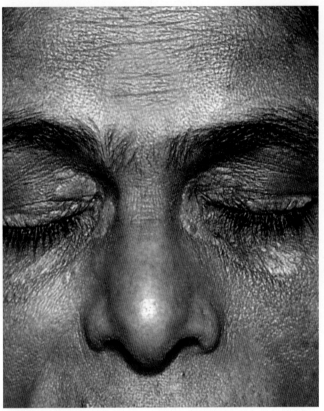

Xanthelasma palpebrarum: bilateral, yellowish plaques on the upper eye lids. Associated with type II hyperlipoproteinemias or normolipemic state.

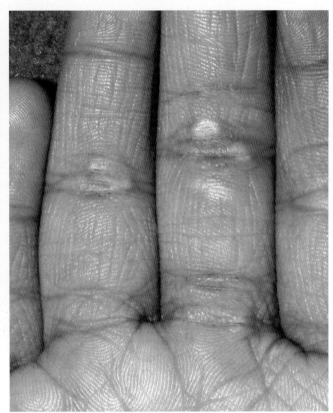

Xanthoma striate palmaris: plane xanthomas in palmar creases. Pathognomonic of type III hyperlipoproteinemia. Patients often also have tuberous xanthomas.

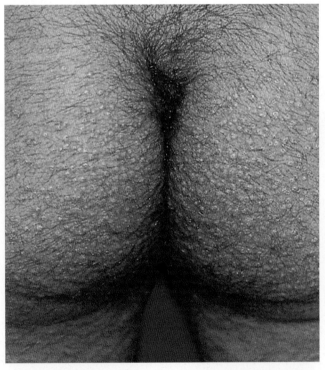

Eruptive xanthomas: multiple reddish yellow papules on buttocks. Also present on elbows. Associated with type I, IV, V hyperlipoproteinemia. Eruptive xanthomas usually subside without residual skin change.

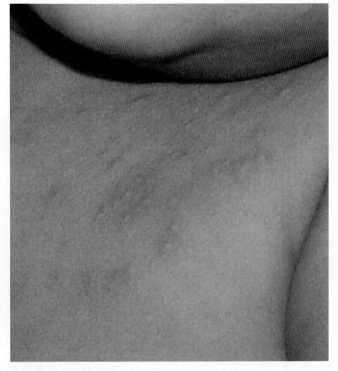

Eruptive xanthomas: multiple yellow-red papules on trunk.

Disorders that manifest with cutaneous lesions as direct or indirect, effect of metabolic abnormalities. Or nutritional imbalances. Environmental factors, such as diet and light, may play an important role.

CUTANEOUS XANTHOMATOSES

Etiology

Primary hyperlipoproteinemia, perhaps genetically determined but influenced by environmental factors particularly dietary. Five classes of hyperlipoproteinemia, classified by **Fredrickson**:
- Type I: chylomicronemia
- Type II: hypercholesterolemia
- Type III: dysbetalipoproteinemia
- Type IV: hypertriglyceridemia
- Type V: mixed hyperlipidemia.

Hyperlipidemia also secondary to systemic diseases such as diabetes mellitus, pancreatic disease, biliary cirrhosis or nephrotic syndrome. Normolipemic xanthomas due to local proliferation of histiocytes with ingestion of lipids. Association between the type of xanthoma and type of hyperlipidemia often not specific, but some associations more frequent.

Epidemiology

Not uncommon.

Clinical Manifestations

Varied morphology: yellowish or reddish yellow papules, plaques, nodules or tumors. Result of collection of lipid-laden histiocytes in skin and/or subcutaneous tissue. Size, shape and distribution variable. Different designations: *plane xanthomas, eruptive xanthomas, tuberous xanthomas* and *tendinous xanthomas*. Hyperlipoproteinemia, a common finding; occasional patient normolipemic.

Plane Xanthomas

Two types described:
Xanthelasma palpebrarum: most common xanthoma. Young or middle aged adults. Upper, lower or both eyelids, often bilaterally involved. Mostly normolipemic. Sometimes associated with hyperlipoproteinemia, commonly type II (familial hypercholesterolemia). Also secondary to diabetes mellitus, biliary cirrhosis.

Xanthoma striate palmaris: plane xanthomas on palmar creases, almost pathognomonic of type III hyperlipoproteinemia. Associated tuberous xanthomas.

Eruptive Xanthomas

Uncommon. Children or adults. Sudden crops of discrete, yellowish or reddish yellow papules. Extensor aspects of the extremities, buttocks, back and trunk affected. Spontaneous resolution without residue usual. Associated increase of triglycerides (Types I, IV and V hyperlipoproteinemia).

Tuberous Xanthomas

Uncommon. Plaques and large, yellowish brown nodules. Elbows, knuckles, buttocks, knees and heels generally involved. Seldom regress. Associated xanthelasma palpebrarum and xanthoma tendinosum. Rule out Type II hyperlipoproteinemia (hypercholestrolemia) and cardiovascular disease.

Tendinous Xanthomas

Asymptomatic or painful. Subcutaneous flat; elongated nodules overlying tendons or ligaments. Severe hypercholestrolemia and elevated levels of LDL (Type II hyperlipoproteinemia).

Investigations

Investigations a must in all xanthomas. Biochemical evaluation for underlying hyperlipoproteinemia. In normlipemic rule out diabetes, liver disease.

Lipid Profile

Xanthoma	Lipid profile	Type of lipoproteinemia
Xanthelasma palpebrarum	Normolipemic* Hypercholesterolemia	Type II
Xanthoma striate palmaris	Hypercholesterolemia Hypertriglyceridemia	Type III
Eruptive xanthomas	Hypertriglyceridemia	Types I, IV and V
Tuberous xanthomas	Hypercholesterolemia	Type II
Tendinous xanthomas	Hypercholesterolemia (severe) Hypertriglyceridemia	Type II

* Rule out diabetes

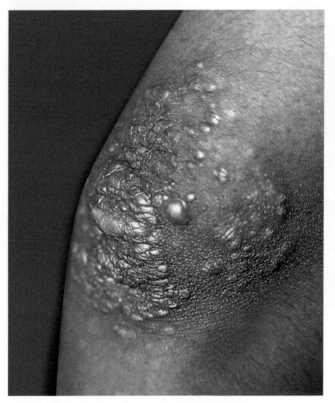

Tuberous xanthomas: papules, plaques and nodules around the knee. Associated with type II hyperlipoproteinemia

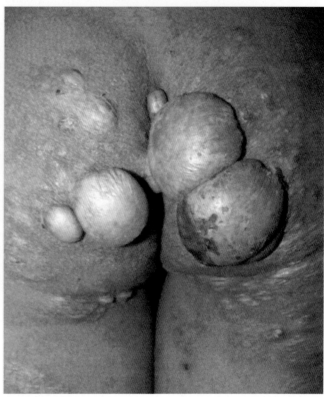

Tuberous xanthomas: large tumorous and flat masses on the buttocks.

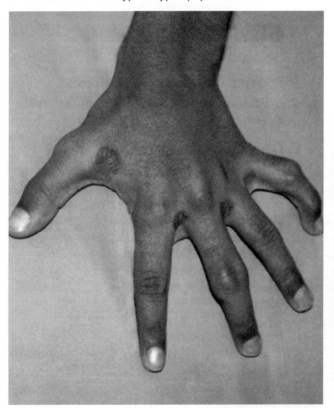

Tendinous xanthoma: deep-seated, pale yellow, flat nodules overlying the tendons. Associated with type II hyperlipoproteinemia (familial hypercholesterolemia). Presence of interdigital web space plane xanthomas pathognomonic of homozygous state.

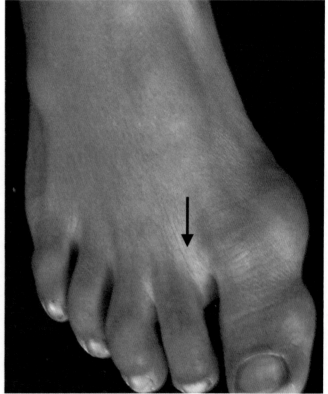

Tendinous xanthomas: yellowish linear, flat nodules, overlying tendons of the foot.

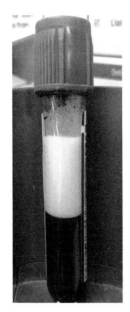

Serum in type I hyperlipoproteinemia: creamy top layer.

Histopathology

Biopsy diagnostic. Foamy, lipid-laden histiocytes (**xanthoma cells**). Large giant cells (**Touton giant cells**) with multiple peripheral and central nuclei present. Admixture of inflammatory cells seen.

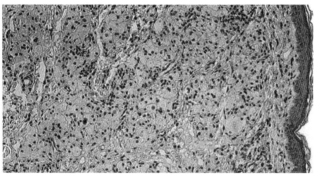

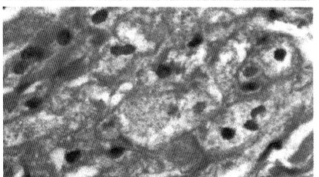

Histopathology of xanthoma: foamy, lipid-laden histiocytes (xanthoma cells). Large giant cells (Touton giant cells) with multiple peripheral and central nuclei present. Admixture of inflammatory cells seen; top (x10), bottom (x40).

Other Investigations

Rule out coronary and peripheral arterial disease in patients with tendinous, tuberous/palmar and web space xanthomas.

Treatment

General Measures

Depends upon metabolic abnormality. Reduce total calorie intake. Low cholesterol and/or low triglyceride and/or low carbohydrate diet. Substitute polyunsaturated for saturated fatty acids. Treat primary disease: diabetes mellitus, hypothyroidism and others.

Specific Measures

HMG-CoA reductase inhibitors (statins) and clofibrate 1.5–2 g/day helpful in some cases. Xanthelasma responds well to topical application of trichloroacetic acid (10–25%), electrodessication, laser therapy (Er:YAG laser) and excision. However, recurrences common.

AMYLOIDOSIS

Dermatoses characterized by deposition of proteinaceous material, amyloid, in dermis. Distinctive tinctorial properties (stains with Congo red and metachromatically with crystal violet). Could be purely cutaneous. Or cutaneous manifestations of a systemic form.

Primary Cutaneous Amyloidosis

Etiology

Normally soluble plasma proteins deposited in the extracellular space in an abnormal insoluble fibrillar form. Probably related to local friction/scratching.

Clinical Features

Macular and papular (lichen) forms; occasionally mixed.

Macular amyloidosis

Uncommon. Young or middle aged adults. Asymptomatic or mildly itchy greyish-brown pigmentation in rippled pattern. Upper back and interscapular areas, forearms and arms affected.

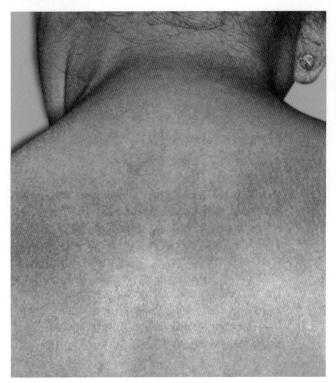

Macular amyloidosis: slate-grey pigmentation on the upper back; ripple pattern is characteristic.

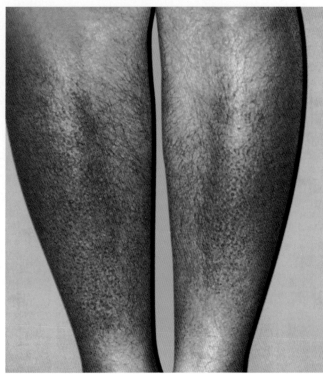

Lichen amyloidosis: dark, hyperkeratotic papules on the shins.

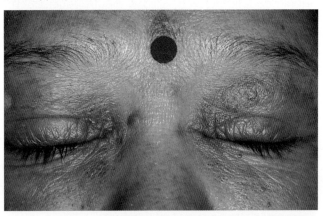

Primary systemic amyloidosis: purpuric lesions on the eyelids (racoon eyes). Note infiltrated waxy plaques.

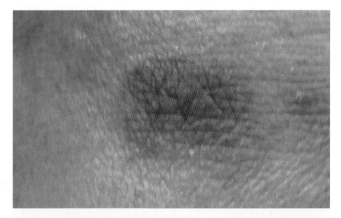

Primary systemic amyloidosis: pinch purpura, which develops after slight trauma.

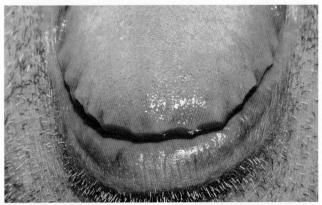

Primary systemic amyloidosis: macroglossia with indentation of teeth.

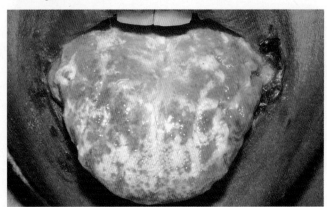

Primary systemic amyloidosis: macroglossia with infiltrated papules and nodules, some hemorrhagic.

Lichen amyloidosis

The papular form. Uncommon. Young or middle aged adults. Intensely pruritic, discrete, hyperkeratotic and warty, greyish-brown papules, plaques or nodules. Often bilateral and symmetrical and arranged in rippled configuration. Chronic, slowly progressive course. Present alone or in association with the macular form (**biphasic amyloidosis**). Extensors of legs, occasionally forearms affected.

Investigations

Usually none required. Biopsy done occasionally.

Histopathology

Variable acanthosis and hyperkeratosis. Deposition of homogeneous eosinophilic material in dermal papillae. Congo red, as special stain gives red-green dichroism observed when tissue viewed under cross-polarized light.

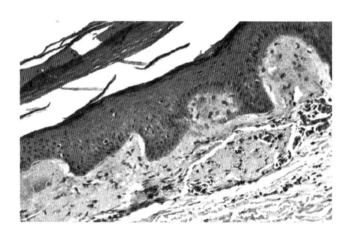

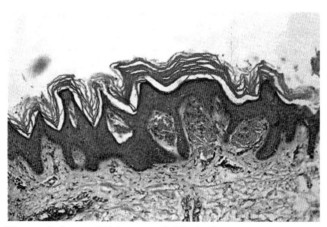

Histopathology of lichen amyloidosis: homogeneous, amorphous eosinophilic material in papillary dermis; H & E (top) and Congo-red (bottom).

Treatment

Potent topical corticosteroids with (for lichen variant) or without occlusion. Topical and systemic retinoids also helpful.

Primary Systemic Amyloidosis

Etiology

Associated with plasma cell dyscrasia, commonly multiple myeloma.

Clinical Manifestations

Systemic disease, with skin involvement being incidental.

Mucocutaneous manifestations

Petechiae and other purpuric lesions; spontaneous or following minor trauma the most common presentation. Shiny, spherical, pale-yellow, almost waxy, translucent, at times hemorrhagic, papular lesions over the central area of the face (nasolabial folds, lips, eyelids). Occasionally trunk, extremities, palms and soles affected. Dry waxy, orange-peel appearance. Non-cicatricial alopecia. Macroglossia and laryngeal involvement. Also soft rubbery swellings in mucosae.

Systemic manifestations

Renal amyloidosis manifests as nephrotic syndrome. Cardiac involvement as restrictive cardiomyopathy. Sensory and autonomic neuropathy common. So also hepatomegaly.

Investigations

Investigate to confirm diagnosis. And to rule out underlying plasma cell dyscrasia. And to find extent of involvement.

Histopathology

Biopsy a suggestive skin lesion. If absent, consider abdominal fat aspiration, rectal or gingival biopsy. In skin biopsy, amyloid deposits seen in dermis and subcutis. Also often found around sweat glands and within blood vessel walls.

Rule out underlying plasma cell dyscrasia

By urine and serum protein electrophoresis and immunofixation electrophoresis. And bone marrow aspirate and biopsy.

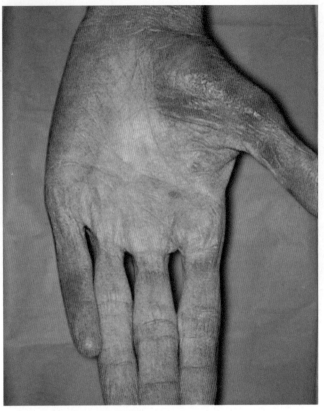

Primary systemic amyloidosis: purpuric lesions on the palms.

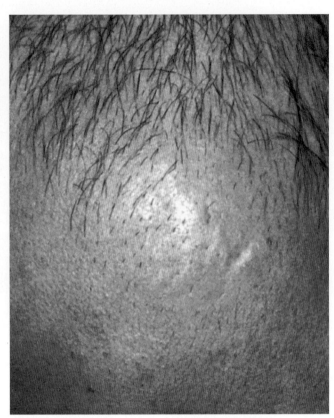

Follicular mucinosis: ill-defined erythematous, alopecic plaque.

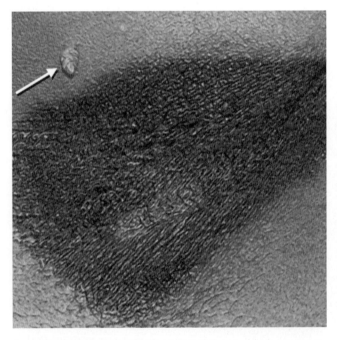

Acanthosis nigricans, obesity related: brown-black pigmentation and papillomatous velvety thickening of axillary skin in an obese individual. Note skin tag.

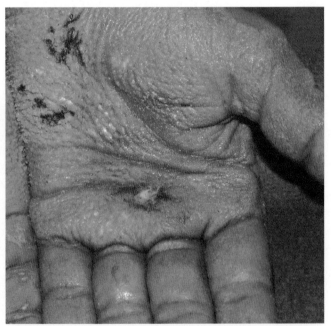

Acanthosis nigricans, malignant: velvety thickening at unusual sites. Manifesting here as tripe palms. This patient also had hyperpigmented velvety plaques in the perioral region.

Find extent of involvement

Rule out cardiac, renal, hepatic and other involvement.

Treatment

No satisfactory treatment available; chemotherapeutic regimens containing melphalan, vincristine, doxorubicin and prednisolone may prolong survival, in some cases. And autologous peripheral blood stem cell transplantation.

FOLLICULAR MUCINOSIS (ALOPECIA MUCINOSA)

Can be primary. Or secondary.

Epidemiology

Rare. Primary seen in children and young adults. Secondary more frequent in older patients.

Etiology

Idiopathic deposition of acid mucopolysaccharides in the hair follicles and sebaceous glands. Or secondary to atopic dermatitis (AD) or cutaneous T-cell lymphoma (CTCL).

Clinical Manifestations

Primary Follicular Mucinosis

Benign form. Presents as an acute or subacute eruption. Single or multiple, erythematous, ill-defined plaques consisting of grouped follicular papules causing alopecia. Seen on face and scalp.

Secondary Follicular Mucinosis

Secondary to AD, CTCL. Larger and more numerous plaques with a chronic clinical course.

Investigations

Histopathology

Done to confirm diagnosis.

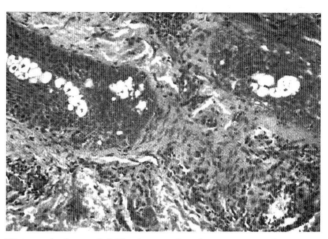

Histopathology of follicular mucinosis: mucinous change in two hair follicles.

Treatment

Spontaneous resolution can occur. Localized form treated with topical or intralesional steroids. The PUVA therapy and topical nitrogen mustard also effective.

ACANTHOSIS NIGRICANS

Uncommon.

Classification

Classified as:
- *Benign:* includes obesity-related (pseudo-acanthosis nigricans), hereditary, syndromic, acral, endocrine, drug-induced forms.
- *Malignant*: associated with tumors, notably gastric adenocarcinoma.

Clinical Manifestations

Obesity-associated most common type.

Morphology

Clinical features (almost!) similar in all. Characteristic velvety thickening with dark brown pigmentation. *Obesity related:* typically with skin tags. *Acral:* on hands especially knuckles. *Malignancy related:* itchy; rapid spread; more pigmented; more extensive involving unusual sites like palms (**tripe palms**) and oral mucosa.

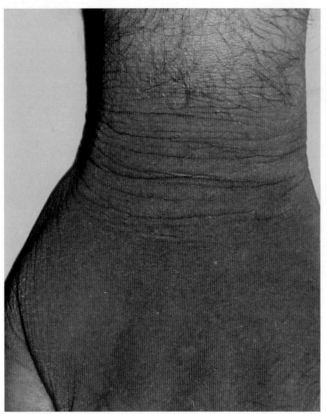

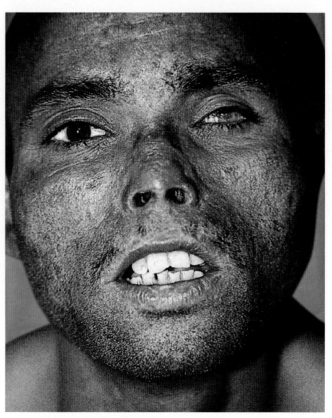

Acanthosis nigricans, acral variant: velvety, hyperpigmented plaques on hands.

Congenital erythropoietic porphyria: evidence of severe photosensitivity, hypertrichosis and scarring on face.

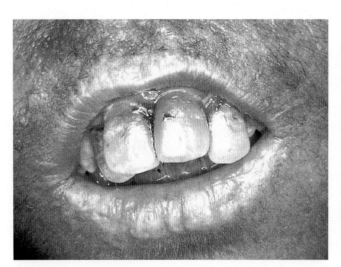

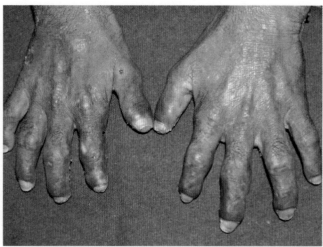

Congenital erythropoietic porphyria: reddish brown teeth (erythrodontia); milia around alae nasi.

Congenital erythropoietic porphyria: mutilated sclerodermoid hands.

Sites of Predilection

Axillae, neck, groins, other flexures, and umbilicus affected.

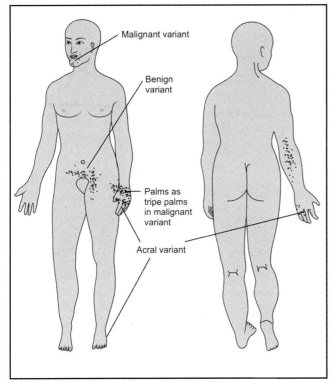

Sites of predilection: acanthosis nigricans.

Course

May progress, remain stationary or regress if primary cause/association corrected.

Treatment

No specific therapy. Weight reduction helps in pseudoacanthosis nigricans. Removal of tumor in the malignant form. Topical retinoids and dermabrasion effective in some patients, but lesions may recur.

PORPHYRIAS

Epidemiology

Rare. One variant porphyria cutanea tarda, also reported to occur as epidemics.

Etiology

Metabolic, (inborn or acquired) absence/dysfunction of one of eight enzymes crucial for heme biosynthesis, which occurs in bone marrow and liver. Results in accumulation of substrate of absent/dysfunctional enzyme. The accumulated substrate (or its metabolic product synthesized through alternate pathways) either circulate in blood, or are deposited in various tissues including skin, or are excreted in urine/feces. Increased deposition of porphyrins in the skin associated with photosensitivity and tissue damage. And in other organs associated with neurological and other extracutaneous manifestations. Alcohol and certain drugs (estrogens, griseofulvin and barbiturates) precipitate/exacerbate certain porphyrias.

Porphyria	Enzyme defect	Inheritance
CEP*	Uroporphyrinogen synthase III	Autosomal recessive
EPP**	Ferrochelatase	Autosomal dominant
PCT***	Uroporphyrinogen decarboxylase	Autosomal dominant Sporadic
VP****	Protoporphyrinogen oxidase	Autosomal dominant
AIP*****	Porphobilinogen deaminase	Autosomal dominant

* Congenital erythropoietic porphyria.
** Erythropoietic protoporphyria
*** Porphyria cutanea tarda
****Variegate porphyria
*****Acute intermittent porphyria

Classification

Porphyrias variously classified as:
- *Erythropoietic*:
  - *Congenital erythropoietic porphyria*
  - *Erythropoietic protoporphyria*
- *Hepatic*
  - *Acute intermittent porphyria*
  - *Variegate porphyria*
  - *Porphyria cutanea tarda*

Or as:
- *Non-acute:*
  - *Congenital erythropoietic porphyria*
  - *Erythropoietic protoporphyria*
  - *Porphyria cutanea tarda*

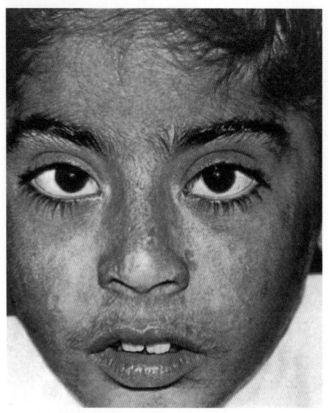

Erythropoietic protoporphyria: marked photosensitivity hypertrichotic forehead; ulcerations and scars on the face.

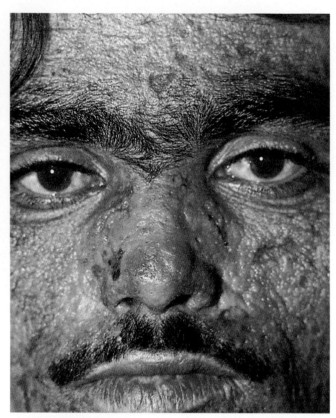

Porphyria cutanea tarda: severe photosensitivity—scars, milia and hypertrichosis.

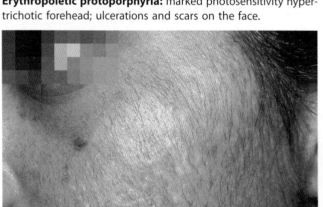

Porphyria cutanea tarda: hypertrichosis and facials scarring.

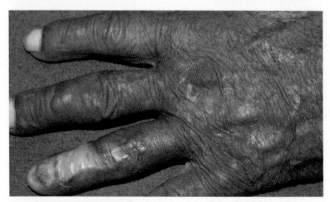

Porphyria cutanea tarda: bullae with clear fluid, erosions and sclerodermoid plaques on hands.

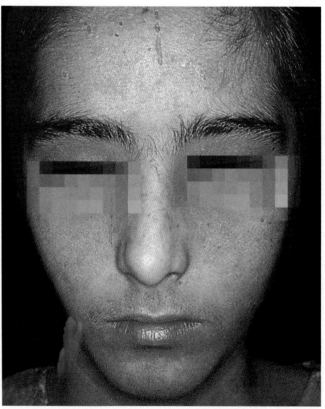

Variegate porphyria: hypertrichosis and superficial ulcerations on the face.

- **Acute:**
  - Acute intermittent porphyria
  - Variegate porphyria

Clinical Manifestations

Congenital Erythropoietic Porphyria (Gunther's Disease)

Rare. Autosomal recessive inheritance; consanguinity in parents common. *Onset:* generally early infancy. *Skin lesions:* Severe photosensitivity, blistering and hyperpigmentation. Hypertrichosis, milia and scarred mutilated look. *Teeth:* dirty reddish brown (**erythrodontia**) — fluorescent orange-red under Wood's light. Red colored urine hallmark of disease. Hemolysis, anemia, splenomegaly.

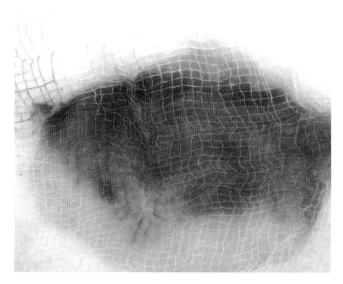

Urine in CEP: red colored, starting at birth. Parents often complain of discoloration (red-brown) of baby's diapers.

Erythropoietic Protoporphyria (EPP)

Relatively common in the West. Autosomal dominant inheritance. Onset in early childhood. Photosensitivity (very symptomatic)—stinging, burning, urticaria, rarely manifest blistering. Hyperpigmentation, hypertrichosis and scarring. Relatively mild course. Death late, often due to liver failure.

Porphyria Cutanea Tarda (PCT)

Genetic (autosomal dominant) sometimes. Usually acquired. Onset late-young adults, often males. Alcohol, oral contraceptive pills and (accidental) ingestion of hexachlorobenzene precipitate/exacerbate the disease. Mild to moderate photosensitivity. Hypertrichosis, scars and milia. Also increased fragility of light exposed skin. Hepatomegaly with deranged liver functions.

Variegate Porphyria (VP)

Common in South Africa. Autosomal dominant inheritance. Clinical manifestations, a combination of photosensitivity (similar to PCT) and episodic neurological manifestations like in AIP, the later in the patient or in another, often a female member of the family. Red urine during acute neurological episodes.

Investigations

Fluorescence of Urine, Stool and Red Blood Cells

Urine and stool fluorescence under Wood's light, a crude method of evaluating presence of porphyrins in the specimen. Similarly look for fluorescence of RBCs.

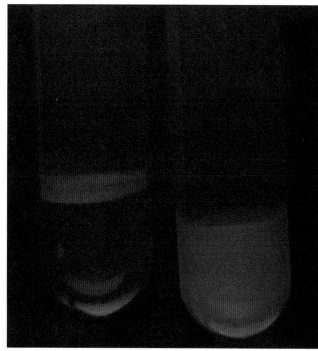

Fluorescence of porphyrins in urine: is positive in CEP, and in acute attacks of VP and AIP

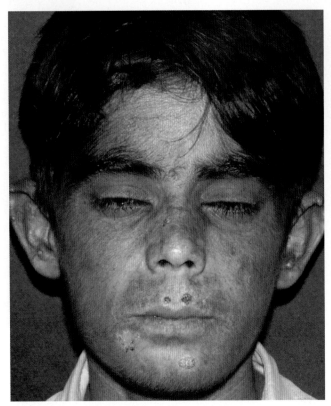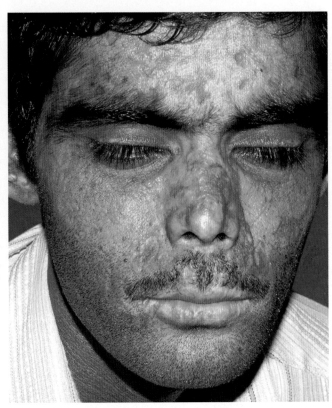

Congenital erythropoietic porphyria: before and six years after a stem cell transplant, which was done at age of 12. Note only a minimal worsening of mutilation.

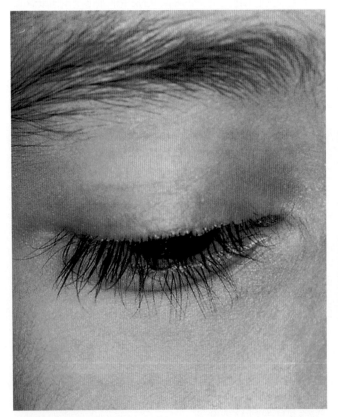

Lipoid proteinosis: characteristic beaded papules on eyelid margins (monilial blepharosis).

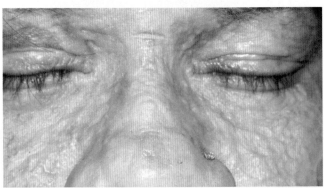

Lipoid proteinosis: varioliform scars. Note moniliform blepharosis.

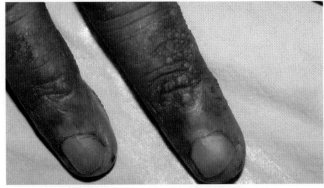

Lipoid proteinosis: waxy papules on dorsae of fingers. Also occur on elbows, forehead.

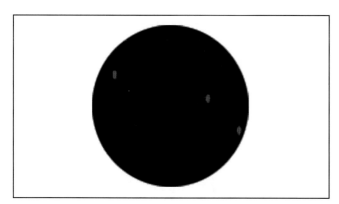

Fluorescence of RBCs in blood: is positive in CEP, and transiently in EPP

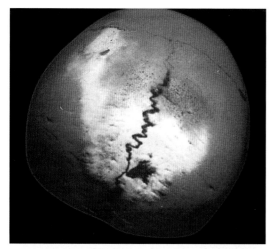

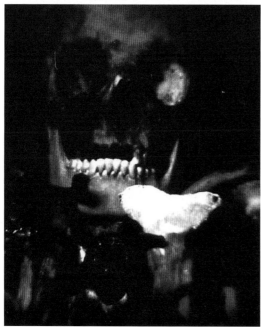

Fluorescence of skull and skeleton: in CEP.

Estimation of Porphyrin Levels

Porphyrin levels are estimated in blood, urine and stool.

	Blood	Urine	Stool
CEP	Plasma: UP & CP RBC: PP	UP, CP	CP > UP
EPP	Plasma: N RBC: PP	N	PP
PCT	Plasma: UP RBC: N	UP > CP (iso)	UP, CP (iso), PP
VP	Plasma: N RBC: N	Attack: PBG, ALA	CP, PP
AIP	Plasma: N RBC: N	PBG; ALA Attack UP: CP	N

UP: Uroporphyrin
CP: Coproporphyrin
PP: Protoporphyrin
PBG: Porphobilinogene
ALA: α levulinic acid
N: Normal

Miscellaneous Tests

Liver function tests
Deranged in PCT

Treatment

General Measures

Photoprotection of paramount importance. Use broad-spectrum sunscreens containing titanium dioxide and zinc oxide. And lifestyle modification.

Specific Treatment

CEP

Unsatisfactory. Hypertransfusions (suppress hematopoiesis) may help. Occasionally splenectomy. Bone marrow transplant results in marked improvement.

EPP

Protect from light. ß-carotene (free radical quencher) 60–180 mg/day, often helpful.

PCT

Avoid alcohol or other triggers. Small doses (125 mg, twice a week) of chloroquine (increases excretion of porphyrins). Or phlebotomy (500 mL, once a fortnight, reduces iron stores) 4–6 times. Or a combination of the two brings about a remission which may last a year or more.

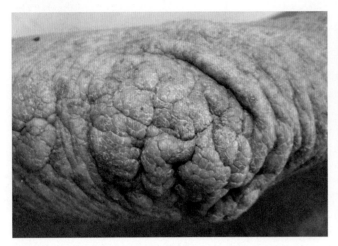

Lipoid proteinosis: verrucous plaques on elbows.

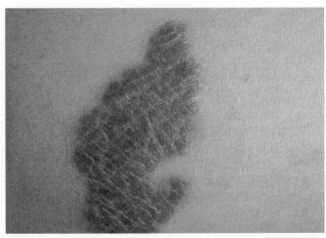

Sarcoidosis, plaque variant: infiltrated papules coalescing to form infiltrated plaque on back.

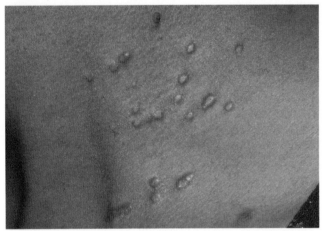

Sarcoidosis, papular variant: asymptomatic, juicy translucent papules on neck.

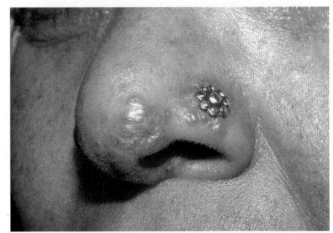

Sarcoidosis, angiolupoid variant: soft, hemispherical well-demarcated plaques with telangiectasia.

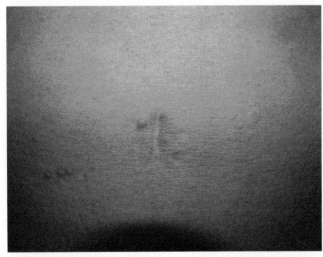

Sarcoidosis: sarcoidal lesion in scar.

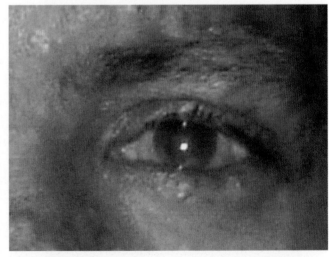

Sarcoidosis: anterior uveitis.

LIPOID PROTEINOSIS

Epidemiology

Rare. Both sexes affected.

Etiology

Autosomal recessive inheritance. Mutation of extracellular matrix protein 1 **(ECM1) gene**. Hyaline deposits in the skin and mucous membranes.

Clinical Manifestations

Onset: infancy or childhood.

Mucosal Manifestations

Hoarseness, a common early and permanent feature due to laryngeal infiltration. Infiltrated tongue—firm and difficult to protrude.

Skin

Two stages recognized. First stage of bullae at sites of trauma. Spontaneous regression with varioliform scars. Second stage of translucent waxy papules or nodules on the free edges of eyelids (**monilial blepharosis**), face, dorsae of hands and feet. Verrucous lesions often develop on extensor surfaces especially on elbows, knees and hands. Light-sensitive lipoid proteinosis patients are those of erythropoietic protoporphyria.

Systemic Associations

Uncommon. Diabetes mellitus, epilepsy.

Treatment

None satisfactory. Oral dimethyl sulfoxide and systemic retinoids may help.

SARCOIDOSIS

Epidemiology

Onset most often in 3rd decade of life. More common in women.

Etiology

Probably a nonspecific granulomatous response to an unknown antigen mediated through antigen presenting cells and antigen-specific T cells.

Clinical Manifestations

Commonly involves lungs and skin. Also lymph nodes, liver and eyes. Less frequently, bones, myocardium, central nervous system, kidneys, spleen and parotid glands.

Mucocutaneous Manifestations

Present in a quarter of patients. And in some, may be the only manifestation.
- *Typically:* Asymptomatic juicy, infiltrated, translucent papules, plaques and nodules. Typically on face and neck. Can occur in scars (**scar sarcoidosis**).
- *Lupus pernio:* Symmetric, violaceous, indurated plaques and nodules on nose, earlobes, cheeks, and digits. Associated with systemic involvement (upper respiratory tract disease).
- *Angiolupoid sarcoidosis:* Pink-violaceus papules and plaques with prominent telangiectasias on face.
- *Less frequently:* Erythroderma, ulcers, alopecia; follicular, verrucous, ichthyosiform, hypomelanotic, psoriasiform and annular lesions seen.

Other system involvement
- *Pulmonary involvement*: Lungs most common (90%) organ involved with sarcoidosis. Though usually asymptomatic and detected radiologically, sometimes symptomatic (dyspnea, cough, chest pain and wheezing).
- *Eye involvement*: Seen in 50%. Usually asymptomatic, but potentially vision threatening. When symptomatic, manifests as redness, burning, itching, or dryness. Uveitis, cataract and glaucoma common. **Heerfordt's syndrome** includes fever, parotid gland enlargement, facial palsy, and anterior uveitis.
- *Others:* Liver involvement usually asymptomatic. Less frequently, bones, myocardium, central nervous system, kidneys, spleen, and parotid glands.

Investigations

Biopsy done to confirm the diagnosis. Radiological evaluation (plain X-ray and HRCT) of chest mandatory, as also ophthalmological evaluation in all patients. Other investigations guided by clinical symptomatology.

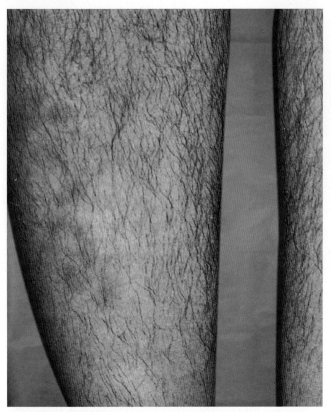

Diabetic dermopathy: erythematous, scaly papules on the shins. Heal with scars.

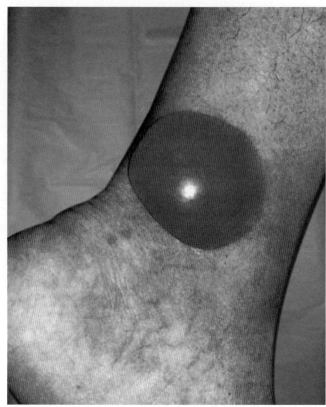

Diabetic bulla: non-inflammatory bulla on the leg.

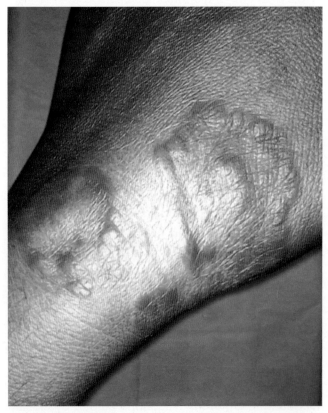

Granuloma annulare: erythematous, well marginated plaques with beaded border and atrophic center.

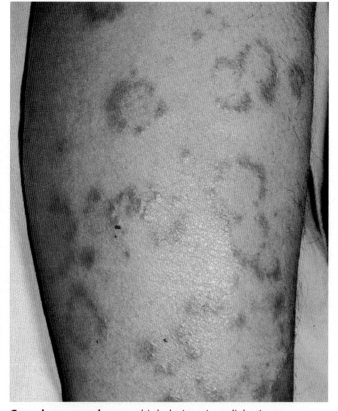

Granuloma annulare: multiple lesions in a diabetic.

Histopathology

Granulomas characteristically monomorphic and naked (devoid of cuff of lymphocytes).

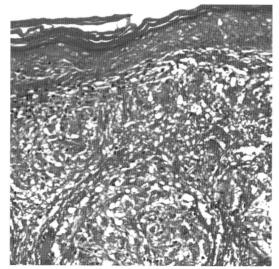

Histopathology of sarcoidosis: granulomas, typically monomorphic and naked (devoid of cuff of lymphocytes).

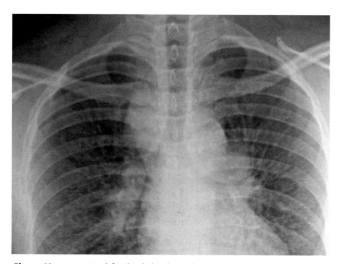

Chest X-ray, sarcoidosis: hilar lymphadenopathy.
Courtesy: Dr Chandan Das, Department of Radiology, All India Institute of Medical Sciences (AIIMS), New Delhi.

Evaluation of Chest

- *Radiological evaluation*: Chest radiograph abnormal in 90% of patients with sarcoidosis. Bilateral hilar adenopathy noted in 75%, while pulmonary parenchymal infiltrates seen in half. CT has a higher pick up.

- *Pulmonary function tests (PFT):* Even if chest radiologically normal, 20–40% show PFT abnormalities.

Treatment

Intralesional steroids for limited skin disease. Oral steroids for extensive cutaneous disease. And for systemic disease. Chloroquine, hydroxychloroquine, isotretinoin, methotrexate, allopurinol, minocycline, and thalidomide useful alternatives. But recurrences common.

SKIN IN ENDOCRINOLOGICAL DISEASES

Several endocrinological diseases manifest in skin.

Diabetes

Diabetes sometimes detected first by dermatologists. Recurrent bacterial infections (carbuncle pathognomonic), fungal infections (tinea, candidal) typical.

Diabetic Dermopathy (Diabetic Shin Spots)

Common, more frequent among elderly diabetic men. Result of microangiopathy. Asymptomatic, multiple, dull red papules or plaques with superficial scaling. Heal with atrophic scars with pigmented halo. Shins commonly affected.

Acanthosis Nigricans

Manifestation of insulin resistance. Brown to gray-black velvety skin thickening along with skin tags. Symmetrically in flexures including posterolateral surface of neck, axillae and groins.

Diabetic Bullae

Cause, uncertain. Non-immunologic, non-acantholytic. Asymptomatic, non-inflammatory, spontaneously occurring, intra or subepidermal bullae. Legs, arms, hands and feet affected. Last several weeks. Heal spontaneously without scarring.

Granuloma Annulare

An uncommon, benign, morphologically distinctive dermatosis. However, not necessarily associated with diabetes.

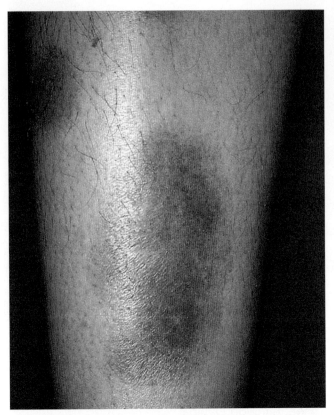

Necrobiosis lipoidica: yellowish, atrophic plaque on the shin with telangiectatic blood vessels.

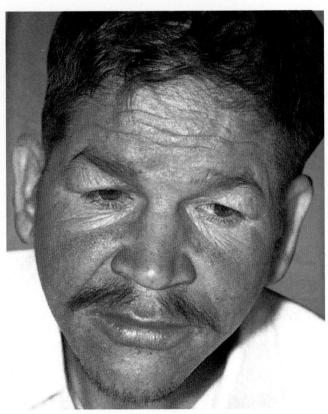

Hypothyroidism: dry, coarse skin; puffy eyelids and a lethargic look.

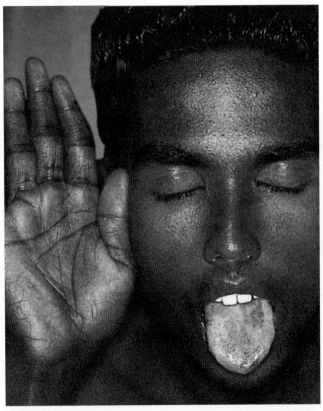

Addison's disease: generalized pigmentation, pronounced in the palmar creases.

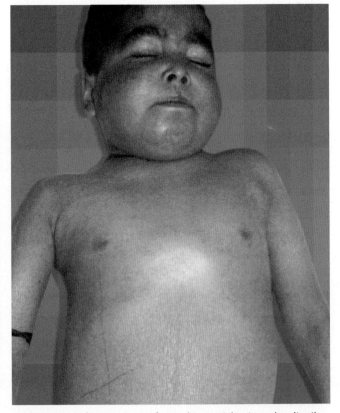

Cushing's syndrome: moon facies, hypertrichosis and redistribution of fat.

Clinical manifestations

Children or young adults. Asymptomatic. Single or multiple, sometimes disseminated; the latter occurring in older women often associated with diabetes mellitus. Skin colored or erythematous annular plaques with flat or depressed center and a characteristic well delineated, beaded border. Variable size. May persist. Or regress spontaneously or with treatment. Single lesions most frequently on dorsae of hands or feet. Multiple lesions on upper and lower extremities and trunk.

Diagnosis

Biopsy taken to confirm diagnosis shows degeneration of the collagen, surrounded by palisading granulomas.

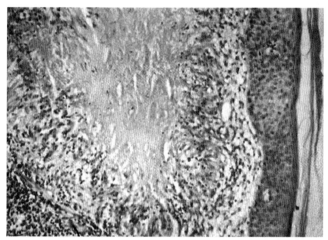

Histopathology of granuloma annulare: foci of degenerated collagen with palisading granulomatous infiltrate at the periphery.

Treatment

May resolve spontaneously. Intralesional or topical steroids and topical tacrolimus in localized disease. PUVA therapy and systemic retinoids for disseminated disease.

Necrobiosis Lipoidica

Frequently associated with diabetes mellitus but uncommon. Not related to its severity, duration or treatment.

Clinical manifestations

Middle-aged women. Asymptomatic, irregular or oval, large, yellowish, shiny, atrophic plaques with telangiectatic vessels and a purple border. Gradually progressive. May occasionally resolve or ulcerate. Shins affected, usually bilaterally symmetrically.

Diagnosis

Biopsy taken to confirm diagnosis shows degeneration of the collagen, surrounded by palisading granulomas.

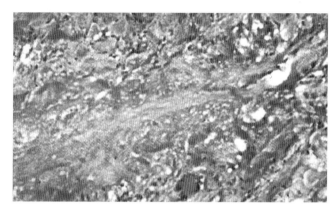

Histopathology of necrobiosis lipoidica: necrobiotic area, mid dermis with surrounding inflammatory infiltrate and a giant cell.

Treatment

Unsatisfactory. Try moderately potent corticosteroids on the active border. Or intralesional steroids.

Hypothyroidism (Myxedema)

Iodine deficiency or idiopathic. Characteristic facies: pale, puffy face with coarse features, lethargic look. Patient feels cold and sweats less. Coarse sparse hair on the scalp; loss of lateral third of eyebrows.

Treatment

Thyroxine replacement therapy.

Addison's Disease

Diminished production of adrenocortical hormones and an increased secretion of melanocyte stimulating hormone (MSH) by the pituitary.

Clinical Manifestations

Uncommon. Young adults. Diffuse brown-black pigmentation, most pronounced in the flexures,

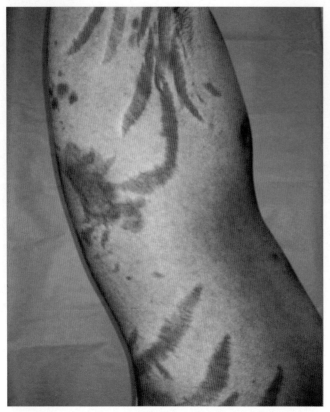

Cushing's syndrome: extensive purple colored striae in a case of recalcitrant pemphigus vulgaris on high dose daily steroids.

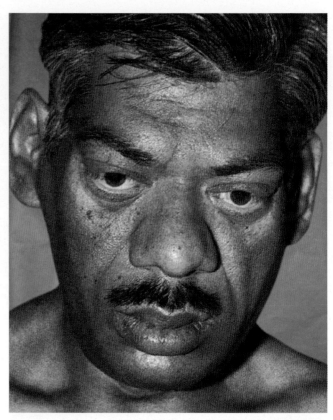

Acromegaly: large face with thick lips, big nose and large jaw.

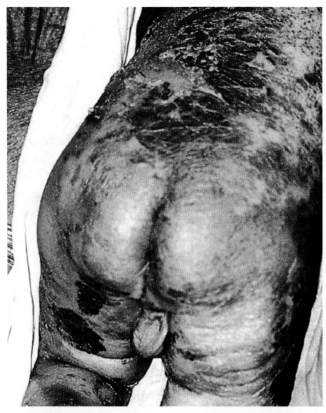

Kwashiorkor: crackled scaly pigmented skin on the trunk and extremities; the latter edematous.

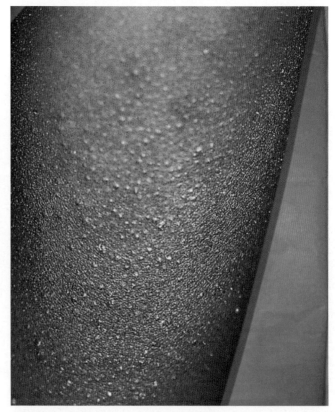

Phrynoderma: keratotic follicular papules.

palmar and plantar creases, genitals and nipples, and light exposed areas of the skin. Buccal mucosal pigmentation almost always present. Occasional vitiligo-like lesions. Systemic manifestations: diarrhea, loss of weight and asthenia due to hyponatremia.

Treatment

Replacement therapy with corticosteroids (7.5–10 mg of prednisolone/day adequate). Advise use of extra salt.

Cushing's Syndrome

Result of excess of corticosteroids in the system. Iatrogenic, exogenous administration. Or endogenous overproduction.

Clinical Manifestations

Cutaneous manifestations due to androgenic influence, catabolic effects and redistribution of fat. Moon facies; buffalo hump on the back; striae distensae; telangiectasia; hypertrichosis/ hirsutism and acneiform lesions. Systemic manifestations include hypertension, diabetes, osteoporosis.

Treatment

Discontinue, if possible, corticosteroid therapy. Or add steroid sparing agents. If cause endogenous treat appropriately.

Acromegaly

Due to overproduction of growth hormone. Results in increased synthesis of collagen and mucopolysaccharides.

Clinical Manifestations

Cutaneous manifestations include coarse facies-large ears and lips. Also large hands and feet. Dilated pilosebaceous pores with an oily skin and acneiform lesions.

Treatment

Bromocriptine. With or without radiation therapy of pituitary. Or surgical excision of eosinophilic adenoma of the pituitary. May spontaneously remit.

CUTANEOUS MANIFESTATIONS OF MALNUTRITION

Cutaneous manifestations result from under (or over) nutrition, food fads, malabsorption, metabolic aberrations, alcoholism or intake of certain drugs. Isolated deficiencies infrequent unless caused by specific factors.

Kwashiorkor

Malignant protein-calorie malnutrition syndrome. Fortunately uncommon now.

Clinical Manifestations

Infants or children. Failure to thrive—mentally and physically. Apathetic, irritable child. *Skin lesions*: erythematous areas with brown-black flaky scales (crackled skin appearance). *Hair*: dry, lusterless, light brown or red, rough and brittle. *Nails*: Softened. *Mucosae:* Cheilitis. Xerophthalmia. *Others:* Edema due to hypoalbuminemia. Progressive course, may be fatal.

Treatment

Prompt treatment with high protein diet; animal products preferred. Maintain with a balanced diet. Correct any parasitosis. As also any other comorbidities/deficiencies.

Vitamin A Deficiency

Common in the developing world. Poor intake of foods particularly animal products (such as milk, eggs, meat) and carotene-rich vegetables

Clinical Manifestations

Children and young adults affected. Dry skin, ichthyosiform scaling; spiny follicular keratosis—**phrynoderma** on buttocks, extensors of elbows and knees affected. Night blindness, xerophthalmia and **Bitot's spots** may be presenting features. Respiratory infections common in children due to poor epithelial maturation.

Treatment

Vitamin A, 50,000–100,000 units per day for several weeks; guard against hypervitaminosis.

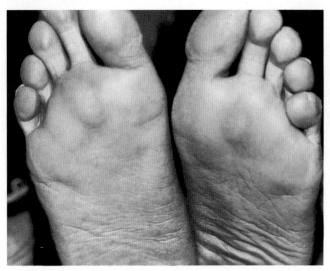

Carotenoderma: orange yellow discoloration.

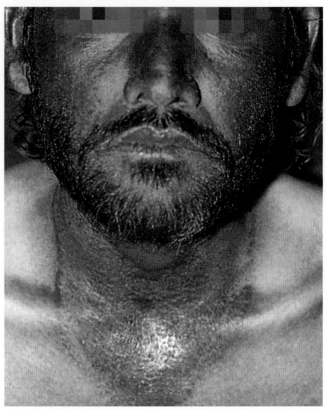

Pellagra: well marginated, dry scaly lesions on the light exposed parts-face and 'V' of neck.

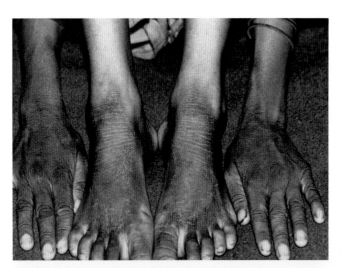

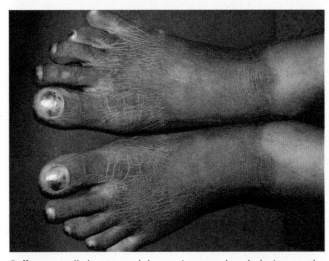

Pellagra: well demarcated, hyperpigmented scaly lesion on the dorsae of hands and feet.

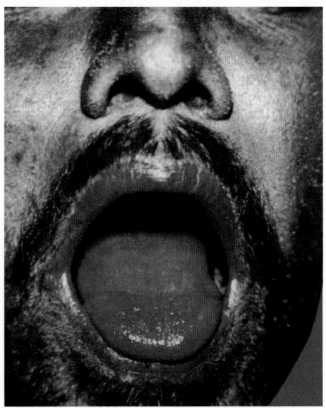

Pellagra: magenta-colored tongue and angular stomatitis.

Hypervitaminosis A

Result of intake of large doses of vitamin A for prolonged periods.

Clinical Manifestations

Skin lesions

Dry, itchy, scaly skin. Alopecia.

Systemic manifestations

Include headaches, insomnia, lassitude, anorexia, bone and joint pains.

Carotenoderma

Due to excessive intake of carrots or other yellow/orange fruits and vegetables.

Clinical Manifestations

Is more easily appreciated in light-complexioned people. Manifests as orange discoloration of skin, most notably on palms and soles which may be the only manifestation in darkly pigmented persons. Sclera are spared (**c.f.,** jaundice)

Pellagra

Uncommon. Adults generally affected. Caused by deficiency of nicotinic acid—nutritional (consuming maize or corn), alcoholism, malabsorptive or due to isonicotinic acid hydrazide (INH) therapy, Hartnup disease or rarely a functional carcinoid tumor.

Clinical Manifestations

Common manifestations dermatitis, diarrhea, dementia—the infamous 3 D's. *Dermatitis*: a photodermatosis; erythema, followed by brown-black, large coarse scales with a peripheral red halo. Sharply delineated to the light exposed areas—face, 'V' of the neck (**Casal's necklace**), dorsa of hands and feet. *Tongue*: atrophic and magenta colored. *Psychotic symptoms*: mild or severe depression or irritability.

Treatment

Larger doses of oral, or preferably parenteral, nicotinamide with a high protein diet. Dramatic response.

12

Disorders of Skin Pigmentation

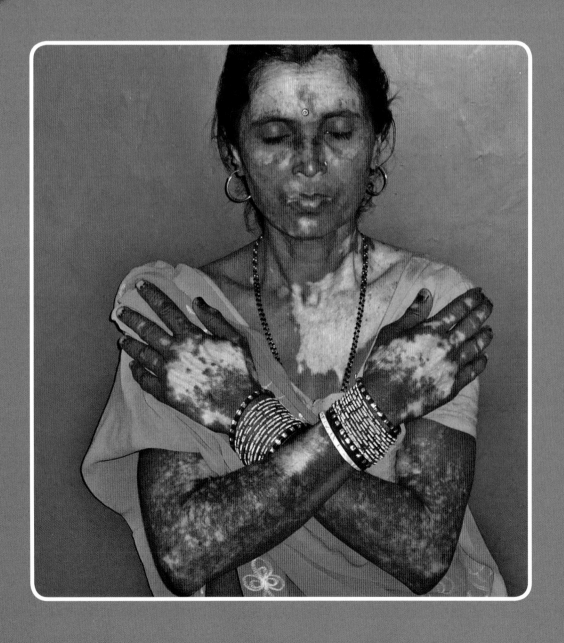

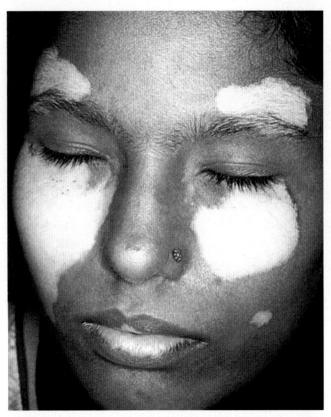

Vitiligo, acrofacial: symmetrical lesions on the face; both lips also affected.

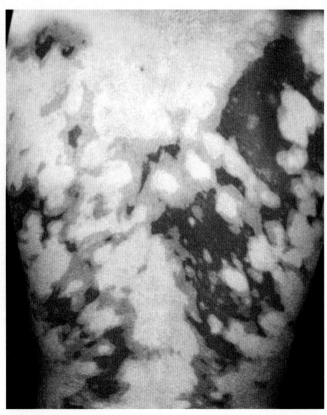

Vitiligo, trichrome: depigmented, hypopigmented and normally pigmented macules.

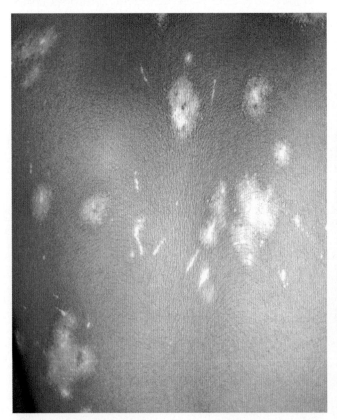

Vitiligo with koebnerization: linear lesions and linear extension of old vitiligo lesions.

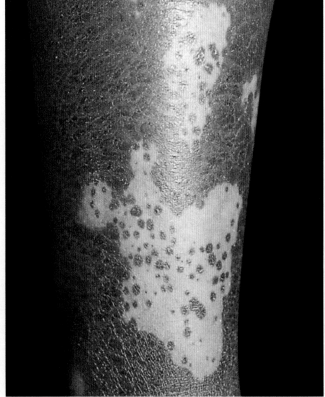

Vitiligo: follicular repigmentation following PUVA therapy.

Dermatoses affecting the skin pigment result from presence of increased or decreased amount of normal pigment(s). Or the presence of abnormal pigment(s). Socially and psychologically devastating. Physiologically not so critical.

DISORDERS OF DECREASED PIGMENTATION

Vitiligo

Acquired depigmentation of the skin.

Epidemiology

Extremely common; Worldwide prevalence approximately 1%. Both sexes equally affected. Considerable psychosocial importance. No age is exempted; the disease frequently starts in children and young adults.

Etiology

Biochemical, neural, autoimmune and genetic are the classic four hypotheses but newer ones include the convergence theory by Le Poole et al, imbalance of epidermal cytokines, melanocyte dysfunction and melatonin theory. As yet etiology is uncertain. Auto-immune hypothesis most widely accepted. Genetic predisposition: autosomal dominant trait with variable penetrance; history of vitiligo amongst first degree relatives in about a fifth; relative risk of developing vitiligo is 7 amongst children whose parents are affected association with other autoimmune disorders and presence of humoral and cell-mediated immune aberrations cited as evidence of autoimmunity. Associations—Type I diabetes mellitus, autoimmune thyroiditis, uveitis, alopecia areata and halo nevi.

Clinical Manifestations

Asymptomatic macules of varied configuration-irregular, oval, circular, linear or punctate. Discrete or confluent. May start as hypopigmented macules on an otherwise normal skin and become depigmented. Depigmentation, hypopigmentation and normal or hyperpigmentation in the same lesion trichrome vitiligo. Koebnerization or isomorphic phenomenon is seen in active disease; lesions develop at sites of trauma or may exacerbate with sunlight.

Work-up for underlying autoimmune disorders done based on relevant clinical and family history.

Sites of predilection

Overlying hair retain pigment. Or turn white (leukotrichia). No autonomic or sensory disturbances. Acute sunburn on light-exposed areas. Or chronic solar damage in long-standing cases. Malignancies seldom seen. Confined to mucocutaneous junctions or acral parts, tacrot aciati or randomly all over the body (vulgaris), or limited to one segment of body, usually unilaterally (segmental). May be generalized or universal. Skin overlying bony prominences particularly affected, sometimes symmetrically.

Course

Unpredictable and capricious. Lesions stationary, self-healing or progressive. Prognosis better in young patients, early lesions and hairy areas. Repigmentation—spontaneous or therapy induced —often caused by repopulation of depigmented skin with melanocytes from hair follicles (perifollicular) or the adjoining normal pigmented skin.

Histopathology

Decrease or absence of melanocytes.
- **Early cases:** May show interface dermatitis with mild lymphohistiocytic infiltrate.
- **Advanced/fully developed cases:** Lymphocyte induced apoptosis of melanocytes. Absence of melanocytes and melanin subsequently. Immunohistochemical staining demonstrates a preponderance of CD4 positive cells.

Treatment

Treatment for vitiligo is difficult and usually pro-longed. Based on body surface area of involvement, topical therapy for vitiligo is usually recommended when depigmentation is less than 10–20% of the skin surface and systemic therapy when exceeding these limits; but when topical therapy of small areas fails or the disease is progressive, systemic treatment may be indicated. With available medical therapies, high repigmentation percentages mostly on facial and neck lesions are achieved, although they are less effective on trunk and limbs and poor on the acral parts of the extremities. Persistence of achieved regimentation

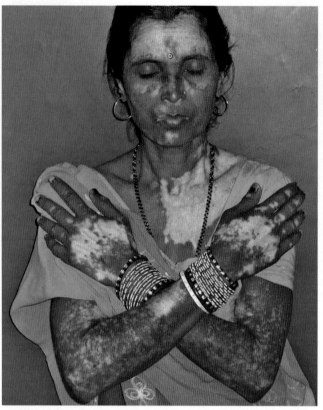

Vitiligo with photo-koebnerization: predominance of vitiligo lesions on sunexposed sites.

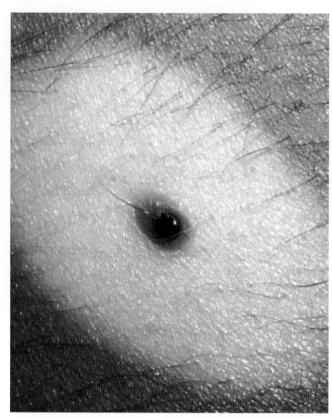

Halo nevus: depigmentation around a pigmented mole.

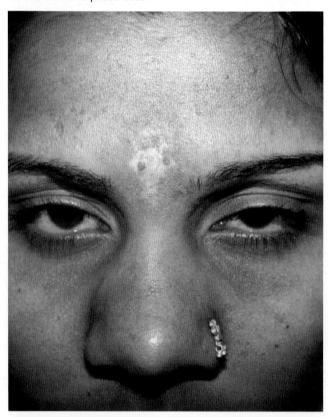

Contact leukoderma: due to adhesive in the 'bindi' worn on forehead by Indian women.

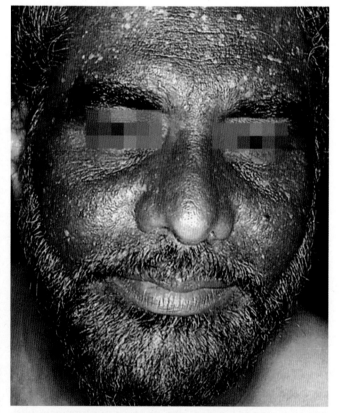

Chemical hypomelanosis: mottled depigmentation caused by monobenzyl ether of hydroquinone.

is variable and an undefined percentage of patients may have variable recurrence. The medical modalities include topical agents such as corticosteroids, calcineurin inhibitors, phototherapy [topical psoralen plus ultraviolet A (topical PUVA), topical psoralen plus sunlight (topical PUVA sol), targeted phototherapy (308 nm excimer laser or light only to involved area)] and systemic agents including immunosuppressives and phototherapy/photochemotherapy [oral psoralen plus UVA (oral PUVA), oral psoralen plus sunlight (oral PUVA sol) and narrow-band ultraviolet B (311+/– 2 nm, NB-UVB)]. NB-UVB has emerged as probably the most effective therapy for generalized disease with superior repigmentation, color match and tolerance as compared to psoralen photochemotherapy. Off late, combination of topical calcipotriol and photo/photochemotherapy have been used with some benefit but the efficacy of topical calcipotriol is as yet questionable. When vitiligo becomes refractory, surgical methods may improve depigmentation as effectively as with medical therapy. Surgical methods include micro punch grafting, split thickness grafting, non-cultured epidermal cell suspension (NCES) and suction blister grafting. NCES is the most well established, and along with SBG, is one of the most common vitiligo surgeries performed. Lately, new technique of follicular outer root sheath cell suspension has also been used with success. In resistant generalized or universal vitiligo, residual normally pigmented skin may be depigmented with 20% monobenzyl ether of hydroquinone. Q switched alexandrite and ruby laser have also been used for depigmenting residual pigmented skin.

Halo Nevus (Sutton's Nevus)

Area of hypopigmentation/depigmentation around a cutaneous 'tumor'. Most commonly halo phenomenon appears around acquired melanocytic nevus but can occur with congenital melanocytic nevi, melanomas and non-melanocytic tumors as well. Usually a marker of resolution of nevus. Appears as a round to oval area of hypo/depigmentation. Leukotrichia may be present in hairy areas. Most common site is back. Lesions

may be single or multiple. Associated with organ specific autoimmune disorders like vitiligo, nevus gradually involutes leaving behind a depigmented area for long time; frequently repigments to normal skin color. No treatment/excision required.

Chemical Leukoderma

Acquired hypomelanosis induced by repeated exposure to chemical substance either by direct contact or from systemic exposure (inhalation, ingestion). Except during early stage, depigmentation is irreversible.

Epidemiology

The incidence of chemical leukoderma has been increasing considerably in recent years due and this is often misdiagnosed clinically as idiopathic vitiligo. Contact/occupational vitiligo is distinct from chemical leukoderma in that the initial cutaneous depigmentation extends from the site of chemical contact and subsequently develops into progressive, generalized vitiligo.

Etiology

Cytotoxic effect to melanocytes more important as opposed to an immunological effect. The compounds known to produce leukoderma are chemically rather similar to tyrosine and DOPA, the endogenous substrates of the melanocyte-specific enzyme tyrosinase. The majority of these chemicals are aromatic or aliphatic derivatives of phenols and catechols. Other contributory toxins are sulfhydryls, mercurials, arsenics, cinnamic aldehyde, p-phenylenediamine, azelaic acid, corticosteroids, tretinoin, otic preparations such as eserine and thiotepa as well as systemic medications such as chloroquine and fluphenazine (prolixin). Subsequently para phenylene diamine (hair dyes), epoxy resins and azo dyes ('alta', lipstick, eyeliner) have also been incriminated.

Depigmentation on contact with articles containing MBH or other depigmenting chemicals, rubber footwear, adhesive coated 'bindi' (adornment worn on forehead by Indian women), rubber gloves, possibly some condoms.

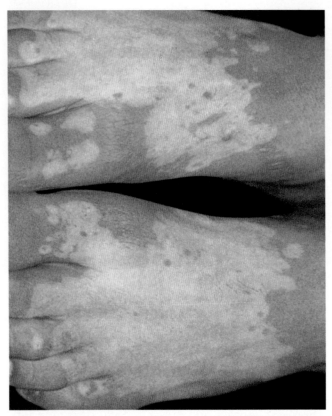

Contact leukoderma: caused by contact with rubber footwear.

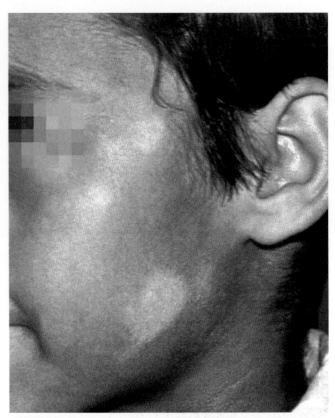

Pityriasis alba: ill-defined hypopigmented macules on the cheek.

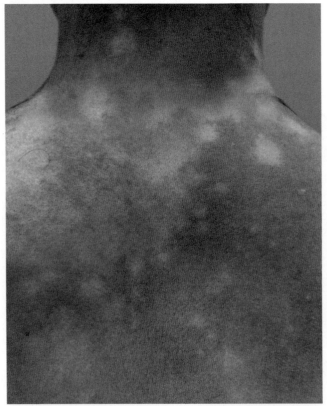

Progressive macular hypomelanosis: hypopigmented discoid discrete and confluent macules over the upper back and nape of neck.

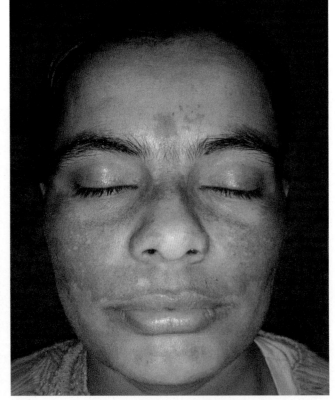

Melasma: predominant centrofacial involvement.

Clinical Manifestations

Depigmentation on contact with materials like rubber footwear, adhesive bindi, 'alta', hair dye, rubber gloves, condoms, leather hand bags/purses, etc. Positive findings of history of repeated chemical exposure (take detail history), hypopigmented macules conforming to sites of exposure, confetti macules (characteristic, although not diagnostic). Pruritus may occasionally present in chemical leukoderma.

Course

Spontaneous recovery possible in many cases on discontinuation of the suspected material. Lesions may progress to distant sites.

Diagnosis

Mainly clinical. Patch testing with the suspected chemicals in proper concentrations considered gold standard but they may produce local allergic reactions followed by development of depigmentation after several month.

Treatment

Topical steroids, tacrolimus, phototherapy/ photochemotherapy often used with variable success.

Pityriasis Alba

Dermatitis of unknown origin—irregular hypopigmented macules with ill-defined margins, fine branny scales. More common in atopics, children and on face; trunk, back and limbs infrequently involved. Mostly asymptomatic; burning or itching sometimes reported.

Treatment

Self-limiting. Hypopigmentation may persist for long. Bland emollients. Mild topical steroids may help in long standing cases.

Progressive Macular Hypomelanosis

Uncommon condition, predominantly affecting trunk. Discrete to confluent, non-scaly, discoid hypopigmented macules. Topical steroids/ antifungals do not work. Spontaneous resolution may occur, may subside with sunexposure/phototherapy.

DISORDERS OF INCREASED PIGMENTATION

Sequence has to be epidemiology, clinical features, histopathology, course, treatment.

Melasma (Chloasma)

Epidemiology

Probably the most common pigmentary disorder, population prevalence varies from 2 to 33% in literature. More common in skin phototypes III and IV pregnant females and those on oral contraceptive pills.

Etiology

Unknown. Probable factors—ultraviolet radiation, estrogen containing birth control pills, estrogen replacement therapy, ovarian or thyroid dysfunction, cosmetics, some photoallergic/phototoxic topical or systemic medications, hormonal disturbances. No exact correlation with serum hormone levels. Genetic predisposition present. Melanocyte activity and dendricity may be increased and not their number. Newer possible pathogenetic mechanisms/molecules—stem cell factor, vascular endothelial growth factor, nerve growth factor, keratinocyte plasmin pathway.

Clinical Manifestations

Commonly three patterns—centrofacial (most common), malar and mandibular. Distribution on light exposed skin-malar eminences, bridge of nose, forehead. Occasionally upper lip affected. Symmetrical, irregularly patterned, rather well-defined, brown macules with or without smaller satellite lesions.

Histopathology

Biopsy may be performed when close differential diagnoses present like drug induced hypermelanosis, exogenous ochronosis, acanthosis. Biopsy shows increased epidermal melanocytes (more dendritic than normal skin) and dermal melanophages.

Course

Chronic. According to a study only 8% patients showed spontaneous remission.

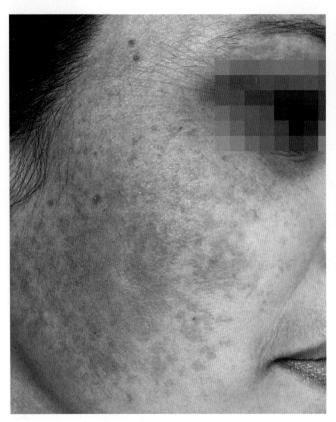

Melasma: predominant malar involvement.

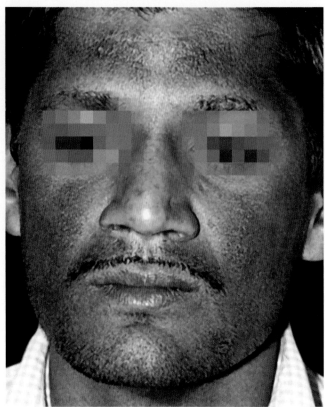

Berloque dermatitis: caused by application of scented cream.

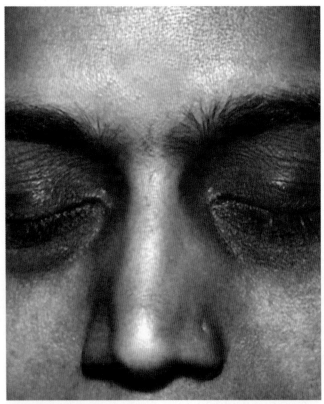

Periorbital melanosis: often familial.

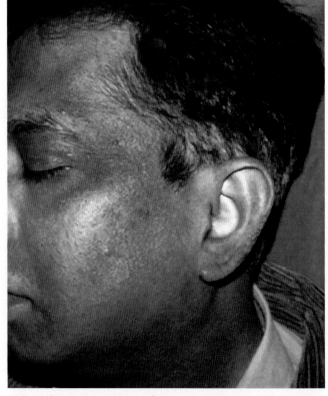

Lichen planus pigmentosus, face: typical slate-grey pigmentation.

Treatment of melasma		
Line	*Main modality*	*Alternative*
First choice	2–4% hydroquinone or triple combination (hydroquinone 4%, tretinoin 0.05% and fluocinolone 0.01%)	Azelic acid 20%
Adjuvant	Ascorbic acid (stable form, 5%)	Kojic acid 2%
Second choice	Glycolic acid peels (starting from 30%)	Tretinoin 1% peel
Third choice	Fractional CO_2, low fluence Q switched Nd:YAG	Intense pulse light
Better studies awaited but hold promise	Tranexamic acid (oral 250–1 gm daily, topical 5% gel, injectable intradermal solution), arbutin, soy extracts, licorice	

Broad spectrum sunscreens to be used several times during day time.

Treatment

Broad spectrum sunscreens needed irrespective of treatment modality. Numerous botanical extracts used but evidence poor for most. Well studied modalities mentioned in table. Diagnosis mainly clinical.

Berloque Dermatitis

Uncommon. Females affected. Distinctive streaky brown-black pigmentation generally on the sides of neck, upper chest or face.

Result of photosensitivity caused by bergapten (5-methoxypsoralen) present in perfumes containing bergamot oil.

Treatment

Protect from sunlight. Avoid contact of perfumes with light exposed parts of the body.

Periorbital Melanosis

Common in certain races-often familial. Dark brown pigmentation around the eyes, accentuated with physical or mental fatigue. Other factors include atopy, vascularity (dermal venules give dark color) and shadow effect (due to loss of periorbital fat and subsequent sunken appearance). Stationary or progressive.

Treatment

No satisfactory treatment but innumerable have been tried. General measures include proper sleep/diet/stress management, photoprotective sunglasses. Sunscreens and mild demelanizing topical preparations like kojic acid/arbutin/vitamin C may provide some relief but evidence poor/lacking. Shadow effect may be mitigated by dermal fillers or autologous fat transfer.

Lichen Planus Pigmentosus

Macular variant of lichen planus. Characterized by slate-grey pigmentation. Common in India; also described from Latin America, Japan and Europe. Differentiation from ashy dermatosis (erythema dyschromicum perstans) is as yet uncertain. Still debatable whether they are distinct clinical entities or part of same spectrum. Differentiation between the two entities (as per the authors' opinion) shown in table. Young adults affected. Asymptomatic or mildly itchy, small or, by confluence, large, irregular or oval macules of slate-grey to blue-black color.

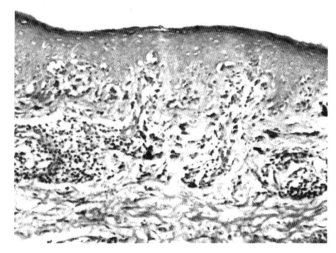

Histopathology of lichen planus pigmentosus: vacuolar degeneration of epidermal cells, incontinence of melanin and focal upper dermal mononuclear infiltrate.

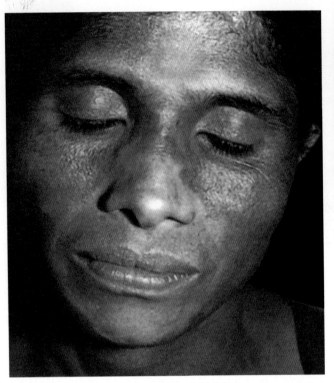

Lichen planus pigmentosus: diffuse bluish-grey pigmentation in a photosensitive distribution.

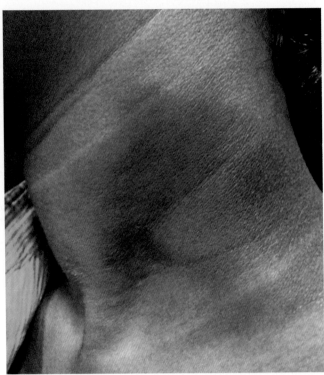

Ashy dermatosis (erythema dyschromicum perstans): solitary slate grey patch with raised erythematous border.

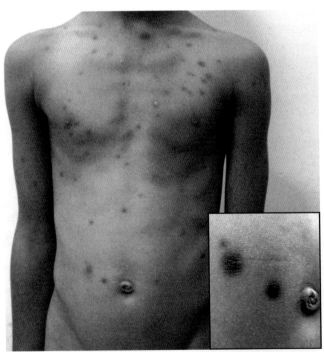

Idiopathic eruptive macular pigmentation: scattered hyperpigmented macules over the trunk; inset shows lesions with velvety surface resembling acanthosis nigricans.
Courtesy: Dr Geeti Khullar, Department of Dermatology, PGI, Chandigarh.

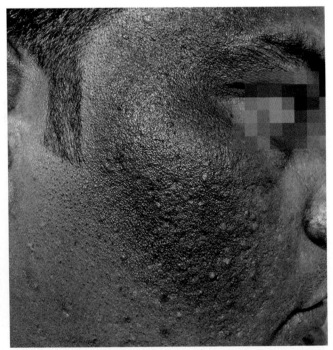

Facial acanthosis nigricans: dark brown-black pigmentation involving the temple and lateral cheek showing subtle velvety texture.

Differences between lichen planus pigmentosus and ashy dermatosis		
Feature	*Lichen planus pigmentosus*	*Ashy dermatosis*
Onset	Abrupt/insidious onset	Insidious onset
Lesion	Discrete to confluent, slate-grey to violaceous pigmentation	Early lesion has peripheral rim of erythema Usually discrete greyish or blue black macules
Reticulate pattern	+/–	–
Margin	Irregular	Round/polycyclic
Sites	Head and neck more than trunk and extremities. Sunexposed/flexural	Trunk more than head and neck
Symptoms	Pruritus +/–	Usually asymptomatic
Oral mucosa	+/–	–
Associated lichen planus	May be there	–
Histopathology	Basal cell degeneration, lichenoid infiltrate, colloid bodies, pigment incontinence in dermis (melanophages)	Less likely to have basal cell damage, colloid bodies and infiltrate, melanophages present
Residual hypopigmented halo	–	+/–

Starts from preauricular region with gradual spread to face, upper extremities, trunk and abdomen. Associated with other, particularly follicular, lichen planus. Mucosal involvement infrequent. Progressive course.

Histopathology

Variable. Active lesions show features of lichen planus. Late lesions—focal incontinence of pigment with mild to moderate lymphohistiocytic infiltrate.

Treatment

Oral course of vitamin A in dose of 1 lac units for 2–3 weeks per month for 8–10 months used in the past with some success. Currently not recommended owing to adverse effect concerns. Topical hydroquinone or triple combinations may be applied to lighten cosmetically important areas. Oral retinoids (isotretinoin) used with promising results in many patients.

Idiopathic Eruptive Macular Pigmentation with Papillomatosis

Rare entity. Asymptomatic brownish-black macules and barely elevated plaques with velvety surface in children and adolescents (peri-pubertal). Appear in crops over face, trunk and proximal extremities. Etiology is unknown. May be form of eruptive acanthosis nigricans. Spontaneous remission over months to years.

Facial Acanthosis Nigricans

Uncommon but increasingly recognized in view of increasing prevalence of insulin resistance, obesity, diabetes. Brown black pigmentation of the facial skin with subtle velvety texture. Sometimes associated with overlying skin tags. Typical sites on face include lateral cheeks, temples, forehead. Although more cases of facial acanthosis in literature reported in association with malignancies but much bigger number is seen with metabolic syndromes and obesity.

Erythromelanosis Follicularis Faciei et Colli

Uncommon condition seen sporadically but few familial cases reported. Erythema, pigmentation and follicular papules present over preauricular area and cheeks, extending to sides of neck. More reported in young men/adolescents. Associations observed—keratosis pilaris, keratosis rubra pilaris. No known treatment. Topical retinoids may help.

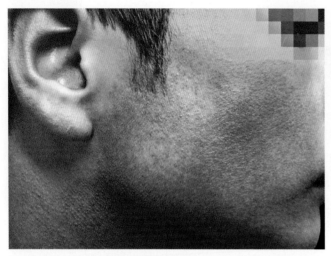

Erythromelanosis follicularis faciei et colli: well-defined erythema, pigmentation over the lateral cheek, ear lobule rim and side of neck, studded with fine follicular papules.

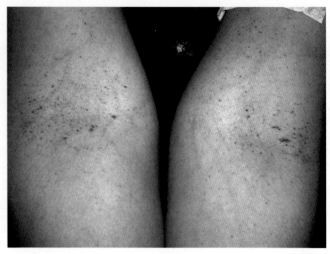

Dowling Degos disease: punctate black spots in bilateral cubital fossae.

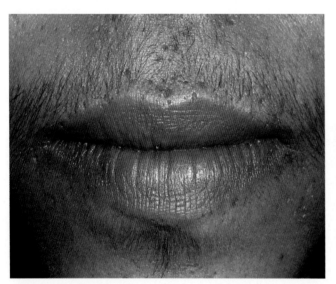

Dowling Degos disease: punctate perioral pits (especially along borders of lips and angles of mouth).

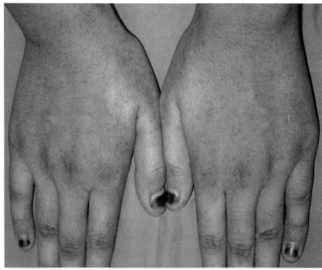

Reticulate acropigmentation of kitamura: punctate dark brown macules over dorsae of both hands.

RETICULATE PIGMENTARY DISORDERS

Uncommon group of disorders characterized by punctate hyperpigmented macules, grouped or discrete and often inherited. The term dyschromatoses is used when such hyperpigmented macules are intermixed with hypopigmented macules. They comprise of various diseases with syndromic associations and are mostly untreatable.

Dowling Degos Disease

Rare autosomal dominant condition caused by loss of function mutation in keratin 5 gene. Sporadic more common. More commonly discrete to grouped macules rather than reticulate pattern. Predominantly flexural (neck, axillae, cubitals, popliteals), head and neck. Perioral pitting, comedo-like papules, epidermoid/trichilemmal cysts. Generalized variant may have erythematous as well as hypopigmented macules and papules in addition.

Histopathology

Shows branching of rete pegs which are pigmented at their tips. Recently, follicular Dowling Degos disease (DDD) has been reported which has tiny hyperpigmented macules, comedonal papules and follicular scars. Lesions show the classic histological changes of DDD limited to follicular epithelium.

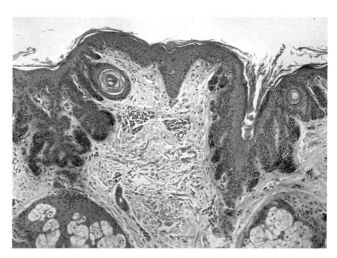

Histopathology of Dowling Degos disease: elongated and branching rete pegs with prominent pigmentation at tips.

Reticulate Acropigmentation of Kitamura

Rare pigmented disorder of autosomal dominant inheritance with same genetic locus as DDD. Atrophic hyperpigmented macules, mainly over the dorsae of hands and feet. Extensors of extremities may be involved. Palmar pits.

Other conditions have been summarized below in the flow chart.

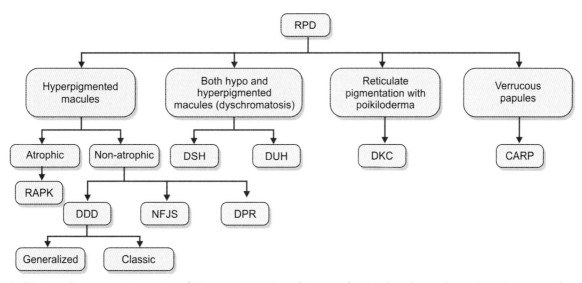

RAPK: Reticulate acropigmentation of Kitamura; NFJS: Naegeli Franceschetti Jadassohn syndrome; DPR: Dermatopathia pigmentosa reticularis; DSH: Dyschromatosis symmetrica hereditaria; DUH: Dyschromatosis universalis hereditaria; DKC: Dyskeratosis congenita; CARP: Confluent and reticulate papillomatosis; RPD: Reticulate pigmentary disorders; DDD: Dowling Degos disease.

13

The 'Connective Tissue Diseases'

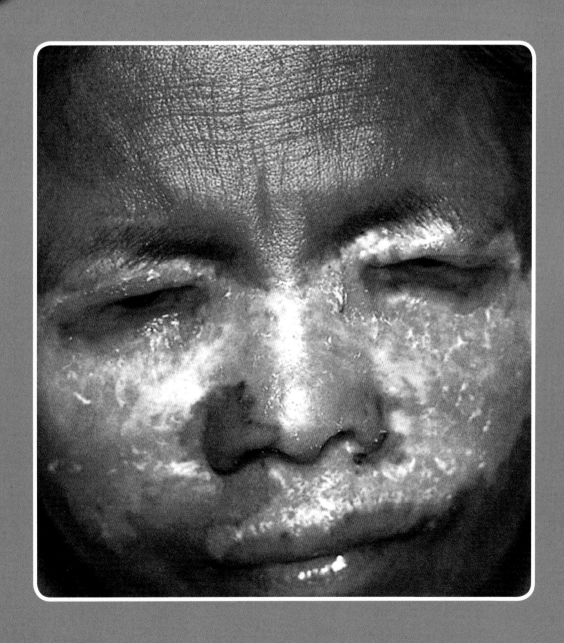

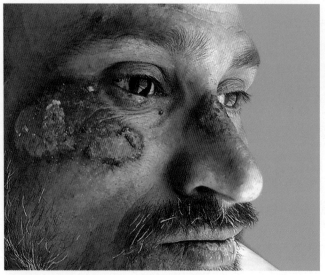

Chronic discoid lupus erythematosus: depigmented scaly plaques over right malar eminence, lower eyelid nasal bridge and lower lip.

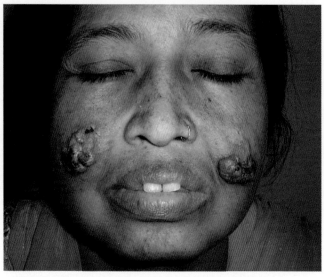

Hypertrophic discoid lupus erythematosus: erythematous verrucous plaques involving both cheeks almost symmetrically.

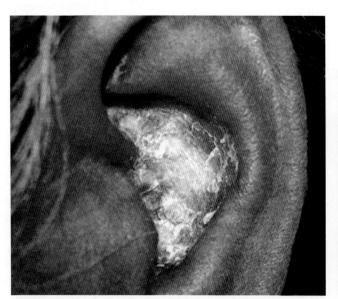

Chronic discoid lupus erythematosus: scaly red plaque involving the ear concha, a typical site.

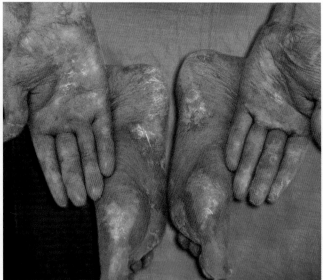

Palmoplantar discoid lupus erythematosus: depigmented scaly plaques with blanchable erythema involving the palms and soles in a patient with disseminated DLE.

The appropriate term to group all these disorders is yet unknown but the term 'connective tissue disorders' has been used in absence of better alternative. Systemic disorders characterized by involvement of connective tissue and blood vessels in different organs and systems. Autoimmune in nature. Immune-complex mediated injury, a dominant feature, though not the only one. Clinical features diverse and yet overlapping. Lot of conditions included conventionally but the ones currently placed together are lupus erythematosus, scleroderma, dermatomyositis, Sjögren's syndrome and rheumatoid arthritis.

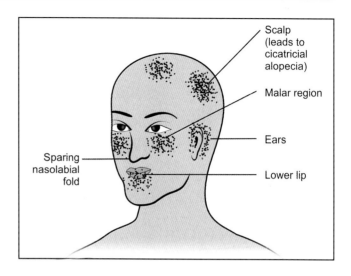

LUPUS ERYTHEMATOSUS

Cutaneous lupus erythematosus (LE) is of three types: acute cutaneous LE (ACLE); subacute cutaneous LE (SCLE) and chronic cutaneous LE (CCLE). Details of the Gilliam classification are given in the table. These subtypes are probably a continuous spectrum.

Discoid Lupus Erythematosus

Chronic. Cutaneous and/or mucocutaneous involvement. No systemic component. Common in young or middle aged adults, more often females. Autoimmune etiology. IgG and complement bound

The Gilliam classification of skin lesions associated with lupus erythematosus	
LE-specific skin disease (CLE)	**LE-non-specific skin disease**
• ACLE – Localized ACLE – Generalized ACLE	• Cutaneous vascular disease – Vasculitis – Vasculopathy – Periungual telangiectasia – Livedo reticularis – Thrombophlebitis – Raynaud phenomenon – Erythromelalgia (erythermalgia)
• SCLE – Annular SCLE	• Non-scarring alopecia – "Lupus hair" – Telogen effluvium – Alopecia areata

• Chronic cutaneous LE (CCLE)
 – Classic discoid LE (DLE)
   i. Localized DLE
   ii. Generalized DLE
 – Hypertrophic/verrucous DLE
 – Lupus profundus/lupus panniculitis
 – Mucosal DLE
   i. Oral DLE
   ii. Conjunctival DLE
 – Lupus tumidus (urticarial plaque of LE)
 – Chilblain LE (chilblain lupus)
 – Lichenoid DLE (LE/lichen planus overlap, lupus planus)
	• Sclerodactyly
	• Rheumatoid nodules
	• Calcinosis cutis
	• LE-non-specific bullous lesions
	• Urticaria
	• Papulonodular mucinosis
	• Cutis laxa/anetoderma
	• Acanthosis nigricans (type B insulin resistance)
	• Erythema multiforme
	• Leg ulcers
	• Lichen planus

CLE: Cutaneous lupus erythematous; ACLE: Acute cutaneous lupus erythematosus; SCLE: Subacute cutaneous lupus erythematosus; CCLE: Chronic cutaneous lupus erythematosus; DLE: Discoid lupus erythematosus; LE: Lupus erythematosus.

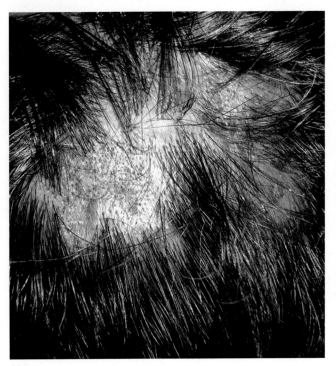

Cicatricial alopecia secondary to discoid lupus erythemato-sus: scaly erythematous plaques with overlying prominent follicular plugging and scarring hair loss.

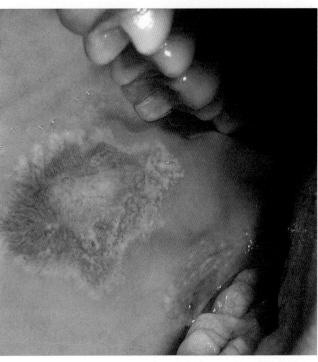

Discoid lupus erythematosus plaque on buccal mucosa: showing central atrophy and peripheral white striations and telangiectasias.

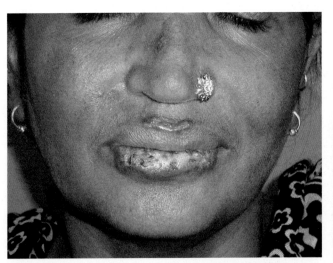

Discoid lupus erythematosus-lichen planus overlap: violaceous plaques over the nose and upper lip suggestive of LP. Dipigmented plaque with peripheral hyperpigmentation over the lower lip.

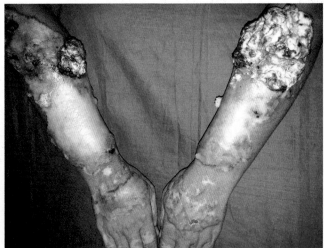

Discoid lupus erythematosus with squamous cell carcinoma: long standing discoid lupus erythematosus plaques with overlying ulcerated and cauliflower like squamous cell carcinoma plaques.

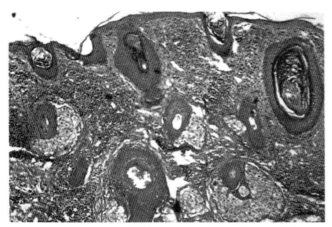

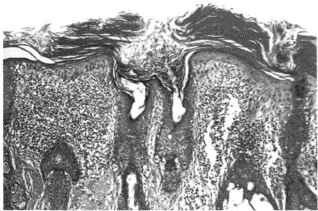

Histopathology of chronic discoid lupus erythematosus: atrophy of the epidermis, keratotic plugs, vacuolar degeneration of basal cell layer, dense inflammatory infiltrate in upper dermis and around the appendages; top (10x). Bottom (10x) shows marked hyperkeratosis in addition to above findings.

to the basement zone of the lesiotial skin (c.f. SLE). Light exposed areas preferentially affected. Commonly affects the face (cheeks, bridge of the nose, forehead), ears, scalp. Less frequently, extremities and trunk, lips and buccal mucosa. Designated disseminated OLE when lesions below neck. Bilateral, often symmetrical; occasionally unilateral. Well-defined, erythematous and scaly plaques with follicular plugs. Scales large and adherent. Removal of the scale reveals adherent follicular plugs at its undersurface and this is known as 'carpet tack' or 'tin tack' sign. Peripheral spread with brownish discoloration; central healing with depigmentation and atrophy or scarring. Scalp: cicatricial alopecia.

Histopathology

Hyperkeratosis with follicular plugging. Irregular atrophy of the stratum malpighii. Liquefactive degeneration of basal cell layer. Periappendageal and perivascular lymphocytic infiltration. Mucin deposition in dermis.

Direct immunofluorescence (DIF): IgG and C3 deposit in basement zone, only lesional skin.

Course

Untreated lesions tend to persist. Scarring in about 2/3rd and pigmentary abnormalities in 1/3rd. Risk of developing SLE 6.5% for localized DLE, 22% for disseminated DLE, 20% for chilblain like LE, and about 50% of lupus profundus have SLE. Long standing DLE lesions may rarely develop malignancies like SCC and occasionally BCC.

Treatment

Protect from sunlight. Sunscreens—organic like benzophenones or inorganic such as titanium dioxide and calamine lotion. Protective clothing. Topical (often potent) or intralesional corticosteroids for small localized lesions. For more extensive lesions, systemic chloroquine (250 mg twice a day for about a month, later once daily) or hydroxychloroquine (200 mg twice a day). Watch for ocular toxicity when on chloroquine therapy. Or corticosteroids (prednisolone 20–40 mg/day or equivalent).

Systemic Lupus Erythematosus

A multisystem disease. Cutaneous involvement, an important, often diagnostic, but not an invariable component. Kidneys, joints, heart, lungs, nervous system and other organs/systems affected.

Etiology

Autoimmune etiology. Organ-specific and non-specific antibodies in circulation. Immunoglobulins and complement bound to the basement zone in the clinically affected and unaffected skin (c.f. DLE). Genetic predisposition perhaps operative. Certain drugs, such as procainamide, sulfonamides, hydantoin and griseofulvin known to precipitate SLE. Young adults; females far more frequently,

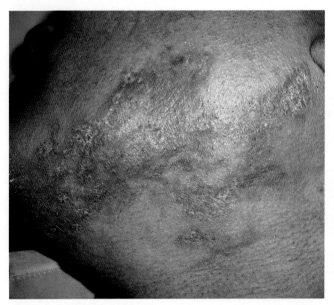

Lupus profundus et hypertrophicus (DLE with LE panniculitis): erythematous scaly plaques with atrophy scarring and fat loss over left mandibular area.

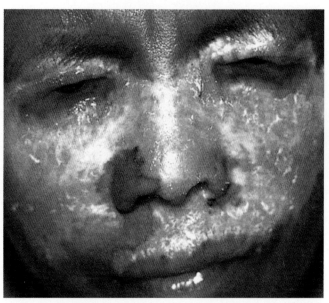

Complement deficiency systemic lupus erythematosus: extensive lesions on the cheeks and nose, upper lip and eyelids with facial scarring and bilateral ectropion.

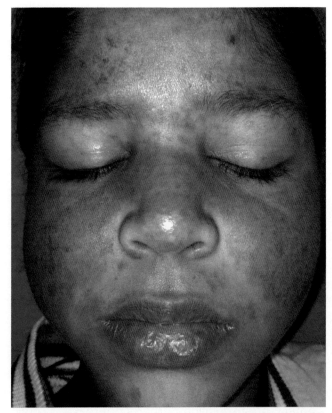

Systemic lupus erythematosus (acute lupus erythematosus): characteristic malar rash, sparing the nasolabial folds, perioral area and eyelids.

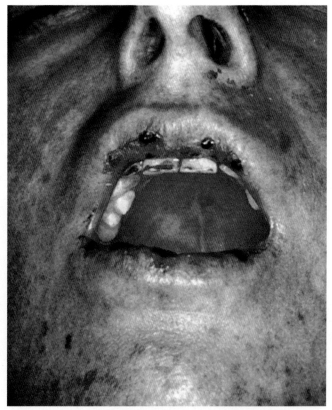

Toxic epidermal necrolysis like lupus erythematosus: hemorrhagic crusting over lips, palatal ulceration with malar rash.

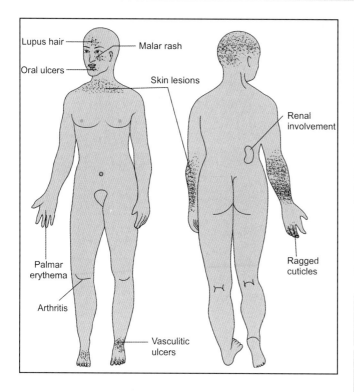

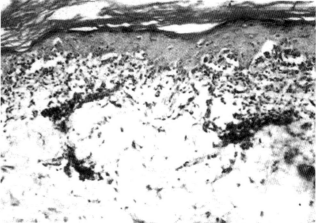

Histopathology of systemic lupus erythematosus: hyperkeratosis, degeneration of epidermis; upper dermal infiltrate.

affected. Smokers at increased risk than non-smokers or ex smokers.

Clinical Manifestations

Classic photosensitive butterfly malar rash on the cheeks; other areas also affected. Erythematous papules or plaques with fine scaling. Occasionally purpuric or ulcerative lesions. Palmar erythema with telangiectasia and atrophic scars. Telangiectasia of nail fold capillaries. Raynaud's phenomenon and chilblains (pernio tic LE). Diffuse or frontal, non-cicatricial alopecia of the scalp. Livedo reticularis on the legs and arms. Occasionally sclerodactyly or DLE type lesions. Mucosal involvement—frequent; superficial ulcerations in the buccal mucosa, palate, gums. Variable extracutaneous manifestations—fever, arthralgia/arthritis. Renal involvement: albuminuria, microscopic hematuria. Serositis. Central nervous system involvement.

Course

Variable-spontaneous or corticosteroid induced remissions. Life expectancy poor in fulminant cases. Death due to renal failure, internal hemorrhage or infection. Prognosis worse in males. Pregnancy variably affects the mother. High fetal and perinatal mortality. Infrequently neonatal LE.

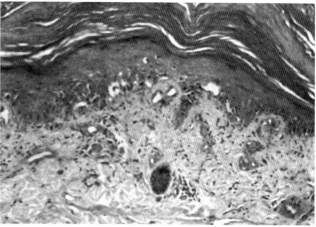

Histopathology of systemic lupus erythematosus: hyperkeratosis with vacuolar degeneration of basal cell layer. Note vessel wall thickening.

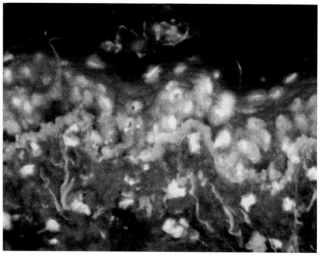

Systemic lupus erythematosus: positive lupus band test.

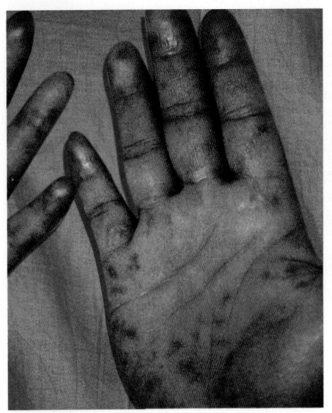

Systemic lupus erythematosus vasculitis: ill-defined erythematous macules on the palms with telangiectasia and superficial ulceration.

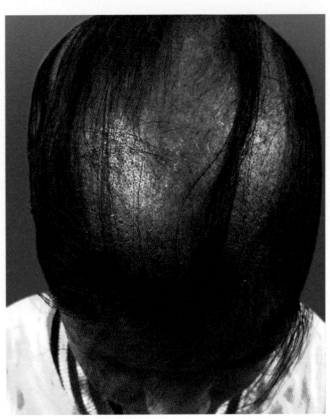

Systemic lupus erythematosus: Severe diffuse alopecia with baldness and short broken hair in anterior hairline (lupus hair).

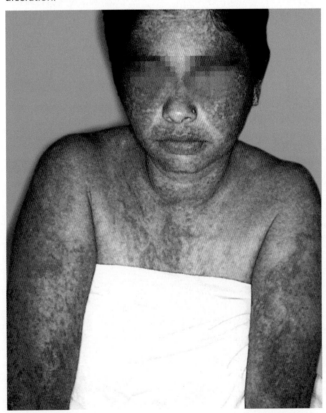

Subacute cutaneous lupus erythematosus: erythematosquamous lesions on face, 'V' of neck, shoulders and extensors of arms.

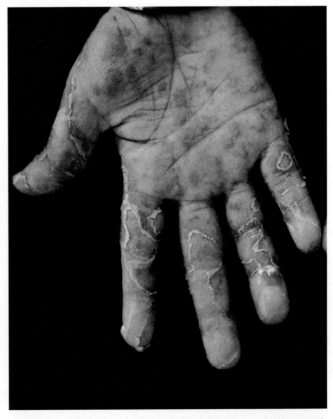

Rowell's syndrome: a typical targetoid lesions subsiding with exfoliation over right palm in a patient of systemic LE.

Histopathology

Hyperkeratosis, basal cell degeneration, upper dermal edema, vessel wall thickening and peri-vascular infiltrate of lymphocytes and histiocytes. On DIF, lupus band in clinically uninvolved skin also. Lupus band test is considered highly specific for SLE if 3 or more immunoreactants (IgG, IgM, IgA, C3) are found at the dermaepidermal junction of non-lesional skin. Positive lupus band test also predicts decreased survival and increased risk of nephritis.

Hematologic Abnormalities

Anemia, leukopenia, thrombocytopenia, pancyto-penia. Elevated sedimentation rate, LE cell phenomenon.

Immunologic Findings

Low complement levels. Auto-antibodies against nuclear antigens and double stranded DNA (associated with lupus nephritis) or single stranded DNA (drug induced lupus). And antibodies against cytoplasmic antigens (Ro) or acidic nuclear proteins (Sm). False positive serologic tests for syphilis.

Diagnosis

SLE was diagnosed on the basis of American College of Rheumatology till now. Recently, new SLICC (systemic lupus international collaborating clinics) criteria have been found to be more sensitive and specific. They include more cutaneous features of LE like acute cutaneous LE (ACLE) and its variants, other variants of DLE, non-scarring alopecia and even nasal ulcers. Photosensitivity is included under ACLE.

Treatment

Mild cases treated with hydroxychloroquine. Corticosteroids, treatment of choice in most patients with severe disease. Methotrexate (for skin lesions) azathioprine, cyclophosphamide, used as adjuvants/steroid sparing agents. Cyclophosphamide also used alone, as 500 mg monthly intravenous pulse, especially in lupus nephritis.

Subacute Cutaneous LE (SCLE)

Relatively uncommon. Young adult females. Cutaneous lesions—photosensitivity. And widespread bilaterally symmetrical lesions face, neck, upper chest, back and upper extremities. Two morphologic patterns—papulosquamous psoriasiform. Or annular; both may co-exist. Discrete or confluent. Heal without scarring but with reversible depigmentation. Diffuse non-cicatricial alopecia on the scalp. Buccal mucosal involvement and periungual telangiectasia infrequent. Systemic involvement—frequent but mild: fever, malaise, arthralgia. Renal involvement infrequent and mild. Laboratory findings—leukopenia, elevated sedimentation rate and positive ANA; antibodies to cytoplasmic antigens (Ro/La) frequently present and suggestive. Course variable and prolonged.

Treatment

Systemic chloroquine, 250 mg twice a day. Systemic steroids, if response inadequate.

Rowell's Syndrome

It is a clinical presentation where targetoid lesions occur in patient with any form of LE with seropositivity for rheumatoid factor (RF) and anti La (SS-B) antibodies.

SCLERODERMA

Purely cutaneous or systemic; the latter designated systemic sclerosis.

Cutaneous disease may be localized or generalized. Systemic sclerosis involves skin, blood vessels, lungs, gastrointestinal tract, kidneys and heart. Excessive synthesis of normal collagen, possibly immune-mediated. Result of complex interplay between endothelial cells, epithelial cells, fibroblasts and lymphocytes. Other factors include trauma, radiation, genetic factors, infections and medications. Blood vessel involvement, an important component—Raynaud's phenomenon, telangiectasia, and ischemic ulcerations. Skin involvement occasionally absent.

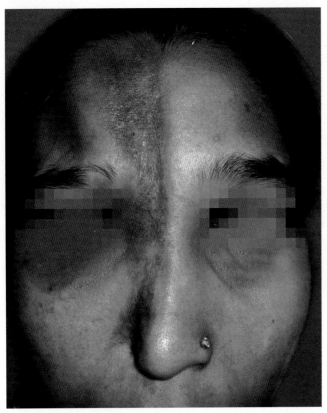

En coup de sabre (linear morphea): linear depressed hyperpigmented plaques involving right side of forehead, eyelids and nose with destruction of right nasal ala.

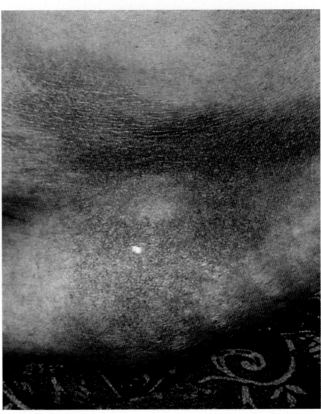

Plaque morphea: discoid, hyperpigmented, bound down plaque on the abdomen.

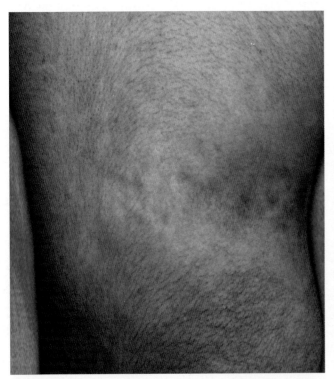

Atrophoderma of pasini pierini: burnt out morphea plaque over flank causing soft tissue atrophy.

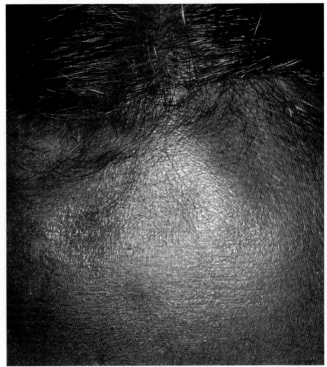

Morphea profundus: multiple depressed plaques with subcutaneous atrophy with overlying normal or slightly pigmented skin seen over the forehead.

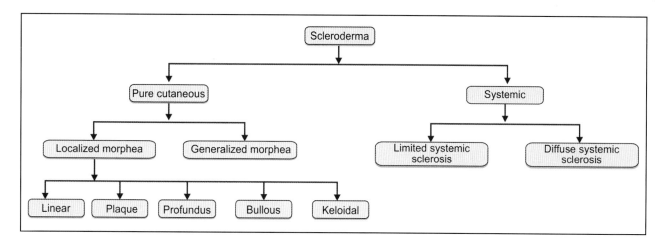

Localized Morphea

Not uncommon. Children or young adults; females 3–4 times more frequently. Trunk, face or extremities involved. Initial lesions—localized pigmented macules or edematous indurated plaques. Later: atrophic, shiny, bound-down and depressed, circumscribed plaques-skin colored or hyperpigmented (lilac ring described on white skin, seldom seen in the pigmented). Loss of hair and sweating. Circular, oval, irregular or linear configuration. Linear bands on extremities or elsewhere; on forehead and scalp called en coup de sabre. May cause hemiatrophy of face—deeper structures (muscles, bones) sometimes involved. No systemic associations. Occasionally indurated atrophic, depigmented papules designated guttate morphea. Variable course-progressive. Or occasionally spontaneous resolution.

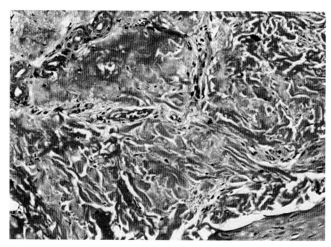

Histopathology of morphea: collagen sclerosis (homogenization) in mid dermis.

Generalized Morphea

Defined as presence of 4 or more plaques, each >3 cms, involving >2 anatomic sites. Rare. Large number of plaques similar to localized morphea. On the trunk, abdomen, upper thighs. Extracutaneous features are rare include arthralgias, Raynauds' phenomenon, CNS symptoms and ocular abnormalities (latter two esp. in en coup de sabre).

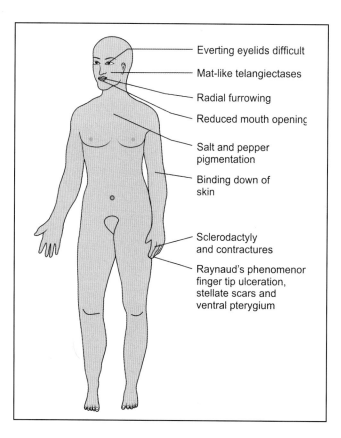

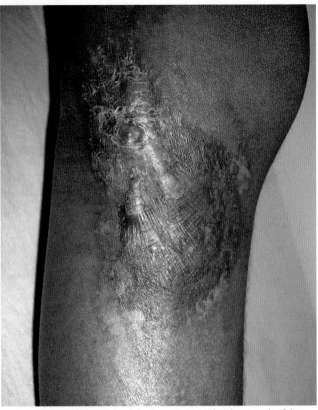

Keloidal morphea: keloidal plaques over background of linear morphea.

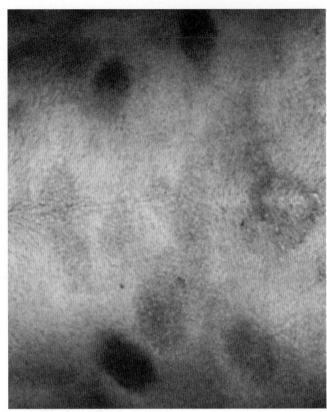

Generalized morphea: multiple, pigmented, atrophic plaques on the trunk.

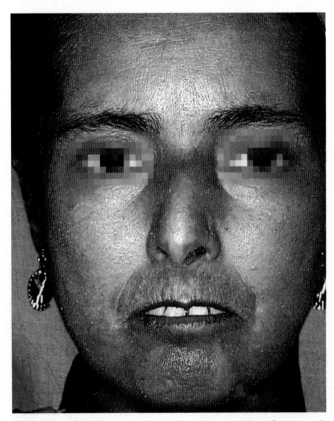

Systemic sclerosis: typically taut expression-less facies with pinched nose.

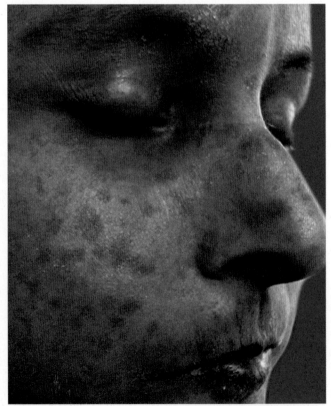

Systemic sclerosis: mat-like telangiectasia over the face.

Treatment

Localized Morphea

Topical tacrolimus is first line agent. Mid potent topical steroids may be used. Further, topical calcipotriol-betamethasone dipropionate combination, topical imiquimod may be given. UVA/UVA sol/NBUVB/MTX in resistant cases.

Generalized Morphea

Phototherapy is first line (UVA/NBUVB). Further methotrexate, systemic steroids and mycopheno-late mofetil may be given.

Systemic Sclerosis

A common multisystem disease. Autoimmune etiology.

Clinical Manifestations

Young adult females affected more frequently. Raynaud's phenomenon, often the first complaint. Skin changes—edematous, thickened and indurated; later, atrophic, smooth, shiny and bound-down. And difficult to pinch. Hands, feet, face affected first. Later (though not always) trunk and proximal parts of extremities. Characteristic fades—expressionless ('mask facies'); ironed out skin folds. Pinched nose. Small mouth with radial furrows on closing. Telangiectasia-'mat-like'—on face and palms. Hands and feet—edematous; pulp of fingers resorbed; sclerodactyly. Painful gangrenous ulceration and flexion deformity of fingers. Pigmentary changes—diffuse generalized hyperpigmentation or depigmentation or both— salt

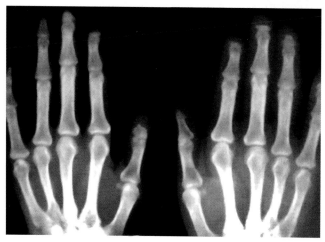

Systemic sclerosis: acro-osteolysis-resorption of terminal ends of distal phalanges.

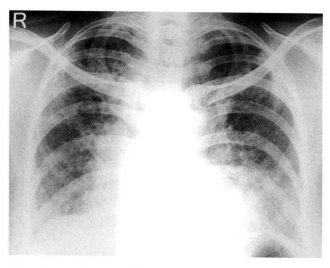

X-ray chest of advanced systemic sclerosis patient: showing extensive interstitial lung diseases and fibrosis, more prominent in bilateral lower lung zones.

Difference between diffuse and limited systemic sclerosis		
Features	Diffuse	Limited
Duration of Raynaud's phenomenon	Short	Long
Skin involvement	Truncal and peripheral	Peripheral only
Calcification and telangiectasia	Uncommon	Common
Pulmonary involvement	Early and common	Late (pulmonary hypertension)
Cardiac, gastric and renal involvement	Frequent	Uncommon
Nail fold changes	Capillary drop-outs	Capillary dilatation
Antibodies • Scl-70 • Anticentromere	 • Frequently positive • Negative	 • Infrequently positive • Positive

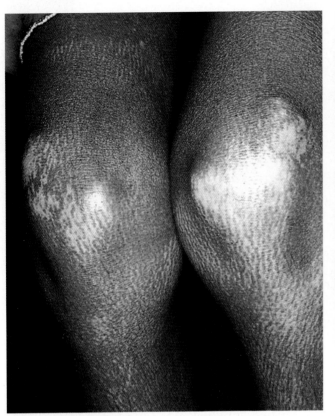

Systemic sclerosis: salt and pepper pigment appearance on lower extremities.

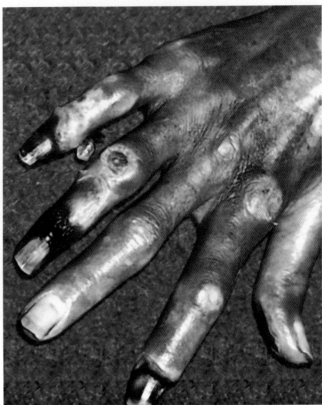

Systemic sclerosis: superficial ulcerations on the knuckles with gangrenous changes on tips of several digits.

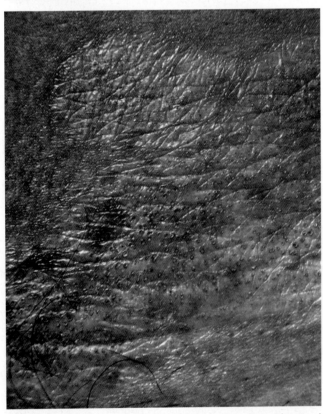

Lichen sclerosus: wrinkled hypopigmented plaque with pitted follicular scars over abdomen.

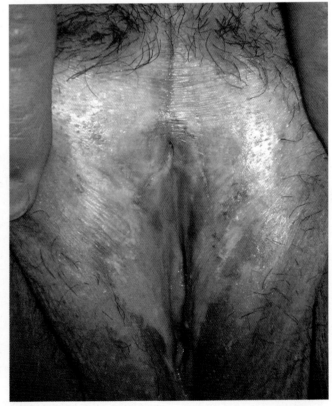

Vulval lichen sclerosus: depigmented plaque involving the vulva causing destruction of clitoris, urethral stenosis and punctate erosions over labia minoria.

and pepper pattern typical. Calcinosis of skin around the joints and stellate scars on finger tips. Systemic involvement—variable, depending on type whether limited variant or diffuse. Arthralgia/ arthritis, dysphagia, alternating constipation and diarrhea. Exertional dyspnea due to pulmonary interstitial fibrosis. Cardiac, renal and skeletal muscle involvement occasional.

Course

Variable, often progressive. Death from intercurrent infections. Or respiratory, cardiac or renal failure. Poorer prognosis in males.

Histopathology

Atrophic epidermis. Hyalinization of the dermal collagen. Fresh collagen laid in the lower dermis or hypodermis. Intimal thickening of blood vessels with perivascular mononuclear infiltrate.

Diagnosis

American Rheumatology Association criteria are sensitive as well as specific. Single major criterion is scleroderma proximal to the digits. At least two of the minor criteria should be met—sclerodactyly, digital pitted scarring and bilateral basal pulmonary fibrosis.

Treatment

None satisfactory. Protect from cold and trauma. Abstain from smoking. Raynaud phenomenon/ digital ischemia—calcium channel blockers (nifedipine) are first line. Others therapies proven useful include intravenous iloprost, oral bosentan (endothelin receptor antagonist), sildenafil/ tadalafil (phosphodiesterase inhibitors), alpha adrenergic blockers. Immunomodulator therapy for internal involvement—cyclophosphamide, methotrexate, extracorporeal photopharesis. Less proven therapies include cyclosporine, mycophenolate mofetil, rapamycin.
Symptomatic management for system wise complaints.

LICHEN SCLEROSUS

Term lichen sclerosus (LS) is preferred in place of lichen sclerosus et atrophicus since all lesions may not be atrophic. Although it is debatable, some authors consider it to be a form of morphea. Because numerous cases of morphea associated with LS exist in literature as well as clinical practice. Uncommon. Etiology unknown. Biphasic age distribution. Children or young adults. Small, discrete or confluent, ivory white, atrophic maculopapules or plaques with central depression. Dilated pilosebaceous orifices with keratotic plugs. Trunk, genitals and perianal region affected. Rarely seen in oral mucosa.

Vulvar lesions—atrophy and shrinkage of the vulva and narrowing of the vaginal introitus. Malignant potential, often debated.

Balanitis Xerotica Obliterans

Uncommon. Penile form of lichen sclerosus et atrophicus. Firm, phimotic, bluish-white, shiny prepuce. Glans—telangiectasia and meatal narrowing.

Course

Variable and unpredictable—spontaneous resolution, stationary or progressive. Malignant potential controversial.

Histopathology of Lichen Sclerosus

Atrophic epidermis with hyperkeratosis and keratotic plugs. Basal cell degeneration. Edema and hyalinization of the upper dermis. Lymphocytic infiltrate below the hyalinized area.

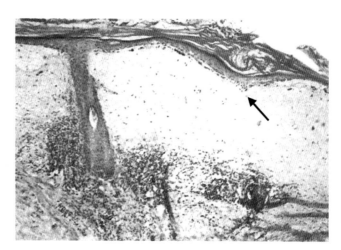

Histopathology of lichen sclerosus et atrophicus: epidermal atrophy, keratotic plugs, edema and hyalinized upper dermis with inflammatory infiltrate in the mid dermis.

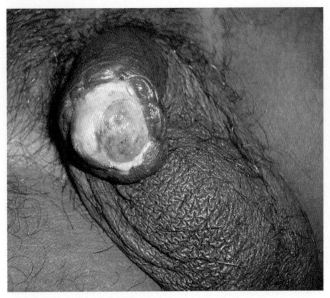

Balanitis xerotica obliterans: hypopigmented glans with a fleshy plaque suggestive of early squamous cell carcinoma and preputial phimosis.

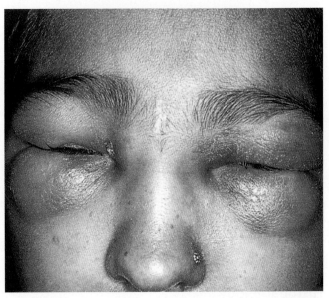

Dermatomyositis: erythema and edema of both upper and lower eyelids.

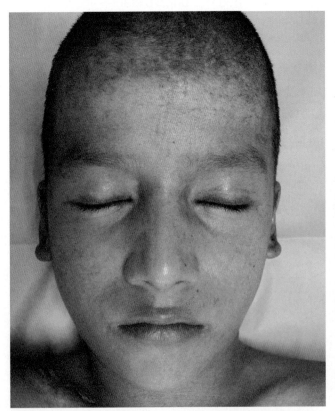

Juvenile dermatomyositis: erythema and telangiectasia over the upper eyelids, forehead and cheeks along with post inflammatory hypopigmentation over forehead.

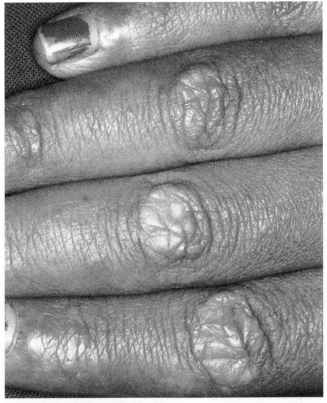

Dermatomyositis: Gottron's papules.

Treatment

None satisfactory. Potent topical corticosteroids give symptomatic relief in genital lesions. Topical tacrolimus may also help. Achronic ulcerated lesion always biopsied, to exclude malignancy.

DERMATOMYOSITIS

Idiopathic inflammatory dermatomyopathies are divided into clinically amyopathic dermatomyositis (CADM), classic dermatomysositis (DM) and polymyositis (PM)/inclusion body myositis. Dermatomyositis is an uncommon condition. Affects muscles with variable cutaneous manifestations. Perhaps auto-immune in etiology.

Clinical Manifestations

Females more frequently affected. Two variants—juvenile and adults. Skin involvement: by definition would involve 100% patients of DM and none of PM patients. Can be non-specific in the beginning and does not reflect severity of the disease. Violaceous erythema (heliotrope) of the face with periorbital edema characteristic. Pruritic confluent macular violaceous erythema of the arms, forearms, back (shawl sign), lateral thighs (holster sign) or other parts of the body. Violaceous, flat topped papules on the dorsa of interphalangeal joints of the hands-Gottron's papules-almost diagnostic. Gottron's sign is linearly arranged violaceous erythema over the dorsae of hands and fingers. Poikiloderma, reticulate pigmentation, telangiectasia and atrophy. Erythema and telangiectasia around the nail folds with ragged nail cuticles. Motor involvement—muscular pains and weakness of proximal muscles of shoulder and hip girdles. Muscles-tender and flabby or firm and fibrotic. Calcinosis cutis more frequent in children prognostically a good feature. Associations—no association with malignancy in children; more often among elderly-lung, breast, stomach, rectum and female genital tract.

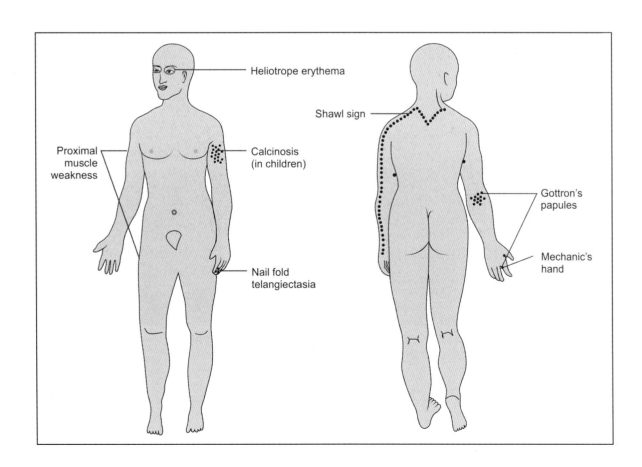

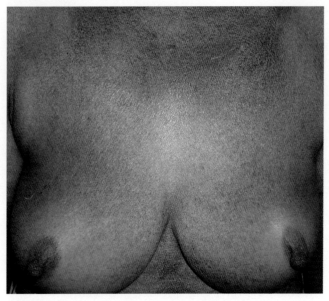

Poikiloderma over chest in an elderly patient of dermatomyositis.

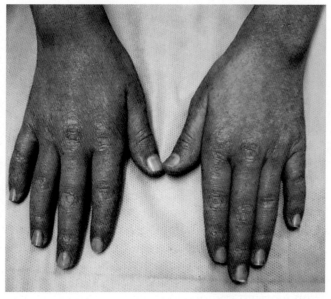

Dermatomyositis: linear violaceous erythema along extensor tendons of hand.

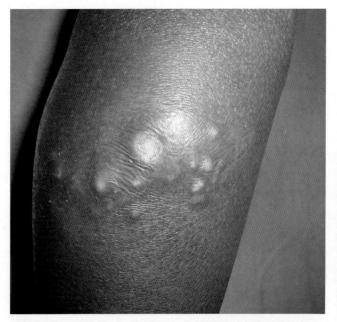

Calcinosis cutis in juvenile dermatomyositis: chalky white papules and ulcers studded over a calcinosis cutis swelling near the elbow.

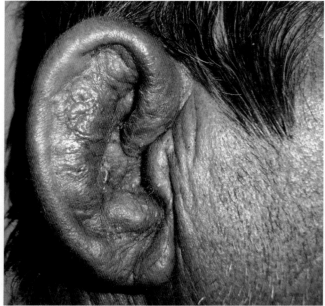

Relapsing polychondritis: swelling involving the cartilaginous part of ear, sparing the lobe.

Hallmark dermatomyositis-specific lesions	
Major	*Minor*
Heliotrope erythema	Confluent macular violaceous erythema
Gottron's papules	Periungual nail-fold telangiectases or cuticular hemorrhagic infarcts
Gottron's sign	Poikiloderma atrophicans vasculare Mechanic's hand Calcinosis cutis Pruritis

Modified Bohan and Peters diagnostic criteria for dermatomyositis
• Hallmark cutaneous lesions of dermatomyositis (2 major + 1 minor or 1 major + 2 minor)
• Symmetrical proximal muscle weakness with or without dysphagia/respiratory muscle weakness
• Elevated serum levels of skeletal muscle-derived enzymes
• Electromyographic features of myopathy
• Evidence of inflammatory myopathy on muscle biopsy
Definite dermatomyositis: 1 + any 3 of the other Probable dermatomyositis: 1 + any 2 of the other Possible dermatomyositis: 1 + any 1 of the other

Course

Variable—juvenile variety self limiting. Adult variety generally progressive. Mechanic's hands associated with poor response to treatment. In cases with associated malignancy, reversed following removal of the tumor. Death due to associated tumor. Or respiratory infections, cardiac failure or debility.

Antisynthetase Syndrome

Patients with antibodies against the aminoacyl tRNA synthetases (PL7, PL12, Jo 1, OJ, EJ) have greater risk of arthritis, interstitial lung disease, Raynaud phenomenon and poor response to therapy.

Treatment

Moderately large doses of systemic corticosteroids (1–2 mg/kg). Immunosuppressives are useful as steroid sparing agents and adjuvants. Methotrexate (primarily for skin manifestations), azathioprine, mycophenolate mofetil, cyclosporine, cyclophosphamide, etc. Newer agents reported to be of use—etanercept, infliximab, rituximab. Calcinosis usually does not respond to any mode of therapy although several agents have been anecdotally found to be useful—alendronate, warfarin, intralesional steroids, colchicine, aluminum hydroxide. Surgical excision may be done for isolated lesions.

Differences between Juvenile and adult dermatomyositis		
Feature	*Juvenile*	*Adult*
Lipoatrophy/panniculitis	Common	Rare
Hypertrichosis	Common	Rare
Vasculitis (skin/gut)	Common	Less common
Arthritis	Common	Less common
Calcinosis cutis	Common	Infrequent
Underlying malignancies	Absent	Present in about one-fourth

RELAPSING POLYCHONDRITIS

Recurrent attacks of chondritis. Most common being auricular (>80%) followed by nasal, respiratory and costochondral. Swelling of ear involves only the cartilaginous portion, sparing the lobe. Repeated attacks cause cartilage loss and sagging. Associated with—arthralgias, ocular inflammation, cardiac manifestations, etc. Treatment depends on system involvement. Usually NSAIDs, colchicine or dapsone sufficient for mild or moderate attacks.

14

Disorders Due to Physical Agents

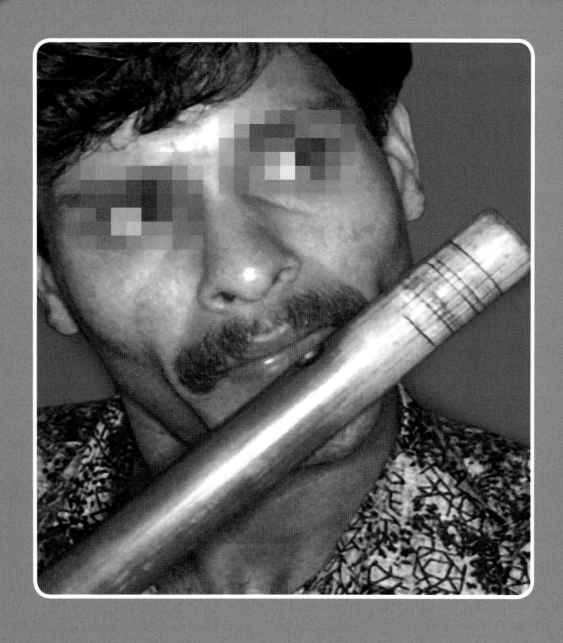

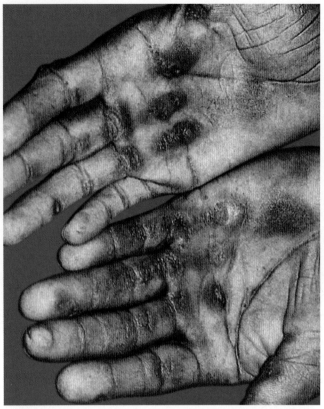

Callosities: on the palms of a manual worker due to intermittent moderate trauma.

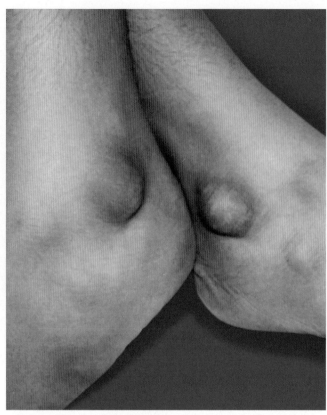

Callosities: due to caliper splints.

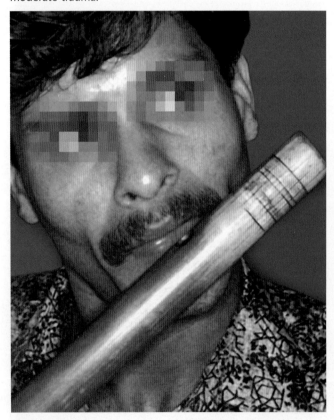

Flutist's chin: flute in contact with the chin and lower lip.

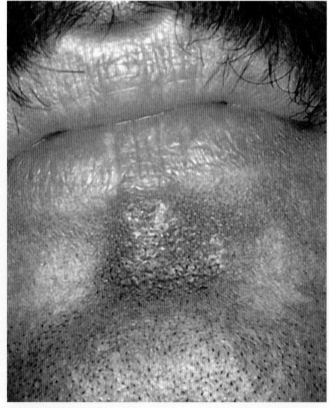

Flutist's chin: hyperkeratotic plaque on the lower lips and chin the site of contact with the flute.

Skin, the mechanical barrier between the body and the environment, responds to various environmental changes-light, heat, cold, mechanical trauma. Physical stimuli variously affect the skin-directly or through vascular changes.

Skin responses depend on several factors: racial, familial and individual differences, the intensity, rapidity and repetitivity of the stimuli and the skin sites affected.

Mechanical trauma such as friction, when mild and repeated, produces thickening of the skin leading to lichenification, callosities and corns. *Acute sudden friction* causes blister formation. In all situations of environmental stress, adaptation plays an important role.

Mild heat causes vasodilatation and sweating. *Severe heat* results in blisters and burns. And *chronic moderate heat* produces erythema, pigmentation, telangiectasia, melanosis, thickening of the skin and malignancies. *Moderate cold* causes vasoconstriction; *severe cold* causes intracellular crystallization and cell death.

Response to light varies with the amount of melanin in the skin. *Acute exposure*, particularly to UVB light, causes sunburn and suntan. *Chronic exposures*: degenerative changes such as solar elastosis and wrinkling and neoplastic changes such as actinic keratoses. And basal and squamous cell malignancies.

DISORDERS DUE TO MECHANICAL INJURY

Callosities

Common. Hyperkeratotic ill-defined plaques at sites of repetitive, intermittent, moderate trauma. Usually painless. Seen on pressure points of hands in manual workers and drivers, on forehead in devout Muslims (prayer nodules), friction of caliper splints in physically handicapped. Or simply habit tics.

Treatment

Removal of trigger. Or padding to buffer pressure. Keratolytics (salicylic acid 6%; urea 10–20%) applied regularly softens area. Paring for faster relief.

Corns

Common. Callosities localized to bony prominences, usually toes. Ill-fitting footwear may contribute. Hyperkeratotic nodule with a central cone shaped hard core directed inwards. Painful and tender.

Treatment

Avoid pressure. Proper wide, pliable footwear. Use topical keratolytic agents—10–40% salicylic acid ointment or 40% urea cream. Pairing, modified instep of footwear sole (cutting out the lesional area sole apposed to the lesion to avoid continuous pressure).

Piezogenic Pedal Papules

Misnomer for a pressure induced condition. Characterized by fat herniation in the dermis induced by weight bearing. Seen in normal individuals, sports persons, Ehler-Danlos syndrome, Prader-Willi syndrome, etc. Yellowish papules and nodules, often asymptomatic but may be painful. Painful lesions helped by excision or orthopedic shoe.

DISORDERS DUE TO TEMPERATURE CHANGE

Erythema Ab Igne

Uncommon. Results from chronic repeated exposure to direct heat-sitting in front of open fire, use of hot water bottles or other heating devices (Kangri in Kashmir). Transient reticulate erythema followed by brownish black pigmentation. Generally lower extremities; occasionally other parts such as the palms, abdomen and back.

Course

Early lesions remit in summer; continued exposure may eventuate in squamous cell carcinoma.

Treatment

Avoid exposure to direct heat. Early lesions, self healing.

Chilblains (Perniosis)

Common. Children or young adults, frequently females. Moderately severe cold and humidity causal.

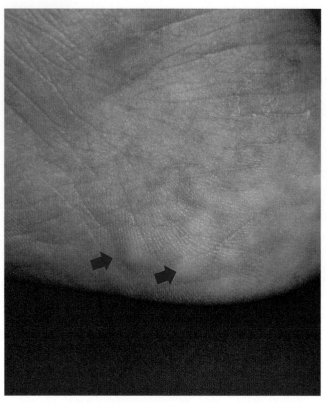

Piezogenic pedal papules: yellowish nodules shown by arroheads on the side of the heel (on putting pressure).

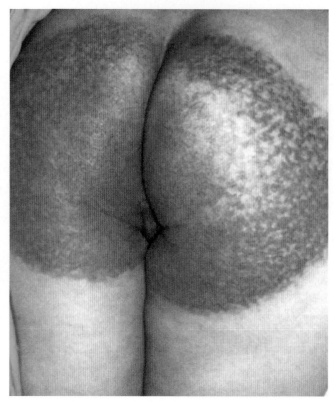

Erythema ab igne: well-defined erythematous telangiectatic plaque due to sitz bath.

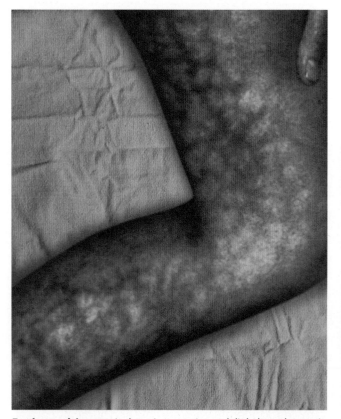

Erythema ab igne: reticulate pigmentation and slight hyperkeratosis.

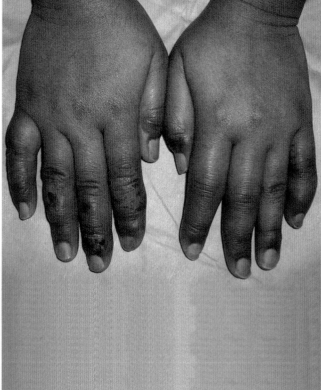

Chilblains: erythematous to dusky edematous plaques over fingers of both hands with focal scaling.

Mechanism uncertain—perhaps an abnormal response or exaggeration of physiological response to cold. Itchy, painful, red or cyanotic edematous nodules on dorsa of the fingers and toes. Vesiculation and ulceration may result. Individual lesion self-limiting clears in 1–2 weeks. Associated acrocyanosis of the hands and feet may be present. Parts feel cold. Remission with warm weather setting in.

Treatment

Prevention is critical. Avoid exposure to cold. Or protect-use adequate clothing and/or heating. Nifedipine helps, usually given if blistering/ulceration present or lesions persistent despite other measures. It may also be given before start of winters in patients who have severe relapses each season. Analgesics, potent topical steroids and antipruritics in established cases for symptomatic relief.

Frostbite

Rare. Result of exposure to extreme dry cold and freezing of the tissues. Seen in mountaineers and troops stationed at high altitudes or other cold conditions. Superficial or deep. Extent of injury apparent only on thawing. *Superficial frostbite:* erythema, edema and vesiculation; deeper tissues feel soft. *Deep:* dry, shrivelled-up, gangrenous peripheral part(s) of the body—the hands, feet, tip of the nose and pinna of the ears. Complete tissue death; dead portion may drop off. Deceptive lack of pain during exposure; thawing painful.

Treatment

Rapid rewarming till erythema returns. Scrupulously avoid further exposure to cold or any trauma and pressure. Analgesics to relieve pain associated with thawing. Surgery of the gangrenous part to be postponed for several weeks until demarcation occurs.

Raynaud's Phenomenon

Can be idiopathic, called raynaud's disease. Most common cause in dermatology connective tissue diseases (scleroderma, SLE, RA, Sjögren's). Other causes trauma, atherosclerosis, neurological or hematological disease. Much more common in women under 40. Precipitated by cold exposure in sequence—pallor, bluish discoloration, erythema.

Treatment

Strict cold protection, calcium channel blockers mainstay (slow release formulations better). Others sildenafil, IV prostacyclins, losarten. Topical nitroglycerin may help.

Livedo Reticularis

It is net like pattern of discoloration usually over the lower limbs which develops as a result of sluggish cutaneous blood flow. Multifactorial. Common causes vasculitis (microscopic polyangiitis, cryoglobulinemic vasculitis), CTDs (SLE, DM, Antiphospholipid antibody syndrome), embolic disease amongst others like endocrine, infections and pellagra. Management of the cause is important.

DISORDERS DUE TO EXPOSURE TO LIGHT

Sunburn

Common. Physiological. Acute inflammatory, response seen 8–10 hours after (over) exposure of the skin to short ultraviolet light (UVB) from the sun or artificial sources. Albinos, skin type I and II (fair skinned, blue eyed, red haired) individuals, and patients with vitiligo more susceptible. More common at high altitudes or sandy beaches because of higher UVB content, (due to reflection); hence amongst mountaineers and trekkers. Face or other exposed areas. Erythema, edema, and vesiculation. Itching, burning or pain. Heal with desquamation and hyperpigmentation. Self-limiting course.

Treatment

Prevent. Avoid overexposure to sunlight. Or use sunscreens or sunblocks. Topical (or systemic) corticosteroids for moderate to—severe cases. Antihistamines help only as antipruritics.

Solar Elastosis

Common among white populations exposed for prolonged periods to sunlight; hence commoner

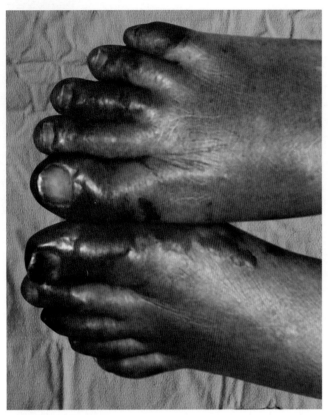

Frostbite: gangrenous tips of toes; erythema and blistering located proximally.

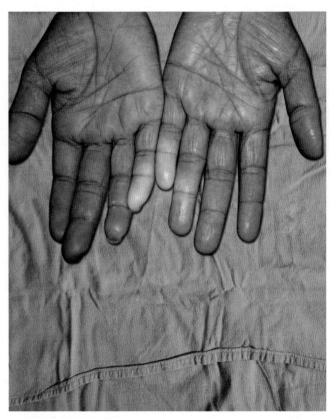

Raynaud's phenomenon: pallor of 2–3 fingers and rest all show bluish discoloration, including the palms.

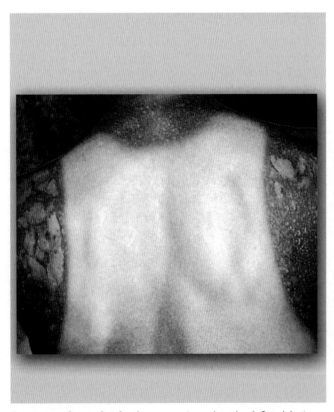

Severe sunburn, back: desquamating, sharply defined lesions; area covered by vest spared.

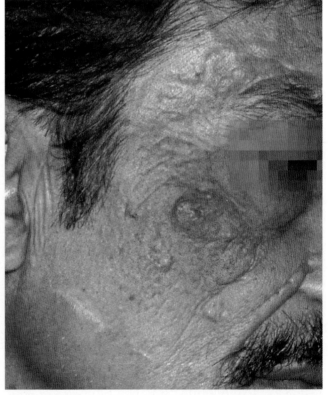

Solar elastosis: skin colored papules and comedones with exaggerated skin markings.

amongst farmers and sailors. Uncommon among colored races except in albinos, mountain dwellers and patients with vitiligo. Middle aged or older individuals. Face (malar areas), neck (nape) and dorsa of the hands generally involved. Several closely related syndromes. Characterized by degeneration of elastic tissue (and atrophy of epidermis). Pale translucent papules with wrinkling or furrowing of the skin. Comedonic lesions on the circumocular areas. Combination of solar elastosis and patulous open comedones known as Favre Racouchot syndrome.

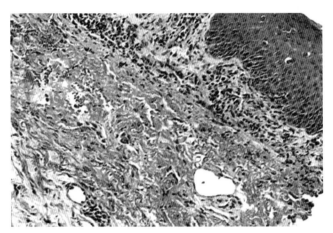

Histopathology of solar elastosis: basophilic, fine, short elastic fibers and amorphous material, upper dermis.

Treatment

Prevention—avoid excessive exposure to sunlight. Use sunscreens—organic. Or inorganic. Topical retinoic acid (0.05–0.1%) may help.

IDIOPATHIC PHOTODERMATOSES

Classification

Polymorphous light eruption
Chronic actinic dermatitis
Solar urticaria
Actinic prurigo
Hydroa vacciniforme

Polymorphous Light Eruption (PLE)

Epidemiology

Most common photosensitivity disorder with an estimated prevalence varying from 1 to 21%.

Etiology

Radiation spectrum—UVA >UVB >UVA + UVB. Possible delayed type hypersensitivity to endogenous cutaneous photo-induced antigen. Genetic predisposition.

Clinical Manifestations

'Polymorphous' designates interindividual variation. Usually there is development of eruption after minutes to hours after sun-exposure. Most commonly appears as grouped erythematous to skin colored papules sometimes coalescing to form plaques. Other variants include micropapular, hypopigmented, eczematous, lichenoid, papulo-vesicular, vesiculo-bullous, insect bite like, EM like, PMLE sine eruptions, etc.

Juvenile spring eruption—Involvement of ear helices of young boys in the form of papules and vesicles.

Photosensitive spongiotic and lichenoid eruption (PSLE) discrete to confluent papules over sun-exposed sites sparing face and histology showing spongiotic and lichenoid reaction patterns.

Investigations

Photoprovocation testing with UVA may be done in case of diagnostic confusion.

Chronic Actinic Dermatitis (Actinic Reticuloid; Photosensitivity Dermatitis; Photosensitive Eczema; Persistent Light Reactivity)

Epidemiology

Relatively uncommon disease. Males are much more commonly affected. More common in 6th to 7th decade.

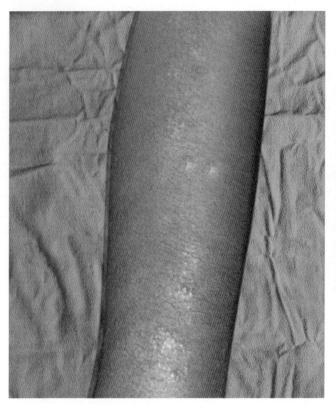

Polymorphous light eruption: lichenoid, micro-papular form, extensors of forearms.

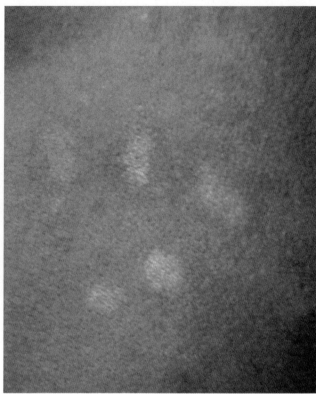

Hypopigmented variant of PMLE: hypopigmented patches over the shoulder.

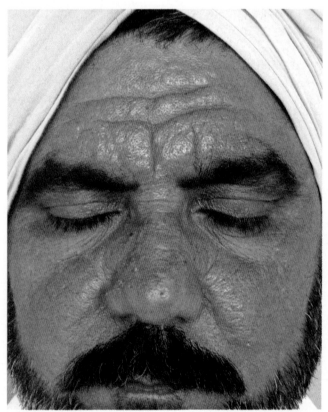

Chronic actinic dermatitis: erythematous infiltrated plaques over face, sparing the periorbital area, part of forehead covered by turban and relatively sparing the nasolabial folds.

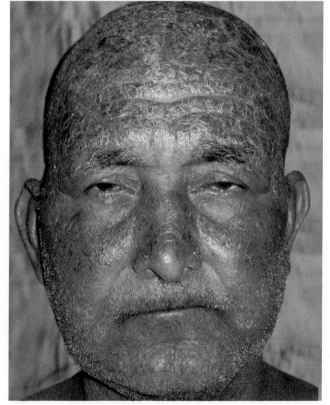

Chronic actinic dermatitis: erythematous scaly plaques diffusely involving face with sparing of the forehead wrinkles, periorbital and perioral area, and the nasolabial folds.

Etiology

Radiation spectrum—UVB >UVA >visible. It is considered a delayed type hypersensitivity response. It is an allergic contact dermatitis like response against UV damaged DNA or a similar or associated molecules.

Clinical Manifestations

Subacute or chronic, extremely pruritic eczema (papules, nodules and plaques) of predominantly sunexposed sites like face, back and sides of neck, upper chest, scalp, and dorsae of hands with clear cut off at lines of clothing. Upper eyelids, skin creases and folds are often spared. In severely affected patients, generalization to covered areas and erythroderma may rarely occur. Lichenification is common in chronic forms and diffuse lymphoma-like infiltration of face ('leonine' facies) may occur in advanced cases. Estimated probability of resolution at 10 years after diagnosis is 1 in 5. In 1990, Norris and Hawk gave unifying concept which considered CAD to be an end stage process which can arise either *de novo* or from photoallergic contact dermatitis, systemic drug induced photosensitivity and or endogenous eczema.

Diagnosis

Clinical. Patch and photopathic testing for allergic and photoallergic contact dermatitis. Histopathology shows variable epidermal spongiosis and acanthosis. Usually there is a deep dermal perivascular moderate to dense mononuclear infiltrate. Eosinophils and plasma cells may also occur. In more infiltrated cases, it may mimic lymphoma.

Solar Urticaria

Rare form of physical urticaria.

Etiology

Action spectrum—Visible >UVA and UVB. It is thought to be mediated through a type I hypersensitivity mechanism.

The IgE antibody is possibly formed against photoproduct of endogenous serum factors which have not been identified till now.

Clinical Manifestations

Appears within few minutes of sun exposure. Very rarely appears after a few hours. Manifest as itching or burning sensation followed by erythema and whealing which subsides within few hours without any sequelae.

Diagnosis

Clinical. Phototprovocation testing helps.

Actinic Prurigo

It mainly affects Mestizo populations of American countries such as Mexico, Central and South America.

Radiation spectrum—UVA >UVB. It has been suggested to be an autoimmune disease associated with an altered epidermal protein antigen. Strong HLA associations. Symmetrical involvement of sun-exposed area of the skin like face (eyebrows, malar, nose, lips), neck, V area of chest, extensors of arms, forearms and dorsae of hands. Lips (in up to 84% patients) and conjunctiva (in upto 45% patients) are commonly involved. Lesions are in the form of erythematous papules, excoriations and lichenified plaques. They heal with dyspigmentation and scarring.

Hydroa Vacciniforme

Very rare photodermatosis of unknown etiology. Action spectrum lies mainly in the UVA region (UVA >UVB). Presents in childhood which sometimes improves in adolescence. Erythema with a burning sensation followed by appearance of tender papules which later become vesicular, umblicated and occasionally confluent and hemorrhagic. Heal within few weeks leaving behind permanent, depressed, hypopigmented pox like scars.

Treatment of Idiopathic Photodermatosis

Shade/sun protective behavior, wide brimmed hats, clothing, glass, sunscreens, specific measures.

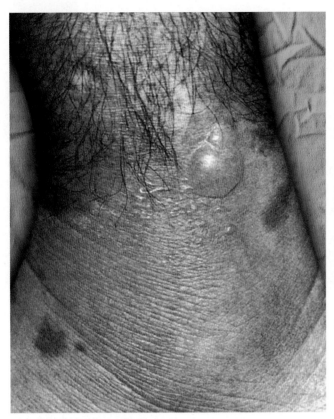

Phototoxic contact dermatitis: topical psoralen induced. The depigmented area affected.

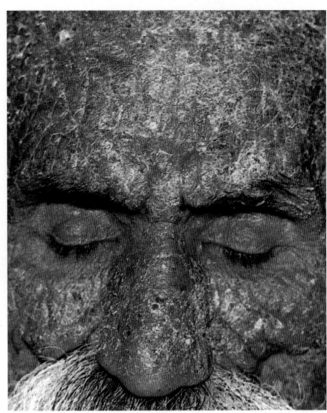

Photoallergic contact dermatitis: due to Parthenium hysterophorus; circumocular area spread.

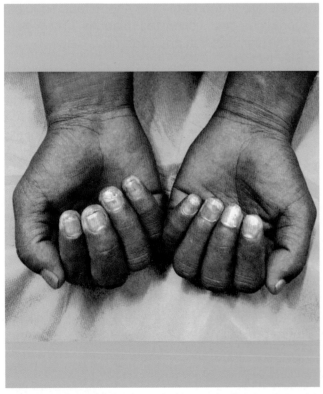

Photo onycholysis: distal onycholysis and adjoining brownish discoloration of a patient on PUVA therapy.

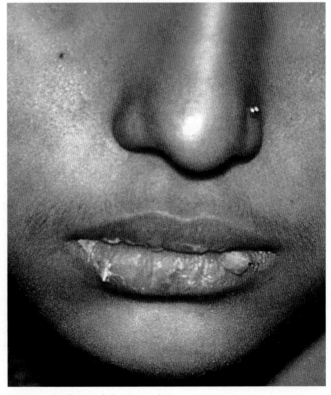

Actinic cheilitis: of the lower lip.

Phase	Polymorphous light eruption	Chronic actinic dermatitis	Solar urticaria	Actinic prurigo	Hydroa vacciniformis
Acute flare	Topical/systemic steroids	Topical/Oral steroids	Photoprotection, H1 antihistamines	Thalidomide	None/symptomatic
Chronic/refractory cases	Antimalarials, Immuno-suppressants	Topical calcineurins, Cs, MTX, AZA, MMF, low dose PUVA	CsA, plasmapheresis/ ECP	Antimalarials, antihistamines, steroids (t/s)	-
Prevention	Sunprotection > Phototherapy	Avoid allergens, UV protective clothing	Sunprotection, UVA/ PUVA desensitization	Sunprotection > Phototherapy	Sunprotection > Phototherapy

Cs: Cyclosporine; AZA: Azathioprine; MTX: Methotrexate; MMF: Mycophenolate mofetil; ECP: Extracorporeal photopheresis; PUVA: Psoralen and ultraviolet A; Steroids (t/s): topical/systemic

Photocontact Dermatitis

Caused by topical contact of the skin with a chemical followed by exposure to light. Mechanistically may be non-immunologic, designated phototoxic contact dermatitis. Or immunologic, called photo-allergic contact dermatitis.

Phototoxic Contact Dermatitis

Light induced counterpart of contact irritant dermatitis. Damage caused by the direct effect of a photo product. Exaggerated sunburn reaction.

Psoralens, tars, dyes and fragrances chiefly responsible. Psoralens employed therapeutically in topical PUVA followed by inadvertent over-exposure to light from sun or artificial sources. Phototoxic contact dermatitis caused by plants (again mostly containing psoralens) called phytophotodermatitis. Heals with hyperpigmentation.

Treatment

Mild cases, soothing lotions. Acute stage—treat with topical or systemic steroids. Can restart after recovery; but with lower concentrations of psoralens and smaller doses of light.

Photoallergic Contact Dermatitis

Immunologically mediated. Light induced (generally UVA) counterpart of allergic contact dermatitis. Confined initially and chiefly to light exposed areas. Later, may spread to light covered areas too. Historically, halogenated salicylanilides important—fortunately not used now. Other potential photocontactants: para-amino benzoic acid (PABA) and its derivatives, buclosamide, fragrances and plants of the composite family—Parthenium hysterophorus in India, Chrysanthemum in the West.

Acute dermatitis infrequently seen. Presents as subacute or chronic lichenified dermatitis on the face, pinna of the ears, 'V' of the neck and dorsa of the forearms and hands. Retroauricular folds and undersurface of the chin conspicuously spared. Sharp margination. Photopatch test positive.

Treatment

Topical or systemic steroids and sunscreens organic and inorganic. Avoid further exposure to photocontactant and sunlight. Methotrexate, azathioprine and cyclosporine useful as steroid sparing agents in severe/extensive disease.

Photosensitivity to Systemic Agents

May induce sunburn-like (phototoxic) or lichenoid, urticarial or papular (photoallergic) responses. Psoralens, tetracyclines, sulphonamides, sulphonylureas, thiazide diuretics, chlorpromazine, NSAIDs often responsible. Pseudoporphyria response (fragility of light exposed skin) also seen. Photo-onycholysis can occur with long-term use of doxycycline and PUVA.

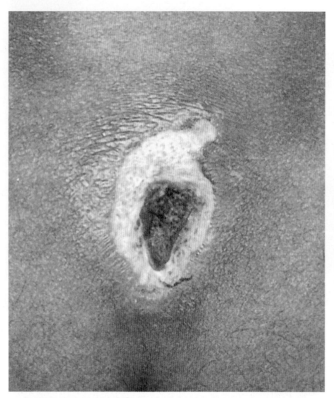

Decubitus ulcer: ulceration with necrotic skin in the middle; sacral area.

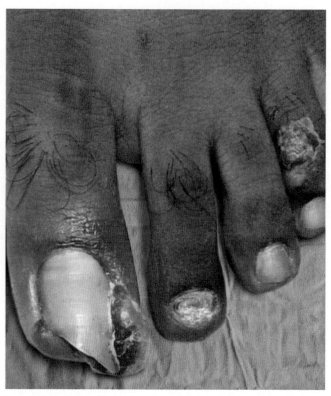

Ingrowing toe nails: mass of granulation on either side of the great toe nail.

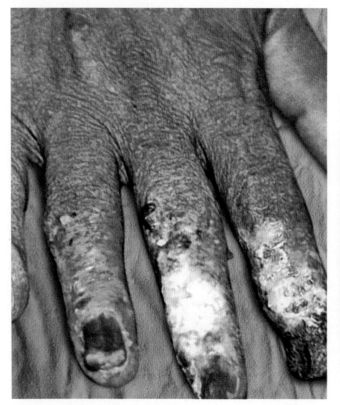

Radiodermatitis: atrophy, depigmentation and ulcerations on the fingers of a radiotherapist.

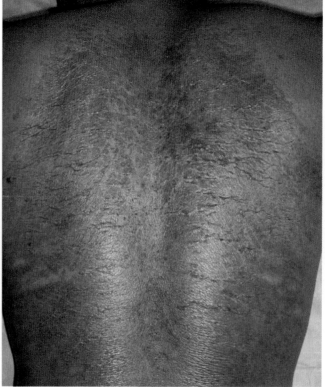

Frictional sweat dermatitis: diffuse but well-defined area of thin polythene like scaling with focal peeling and fissuring over the back in area apposed to the vest (please note that shoulders and nape of neck and adjoining upper back are free).

Treatment

Discontinue the drug. Avoid exposure to sunlight. Topical or systemic steroids and sunscreens.

Actinic Cheilitis

Uncommon. Lower lip affected. Secondary to prolonged exposure to sunlight. Or a manifestation of actinic prurigo or xeroderma pigmentosum. Asymptomatic redness and swelling; later, scaling, fissuring, crusting and thickening of the lower lip. Long standing cheilitis becomes verrucous and may become malignant.

Treatment

Avoid further sunlight exposure. Topical application of retinoic acid or 5-fluorouracil (5 FU). Combination of 5 FU with a potent steroid reduces inflammation.

DISORDERS DUE TO EXPOSURE TO MISCELLANEOUS PHYSICAL STIMULI

Decubitus Ulcer

Occurs amongst the immobilized or bedridden patients. Elderly individuals. Diabetics, paralytics and patients with urinary and/or fecal incontinence, more prone. Persistent pressure results in ischemia, necrosis and ulceration. Sacral area most commonly affected; less frequently other pressure sites overlying bony prominences. Ulcers with undermined edges, variable in depth, and covered with necrotic, sloughed tissue. Surrounding area red and edematous.

Treatment

Prevent. Relieve pressure—by early mobilization, frequent change of postures and use of water or rubber air mattresses. Efficient nursing, key factor.

Treat with debridement, relief of pressure and covering with topical antibiotic dressings.

Ingrowing Toe Nails

Common. Caused by intrusion of an edge or a spicule of nail plate into the lateral nail fold. Ill-fitting shoes or faulty clipping of nails. Painful and tender. Mild erythema followed by swelling, pus formation and sometimes mass of granulation tissue on the medial, lateral or both sides of great toe(s).

Treatment

Appropriate wide footwear. Excise nail spicules. Treat granulation mass with warm compresses and topical or systemic antibiotics or chemical cauterization. In recurrent and severe cases— nail splinting (using cover of butterfly IV cannula, kept in place for 2–6 weeks), lateral matricectomy (chemical-using phenol; surgical excision).

Radiodermatitis

Uncommon. Accidental or injudicious administration of high doses of ionizing radiation. *Acute reactions:* erythema, edema and blistering that heal with scaling and pigmentation. *Chronic radiodermatitis:* atrophy, telangiectasia, loss of pigmentation, ulceration, necrosis. Malignancies may appear after several years.

Treatment

Unsatisfactory. *Acute reactions:* topical corticosteroids. *Chronic dermatitis:* emollients. Avoid trauma. Biopsy, if suspicion of malignancy.

Frictional Sweat Dermatitis

It is an entity characterized by involvement of the area beneath the undergarments or other apparels in direct contact with the skin. Occurs in the hot and humid seasons and lesions are in the form of barely elevated plaques with a shiny wrinkled surface. Mild erythema and fissuring may also be present. Lesions usually scales of in 1–2 weeks without any sequelae. Avoidance of hot temperature, cold water bathing leads to subsidence but in very symptomatic patients, topical steroid may be helpful.

15

Diseases of the Skin Appendages

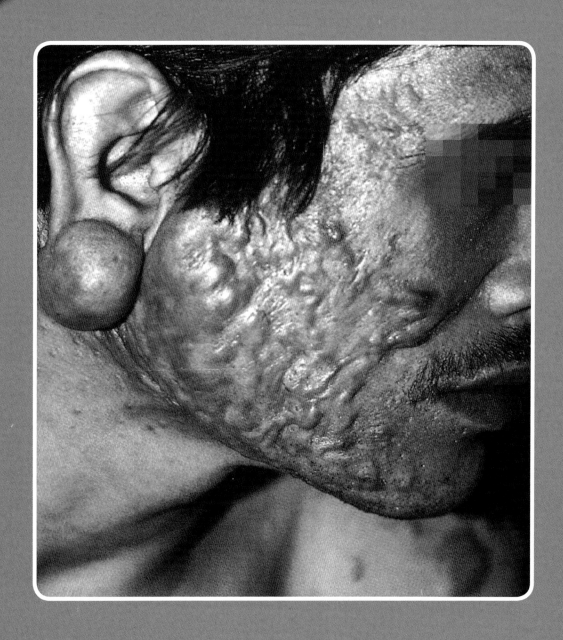

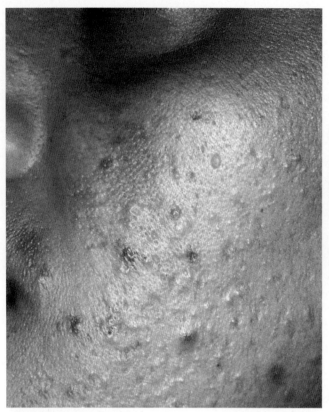

Acne vulgaris: comedones, inflammatory papules and some pitted scars.

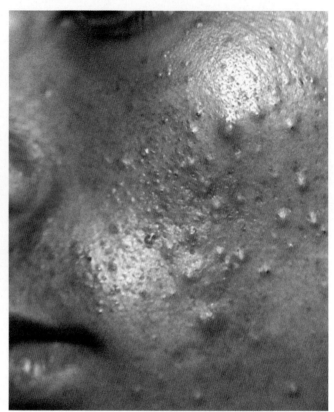

Acne vulgaris: comedones and inflammatory papules.

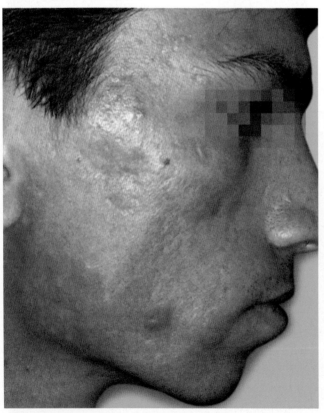

Acne vulgaris, healed: atrophic and pitted scars; occasional papules.

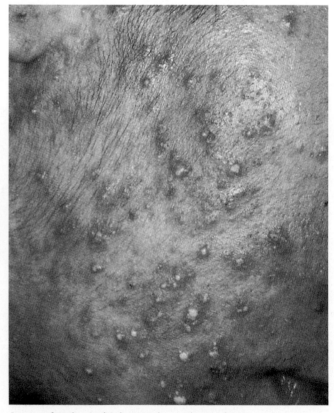

Acne vulgaris: multiple papules and pustules.

Hair, nails, sebaceous and sweat (apocrine and eccrine glands) constitute skin appendages. All derived from the epidermis. Eccrine sweat glands, efficient cooling system; other appendages relatively unimportant. Hair serve aesthetic and psychological functions predominantly, along with its protective function at sites like anterior nares, eyebrows and eyelashes. Nails not only protect the dorsal aspect of finger and toe tips but also provide the precision in picking-up small objects. They also serve aesthetic function. Hair, sebaceous glands and apocrine sweat glands exist in intimate anatomical relationship. Eccrine sweat glands open independently on the skin surface.

Dermatoses affecting appendages heterogeneous and of varying importance; those affecting sebaceous glands and hair frequent and most significant.

DISORDERS OF SEBACEOUS GLANDS

Common dermatoses affecting the pilosebaceous unit. Primary lesion, a *comedone*, a non-inflammatory papule produced by obstruction of the pilosebaceous passage. Obstruction on the surface or within the skin; the comedone respectively, called an *open* (black head) or *closed comedone* (white head). Most common acneiform dermatosis, *acne vulgaris*. Several others—drug induced, due to topical applications or unrelated factors.

Acne Vulgaris

Epidemiology

Probably most common disease affecting human beings, usually more senesce in males.

Etiology

- *Seborrhea:* Excessive androgen production or availability of free androgens or intracellular binding capacity.
- *Comedo formation:* Increase keratinocyte proliferation and decrease desquamation.
- *Propinobacterium acnes colonization*
  - Enzymes may promote follicular wall rupture.
  - Heat shock proteins promote inflammation.
  - Porphyrins may lead to adjacent tissue damage.
  - Toll like receptor-2 binds to *P. acnes* and leads to release of proinflammatory cytokines IL-8 and IL-12.
- *Inflammation*
  - Local perifollicular CD4 T-cells and IL-1 levels
  - Increased neutrophils → pustules
  - Increase lymphocytes and foreign body giant cells → papules, nodules and cysts.

Other factors

- *Diet:* Still unclear. Few studies established causation with high glycemic diets and dairy products.

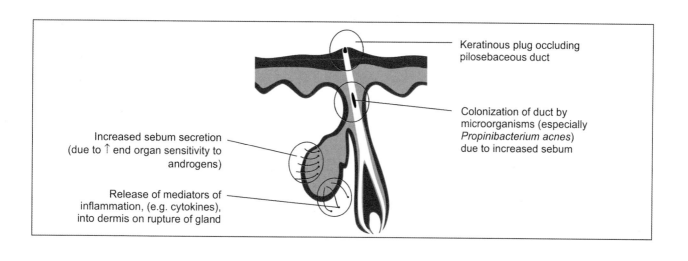

Keratinous plug occluding pilosebaceous duct

Colonization of duct by microorganisms (especially *Propinibacterium acnes*) due to increased sebum

Increased sebum secretion (due to ↑ end organ sensitivity to androgens)

Release of mediators of inflammation, (e.g. cytokines), into dermis on rupture of gland

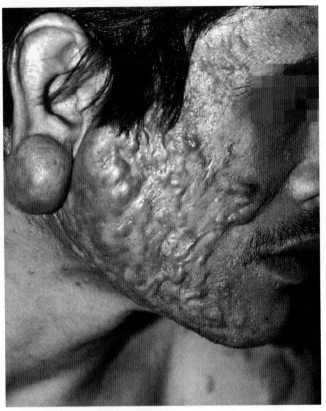

Acne vulgaris, healed: disfiguring hypertrophic scars.

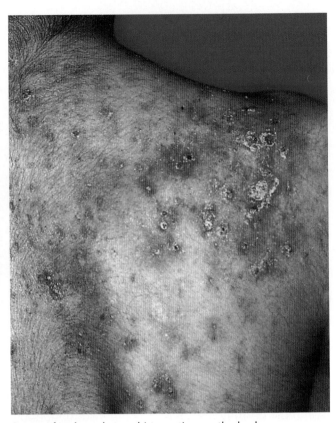

Acne vulgaris: polymorphic eruption on the back.

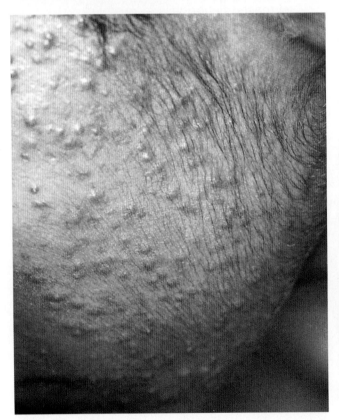

Drug-induced acne: monomorphic papules.

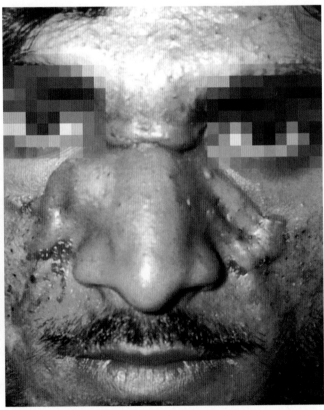

Acne conglobata: interconnecting sinus tracts with nodulocystic acne.

- Premenstrual flare in upto 70%.
- *Pregnancy:* Usually acne improves.
- *Facials:* Acne worsen.

Clinical Manifestations

- Face involved in 99%, back involved in 60%, chest in 15%.
- *Noninflammatory lesions:* Comedones, macrocomedones, submarrine comedones
- *Inflammatory lesions:* Papules, pustules, nodules, erythematous nodules
- *Scars:* Atrophic (Icepick, boxcar, rolling). Hypertrophic (keloid, papular, bridging).

Investigations

- Usually none are required
- Endocrine evaluation may be required in following situations
  - Late onset (>25 years of age)
  - Therapy resistant acne
  - Hyperandrogenism
    - Irregular menses
    - Hirsutism
    - Perioral lesions
    - Hyperseborrhea
- Endocrine evaluation includes
  - Testosterone, SHBG, DHEAS, FSH, LH, PRL, thyroid profile
  - Bld Sgs(F), HOMA-IR
  - Dexamethasone suppression test (for Cushing's)

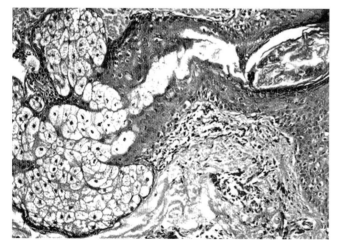

Histopathology of acne vulgaris: keratotic plug in the duct with dilated sebaceous glands; infiltrate in upper dermis.

- Evaluation for PCOS (Polycystic ovarian syndrome)

Treatment

General Measures

Aimed at removing the keratotic plug, decreasing the bacterial population and reducing the size and activity of sebaceous glands. Evidence in literature supporting uses of facial cleaners in treatment of acne is of poor quality.

Specific Treatment

Combination of topical retinoids and tetracyclines (oral) is better than either when given alone. Topical fixed dose combination also better than either alone.

Topical therapy

Depending on severity. Frequent soap and water washes; *avoid* vigorous scrubbing. Topical application of retinoic acid (tretinoin), 0.025, 0.05 or 0.1%, cream/gel, preferably at bed time. Acts as a keratoplastic and keratolytic agent. Start with low concentrations and graduate to higher. Mild irritation not uncommon; if severe, discontinue therapy. Causes photosensitivity in some. Adapalene (0.1%), a newer tretinoin-like agent, causes less irritation and is as effective as 0.025% tretinoin. Tazarotene (0.05%, 0.1%) also effective.

Topical antibiotics—1–2% erythromycin or clindamycin lotion/cream. Benzoyl peroxide, 2, 5 or 10% lotion or cream. Act against *P. acnes*. Azelaic acid, 10–20% a more recent antibacterial agent. Dapsone 5%, recently introduced, also effective.

Systemic therapy

Several antibiotics used—tetracyclines and macrolides. Given for moderate-severe disease. Repeated courses of systemic antibiotics act against microbes and their enzymes; tetracyclines also acts as antiandrogenic. Minocycline, perhaps the most effective tetracycline. Erythromycin may also be useful. Can use full therapeutic doses or small doses over long periods.

Isotretinoin, a retinoid (vitamin A derivative) extremely useful in moderately severe and severe acne including nodulocystic variants. Dose 0.5–1 mg/kg/day for 16–20 weeks.

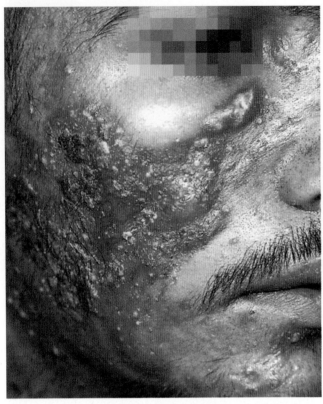

Acne conglobata: multiple inflammatory cysts and burrowing sinuses.

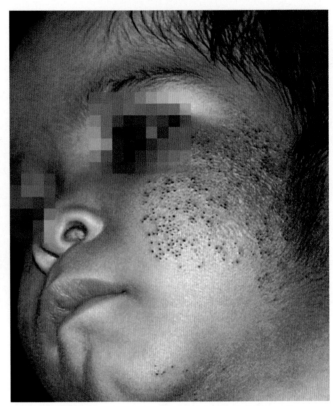

Acne venenata: comedones due to application of vegetable (mustard) oil.

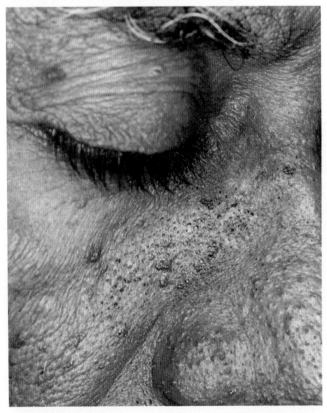

Senile comedones: note associated wrinkling of skin due to solar elastosis.

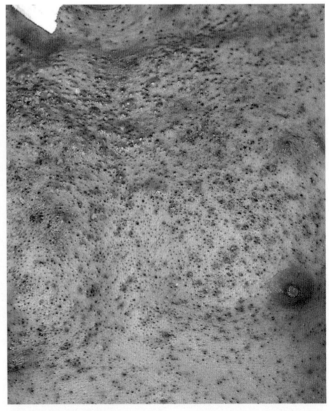

Acne venenata, chest: comedones and inflammatory papules on contact with cutting oils.

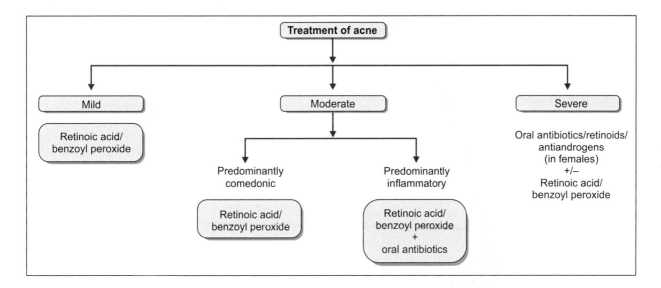

In each course, 120–150 mg/kg can be given. Potentially teratogenic, hyperlipidemic and mildly hepatotoxic. Cheilitis, dryness of skin and eyes, dry mouth and nose universal. *Contraception mandatory* in females of childbearing age. Single course generally adequatea—second course only in case of severe relapse.

ACNE VARIANTS

Acne Conglobata

Suppurating acne. Chronic. Relatively uncommon. Young males affected. More frequent on back, chest and shoulders; occasionally on buttocks and thighs. Double or triple comedones, inflammatory papules, nodules and cysts; burst on the surface. Or burrow within the skin, forming interconnecting sinus tracts. Heal with disfiguring scars. Acne conglobata, part of follicular retention triad; hidradenitis suppurativa and dissecting folliculitis of the scalp.

Treatment

Appropriate systemic antibiotics with or without steroids. Isotretinoin, in doses of 1–2 mg/kg/day for 4–5 months, drug of choice.

Acne Venenata

Occupational hazard in people exposed to halogenated hydrocarbons, cutting oils, crude petroleum. Use of cosmetics, vegetable oils or topical corticosteroids responsible in some.

Lesions chiefly open comedones, with or without inflammatory papules or papulopustules. Site depends on area of contact.

Treatment

Mild lesions resolve spontaneously. Or with topical retinoic acid. Severe disease may need systemic isotretinoin.

Acne Fulminans

Adolescent males, most commonly trunk, abrupt/rapid onset over mild to moderate acne, associated with fever, polyarthropathy, leucocytosis, malaise, bony pain, etc. Lesions become nodular, painful, ulcerate and heal with scarring. Triggers include-testosterone, anabolic steroids, isotretinoin, seasonal infections like EBV, propioniobacterium acnes. Pus and blood culture usually sterile.

Treatment

Oral prednisolone. 0.5–1 m/kg/day slowly tapered and stopped over 2–3 months. Crust removal using emollients and antibiotic creams.

Infantile and Neonatal Acne

Neonatal acne—presents at 2–3 years of age as erythematous papules over nasal bridge. Infantile acne—presents at 3–6 months of age usually as comedones.

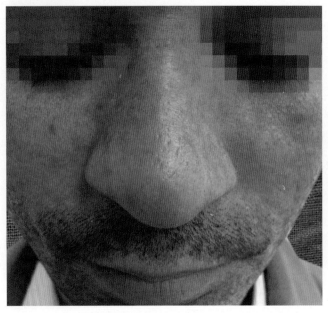

Erythemo-telangiectatic rosacea: diffuse erythema and telangiectasias over cheeks and nose.

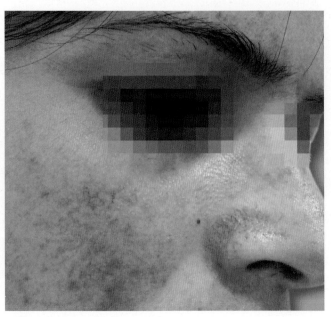

Topical steroid induced rosacea: telangiectasias over cheek and nasal ala after chronic use of topical steroid for melasma.

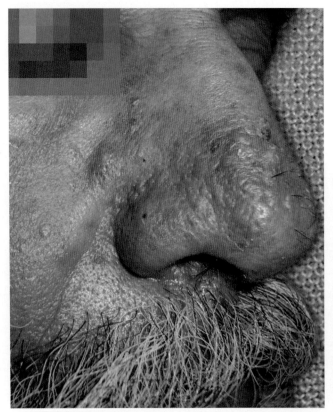

Papulo-pustular rosacea: diffuse erythema over nose with mild rhinophymatous change, studded with papules and pustules.

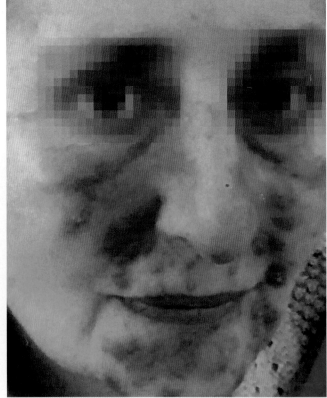

Rosacea fulminans: confluent erythematous plaques, nodules and pustules over the nose and adjoining cheeks.

Courtesy: Prof AJ Kanwar, Dermatologist, Noida.

Senile Comedones

A cluster of pure comedones. Commonly associated with solar elastosis (combination also known as Favre Racouchot syndrome). Elderly individuals, males more often. Periorbital area generally involved.

Treatment

Topical retinoic acid, 0.025–0.05% gel or cream, but with caution!. Comedone extraction.

Rosacea

Epidemiology

Both men and women affected, onset usually after 30 years of age.

Etiology

Multifactorial, uncertain. Altered facial vascular reactivity, microbial colonization, connective tissue structure, pilosebaceous. Triggers include temperature, sunlight, spicy food, alcohol, emotions, cosmetics, irritants, etc.

Clinical Manifestations

Four subtypes—erythemo-telangiectatic (ET), papulo-pustular (PP), phymatous and ocular.

Subtypes may or may not be sequential. Symptoms of facial burning, stinging, roughness, sensitivity, etc. Variable severity. ET type has persistent facial erythema, flushing, telangiectasias, edema. PP has papules and pustules over convexities of face. Phymatous type named according to site—rhinophyma (nose), metophyma (forehead), gnathophyma (chin), blepharophyma (eyelid) and otophyma (ear). Tortuous soft tissue hypertrophy, nodular, thickened skin and patulous follicular ostia. Ocular includes blepharitis, conjuctivitis, keratitis. Granulomatous rosacea is true variant. It has monomorphic erythematous papules and nodules over cheeks and periorificial area. Granuloma seen on histopathology.

Treatment

Erythemo-telangiectatic—Topical antimicrobials (1% metronidazole gel, 1% clindamycin gel). Oral doxycycline/minocycline 100–200 mg/day for several weeks. Topical retinoids. Vascular lasers like PDL, IPL.

Papulo-pustular—In addition to above, oral low dose retinoids and topical retinoids. Occasionally a few day course of low dose oral steroids may be needed to tide over acute inflammatory edema/pustulation.

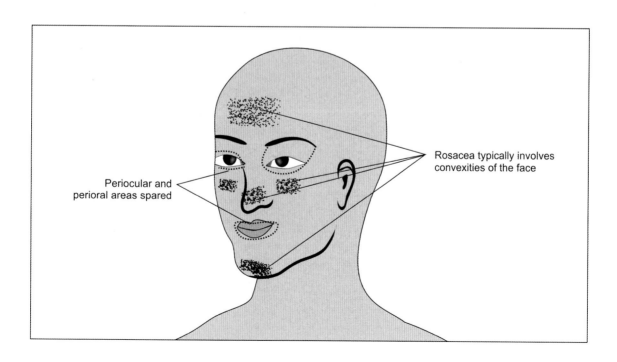

Rosacea typically involves convexities of the face

Periocular and perioral areas spared

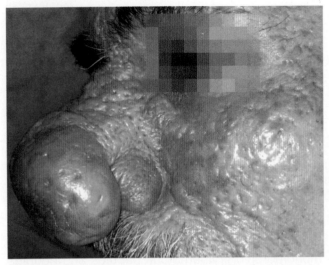

Rhinophyma: marked soft tissue hypertrophy of nose causing distortion of shape and obstructing the external nares.

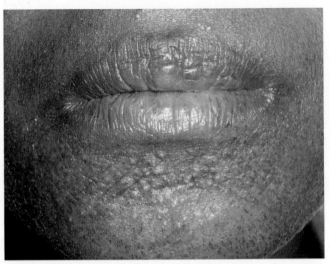

Perioral dermatitis: erythematous papules and few vesicles over background xerosis in perioral distribution.

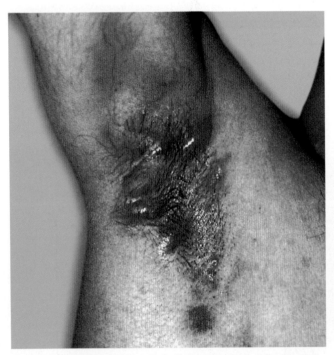

Hidradenitis suppurativa, early lesion: multiple 'blind' boils.

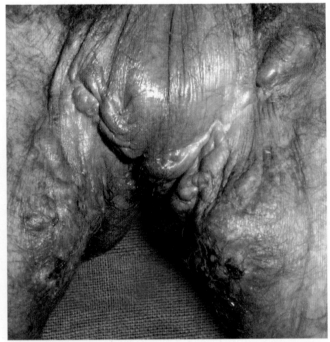

Hidradenitis suppurativa: multiple abscesses, bridging sinuses and scarring.

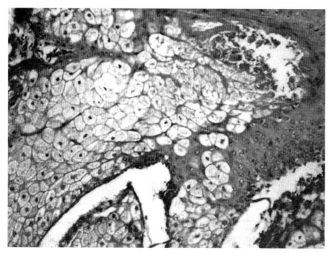

Histopathology of rhinophyma: dilated sebaceous glands.

Rhinophyma

Uncommon. Elderly males generally affected. Caused by hyperplasia of sebaceous glands and connective tissue. Skin colored or reddish, often lobulated swelling of the tip and distal part of the nose. Patulous pilosebaceous orifices. Foul smelling cheesy material expressed on pressure. Often end result of long standing/untreated rosacea. Huge nasal swelling may cause obstruction to breathing. But complaints is usually of cosmetic and social nature.

Treatment

Mild initial swelling/nodulation may respond to oral isotretinoin but fully formed lobulated swelling requires surgical interventions like CO_2 laser. Electrosurgery and blade surgery followed by flap repair.

Perioral Dermatitis

Correct term should be periorificial dermatitis, perioral, perinasal, periorbital. Most common trigger topical fluorinated steroid use/abuse. Idiopathic in children (esp. granulomatous variant). Other lesions papules, vesicles/pustules.

Treatment

Topical Therapy

- Metronidazole, clindamycin, erythromycin.

Systemic Therapy

- Tetracyclines, erythromycin.

DISORDERS OF APOCRINE GLANDS

Hidradenitis Suppurativa (also known as Acne Inversa)

Epidemiology

- Onset usually in young adults.
- More common in females.

Etiology

- Initially thought primary apocrine inflammation but now postulated apocrine glands become secondarily involved.
- Follicular oulusion.
- Familial tendency may be there.
- Bacterial infection as a cause is +/–.
- Smoking may worsen.

Clinical Manifestations

- *Intertriginous area:* Axillae, inguinal, perineal, thighs.
- *Hurley staging*
  - Stage I: Isolated abscesses
  - Stage II: Sinuses with bridging scars.
  - Stage III: Chronic discharge, bridging scars, sinuses and fibrosis, soft tissue hypertrophy.
- Initial lesion a tender, painful, erythematous, intracutaneous nodule a 'blind' or 'closed' boil. Bursts on the surface with seropurulent discharge. Or burrows within the skin to infect adjoining glands and form interconnecting sinus tracts. Recurrences common. Simultaneous appearance of fresh lesions and scars continues for months or years.
- *Complication:* Anal/urethral/rectal strictures.

Investigations

- Pus cultures from abscesses/deep part of sinuses.
- MRI to see complete event of scarring, sinuses and abcesses.
- *Histopathology:* Folliculitis/perifolliculitis suppuration granuloma.

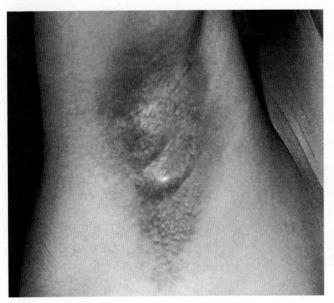

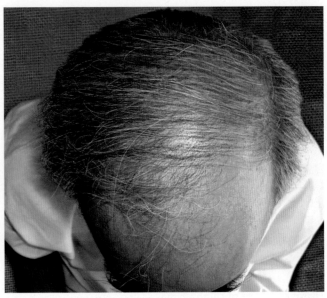

Fox-Fordyce disease: follicular papules of fox-fordyce disease (below the furuncle in axilla).

Androgenic alopecia male, advanced: frontoparietal and occipital baldness.

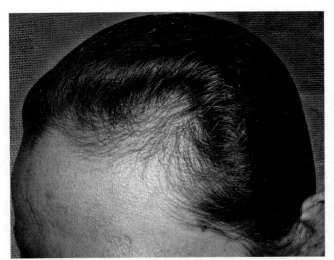

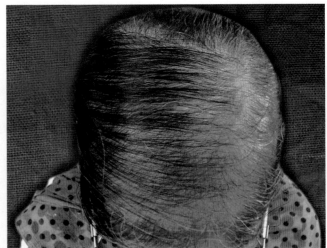

Female pattern hair loss, hamilton type: bitemporal recession and early baldness.

Female pattern hair loss, advanced: diffuse hair loss and baldness.

Treatment

General Measures

Proper cleaning, keeping dry.

Specific Treatment

- *Hurley stage I:* Topical clindamycin/erythromycin. Oral antibiotics (clindamycin, rifampicin, minocycline/doxycycline)
- *Hurley stage II:* As for stage I + localized excision.
- *Hurley stage III:* As for stage II + wide excision, biologicals (infliximab).

Fox-Fordyce Disease

Uncommon. Etiology unknown. Young adult females affected. Results from obstruction and rupture of ducts of apocrine glands—*apocrine miliaria*. Discrete, dome-shaped, skin-colored follicular or parafollicular papules. Extremely pruritic. Chronic course. Pregnancy and use of contraceptive pills induce remission. Axillae most commonly affected, followed by pubic area and perineum, areolae and periumblical area.

Treatment

It is difficult.

Topical Therapy

- Topical clindamycin, tretinoin. Topical steroids give symptomatic relief.

Systemic/Surgical Therapy

- Oral contraceptive pill may induce remission.
- Surgery may be required in cases with intractable pruritus. Excision, electrosurgery, liposuction.

DISORDERS OF HAIR

Alopecia

Thinning, loss or involution of hair. Cicatricial or non-cicatricial. Cicatricial alopecia associated with scarring and thus destruction of hair follicles, hence irreversible.

NON-CICATRICIAL ALOPECIA

Non-cicatricial may be reversible or irreversible. Several types—androgenetic, alopecia areata, telogen effluvium, anagen effluvium, systemic disease such as SLE or local disease such as tinea capitis.

Androgenetic Alopecia (AGA, also known as Patterned Hair Loss)

Epidemiology

- Most common form of hair loss.
- > 50% men (lesser portion of women) develop it by 5th decade, family history strong contribution in males.

Etiology

- Males—Androgen dependent, genetic factor.
- Female—Androgens contribute but association not very clear.

Clinical Manifestations

Males—Hamilton Norwood classification from grade I and VII, starts with bitemporal recession, progresses to frontal/vertex thinning.
Females—3 patterns:
1. Male type (Hamilton)
2. Frontal accentuation of parting (Olsen)
3. Diffuse (Ludwig).

Course

Invariably progressive (slow/rapid).

Investigations

- Diagnosis usually clinical.
- In cases suspected of hyperandrogenism—Free and total testosterone, DHEA-S, LH/FSH, PRL, USG ovaries/adrenals.

Treatment

- Males
  - Mild disease (grade II and III)—Minoxidil 5% or oral finasteride 1 mg
  - Severe AGA (> grade III)—Hair transplant + minoxidil/Finasteride
- Female AGA treatment
  - Premenopausal
    - Hyperandrogenism—finasteride, cyperoterone acetate, spironolactone
    - No hyperandrogenism—minoxidil 2%
  - Postmenopausal—Hormone replacement therapy + 2% minoxidil.

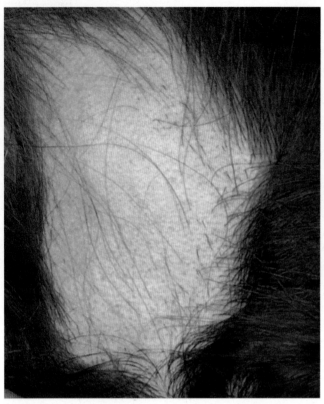

Alopecia areata: localized lesion scalp; note 'exclamation' mark (!) hair.

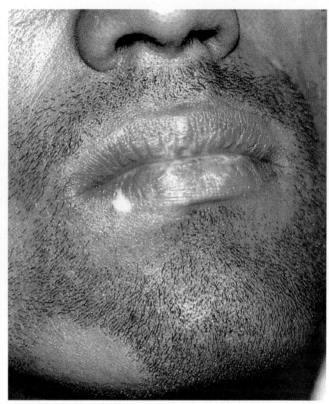

Alopecia areata, chin: well-defined patch of non-cicatricial alopecia; vitiliginous lesion on the lower lip.

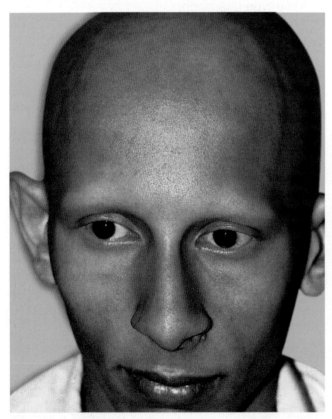

Alopecia universalis: loss of hair from scalp, eyebrows and rest of body.

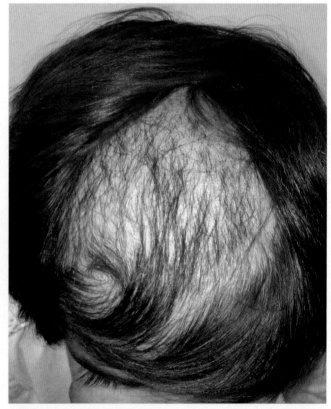

Trichotillomania: solitary alopecic patch on frontal scalp with broken hair of variable lengths.

Alopecia Areata

Epidemiology

- Life time estimated prevalence between 1 and 2%.
- Incidence more in children.

Etiology

- Autoimmune disease—Autoreacting CD8 T-cells.
- Genetic factors—Family history (+) in many cases.

Associations

Certain associations—vitiligo, atopy, uveitis, diabetes mellitus, Down's syndrome.

Clinical Manifestations

Morphology

- Patterns
  - Patchy
  - Ophiasis (band like)
  - Reticular
  - Ophiasis immunesus
  - Diffuse
- Extent
  - Patchy – Areata
  - Total scalp – Totalis
  - Total body – Universalis
  - New subtype – Acute diffuse and total alopecia.

Generally sudden onset. One (or a few), well-defined, oval or circular area of total loss of hair. Exclamation mark (!) hair at the periphery. Underlying scalp (or skin) normal in color and texture; occasionally shiny and mildly wrinkled. Recovery, often with regrowth of white hair, later regain pigment. Associated nail changes—pitting, dystrophy.

Sites of Predilection

Scalp, beard, upper lip, eyebrows, eyelashes or other hair—bearing regions affected.

Course

Unpredictable. Spontaneous recovery common in solitary lesions. May show gradual or rapid progression. Remitting and relapsing course. More favorable course in mild cases < 25% of area involved. May progress to involve the total scalp (*alopecia totalis*) or the whole body (alopecia universalis). Poor prognostic factors—Ophiasic pattern, reticular pattern, family history, atopy, age at onset < 10 kg, extensive disease (totalis/universalis).

Investigations

Usually clinical is sufficient.
- Hair pull test usually negative.
- KOH mount—to rule out tinea capitis.
- Biopsy lymphocytic infiltrate in perifollicular and intrafollicular area esp. around the hair bulb ('Swarm of Bees' appearance).

Treatment

Hair loss < 50% of scalp/localized
- Topical or ½ steroid
- Minoxidil 5%
- Topical dithranol.

Hair Loss > 50% of Scalp/Extensive
- Contact immunotherapy (DPCP).
- Minoxidil 5% + topical steroid/anthralin.
- PUVA
- Systemic steroid—oral mini pulse.
Experimental therapy—JAK inhibitors (ruxolitinib, tofacitinib).

Trichotillomania (Hair Pulling Tic)

An impulse control disorder.

Epidemiology

- More common in children.
- Overall, more common in females.
- In adults, it may be associated with mood disorders.

Etiology

- **Children:** Lack of attention, sibling rivalary, learning disability, unhappiness.
- **Adults:** Anxiety, mood disorders, mental retardation.

Clinical Manifestations

- Most commonly scalp is affected, other uncommon like the eyebrows/beard.

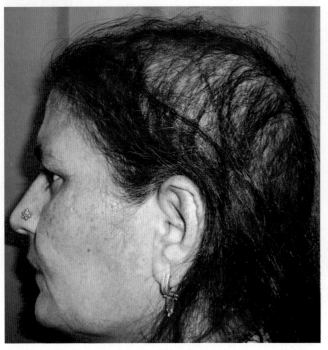

Trichotillomania, tonsure type: diffuse alopecia over scalp with sparing of a rim of long hair along the hairline.

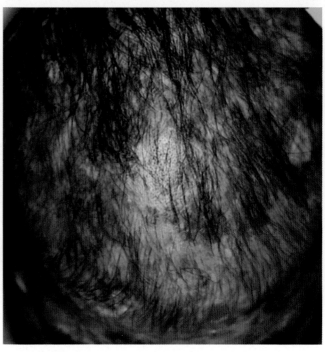

Anagen effluvium: due to cyclophosphamide therapy.

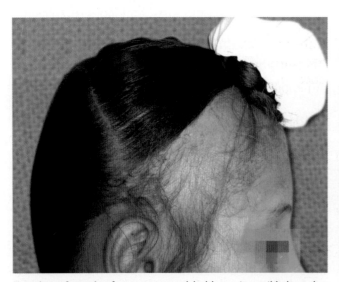

Traction alopecia: fronto-temporal baldness in a sikh boy due to hair tying for turban.

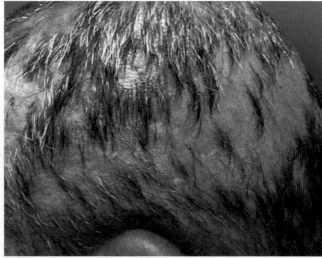

Pseudopelade of Brocq: discrete to confluent skin colored patches of hair loss, sparing intervening hair. Some oval patches appear in line suggestive of 'foot prints in the snow'.

- Tonsure alopecia—Full scalp involved, hair remaining only over the margins of scalp.
- Trichophagia +/–.
- Hair are of uneven length over the alopecic area of appear broken off.

Investigation

- KOH—To rule out tinea capitis.
- Biopsy—Empty hair follicles, perifollicular hemorrhages, trichomalacia, pigment casts.

Treatment

- Referral to psychiatrist.
- Selective serotonin reuptake inhibitors, low dose neuroleptics, lithium.
- Most important—Behavioral therapy.

Telogen Effluvium (TE)

Diffuse hair loss of terminal hair which causes baldness only in advanced cases.

Epidemiology

- More common in females.
- 2nd most common cause of hair fall after AGA.
- Can coexist with AGA.

Etiology

Multifactorial and still poorly understood.
- Endocrine
- Systemic illness
- Stressful events
- Nutritional
- Intoxication
- Drugs
- Inflammatory scalp dermatoses.

Clinical Manifestations

Patterns

- Acute/classic (duration < 6 months).
- Chronic (> 6 months)—idiopathic.
- Chronic diffuse telogen hair loss (> 6 months)—2° to above factors.

Complain of bunches of hair coming out on combing. Baldness in advanced cases only.

Investigations

- Hair pull test—Positive in acute and active stage of chronic TE.
- Trichogram—Anagen to telogen ratio reduces.
- Biopsy—Increase % of telogen hair to 8 to 3:1 (normal value 12—14:1).

Treatment

- Acute—Counseling.
- Chronic—Minoxidil 2% solution, oral iron and multivitamin supplementation, treatment of underlying cause if found.

Anagen Effluvium (AE)

Caused by drugs; generally anticancer cytotoxic drugs, radiotherapy. Alopecia usually complete within 1–2 months of starting chemotherapy. Reversible within 3–6 months of stopping. Risk factors for permanent loss—old age, chronic graft versus host disease (GVHD), radiotherapy.

Treatment

Minoxidil 2% may reduce the severity and duration of anagen effluvium.

Traction Alopecia

Caused by chronic, almost continuous 'pull' due to hair dressing styles of special groups of people, such as the blacks or wearing of special head gear (turban-wearing Sikhs) or beardstring (worn by Sikhs to keep the beard in place). Initially non-cicatricial, later scarred alopecia.

Treatment

Relieve traction. Reversible in early stages.

CICATRICIAL ALOPECIAS

Permanent hair loss, replacement of follicles by firosis. Starts in a patchy manner. Classification shown in Table.

Pseudopelade of Brocq

Uncommon. More in adults/young adults than children. Nosological status uncertain. Variably

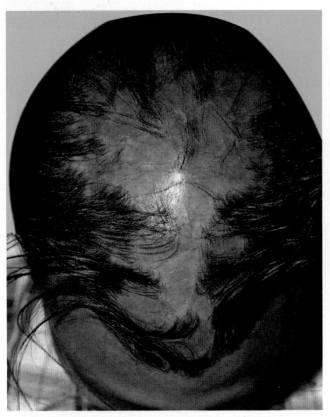

Pseudopelade: crab-like cicatrical alopecia.

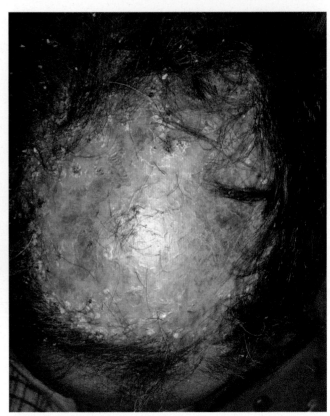

Folliculitis decalvans: shiny atrophic scaly area of scarring hair loss, follicular pustules and crusting in the periphery.

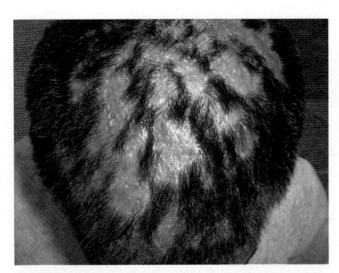

Dissecting cellulitis of scalp: boggy scalp skin with scarring alopecic patches, subtle interconnecting abscesses. Also note depressed follicular scars.

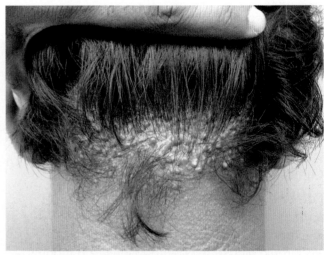

Acne keloidalis of nuchae, early: grouped follicular erythematous papules and pustules. Mild sparsening of hair.

Classification of cicatricial alopecias

Primary	Secondary	Biphasic
Lymphocyte-associated	**Infection**	**Late-stage non-scarring alopecias**
• Chronic cutaneous lupus erythematosus	• Fungal (tinea capitis)	• Alopecia areata
• Lichen planopilaris	• Bacterial	• Patterned hairloss
- Classic lichen planopilaris	• Viral (e.g. herpes zoster)	• Traction alopecia
- Frontal fibrosing alopecia		
- Graham-Little syndrome	**Immunologic**	
• Classic pseudopelade (Brocq)	• Sacroidosis	
• Central centrifugal cicatricial alopecia	• Necrobiosis lipoidica	
• Alopecia mucinosa	• Morphea	
• Keratosis follicularis spinulosa decalvans	• Graft-versus-host disease	
Neutrophil-associated	**Malignancies**	
• Folliculitis decalvans	• Alopecia neoplastica	
• Dissecting cellulitis/folliculitis	• Lymphoproliferative	
(perifolliculitis abscendence suffodiens)		
	Exogenous factors	
Mixed inflammatory infiltrate	• Radiation	
• Folliculitis (acne) keloidalis	• Burns	
• Folliculitis (acne) necrotica	• Drugs	
• Erosive pustular dermatosis		
	Dermatoses	
Non-specific	• Psoriasis	
	Bullous disorders	
	• Cicatricial pemphigois	
	• Epidermolysis bullosa	
	Hamartomas	
	• Organoid nevus	
	Miscellaneous	
	• Lipedematous alopecia	

thought as either a distinct entity or an end stage sequela of lichen planopilaris or discoid lupus erythematosus. Other possible causes—auto-immune, senescence of follicular stem cells, etc. Asymptomatic. Mainly over scalp, rarely elsewhere. Flesh colored or tan oval/round or reticulate or large patches of scarring hair loss with or without epidermal/dermal atrophy. No sign of inflammation. Stray hair present in the patches. Scattered oval patches may give appearance of 'foot prints in the snow'.

Histopathology

Non-specific mild lymphocytic infiltrate around infundibulum. Advanced cases show follicular fibrosis and absence of sebaceous glands.

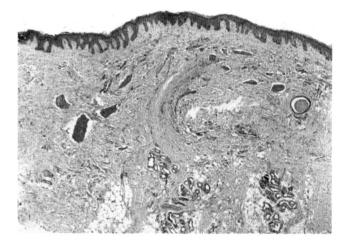

Histopathology of pseuodopelade of Brocq: Unremarkable epidermis with paucity of pilosebaceous units and no dermal inflammation. A linear scar replacing the follicle completely (running perpendicular to the epidermis) and surrounded by atrophic arrector pili.

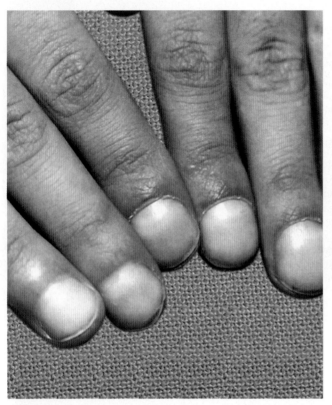

Clubbing of nails: angle between the nail plate and nail fold reduced.

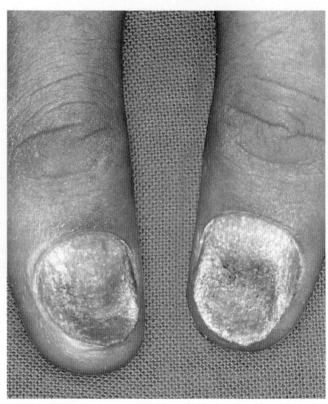

Nail pitting: fine nail pits in patient with alopecia areata.

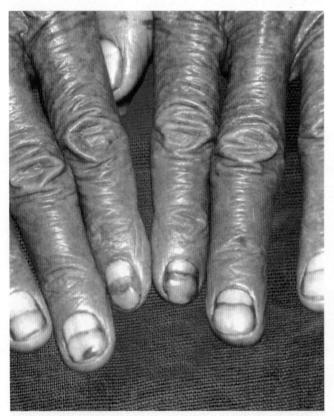

Beau's lines: horizontal furrows uniformly on all nails indicating cessation of nail plate formation.

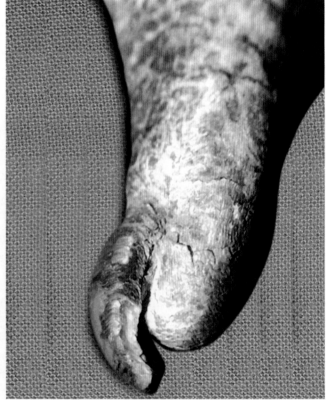

Onychogryphosis: thickening and curving of the nail plate. Patient had pityriasis rubra pilaris.

Treatment

Frustrating. Topical steroids with or without intralesional steroids. If progressive, oral prednisolone, oral minipulse (betamethasone), HCQs.

Dissecting Cellulitis of Scalp (also known as Perifolliculitis Capitis Abscedens et Suffodiens)

Very rare. Mainly in dark skinned/Afro-American individuals. Adults.

Etiology

Unknown. Abnormal follicular keratinization leading to obstruction, secondary bacterial infection, and follicular destruction probable.

Clinical Manifestations

Distinctive clinical appearance. Painful fluctuant/boggy nodules, abscesses and interconnecting sinus tracts with scarring alopecia. May give cerebriform appearance to scalp. Associations: Follicular occlusion triad—(with acne conglobata, hidradenitis suppurativa) and tetrad (as above along with pilonidal sinus).

Treatment

Resistant disease. Oral isotretinoin (starting with 1 mg/kg/day then slow tapering over 1–2 years) treatment of choice. Oral antibiotics—tetracyclines (mino and doxy), cloxacillin, erythromycin. Spiration of abscesses and intralesional steroid.

Acne Keloidalis of Nuchae

Not so uncommon inflammatory condition. Young post pubertal males, more in dark skinned people.

Etiology

Uncertain but possibly multifactorial-racial differences in pilosebaceous units, friction, seborrhea, infection, autoimmunity.

Clinical Manifestations

Smooth, firm follicular papules and pustules that may coalesce into plaques and destroy hair. Most common on occipital scalp near posterior hairline, may also affect vertex.

Histopathology

Perifollicular mixed infiltrate around isthmus and sebaceous gland region of hair.

Treatment

Initially, class I and II topical steroids with or without intralesional steroids. Oral or topical antibiotics (tetracyclines) may help. In advanced cases surgical excision upto muscle fascia and healing with secondary intention or staged excision and primary repair.

Folliculitis Decalvans

Rare, progressive purulent folliculitis. May involve any hair bearing site but mostly over vertex of scalp. Adults only mostly. Etiology unknown. Many cases show isolates of *Staphylococcus aureus*. May be localized immune deficiency against the bacterium.

Start as isolated pustules but progress to form miliary follicular abscesses followed by scarring in center and centrifugal spread. Tufting of intervening hair may be seen.

Histopathology

Dense intra- and perifollicular neutrophilic infiltrate, centered over upper and middle parts of hair.

Treatment

Oral antibiotic with/without topical antibiotic. Oral erythromycin, minocycline/doxycycline, clindamycin, rifampicin, fusidic acid. Long-term control needs intermittent therapy. Dapsone also useful.

DISORDERS OF NAILS

Caused by local factors—trauma, infections, other local diseases or part of a generalized (systemic or cutaneous) disease. One or a few nails involved in local diseases, many or all in generalized disease. Direct nail plate involvement. Or secondary to involvement of nail matrix.

Clubbing

Obliteration or reversal of the angle between the nail plate and posterior nail fold. Hereditary or

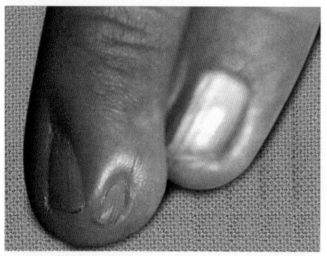

Pterygium unguis: posterior nail fold adherent to the nail bed; note the split in the nail plate.

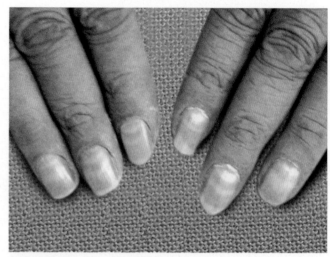

Muehrcke's pair white bands: paired white bands with intervening pink bands.

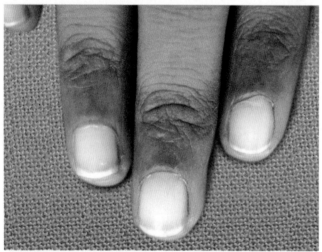

Apparent leukonychia: diffuse whitening of the nails in an anemic (Hb = 7 gm/dL) patient.

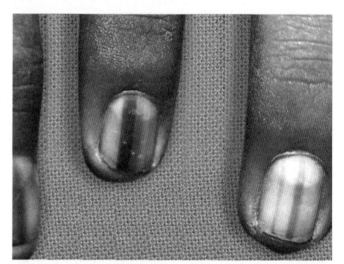

Pigmented longitudinal bands, nails: normal.

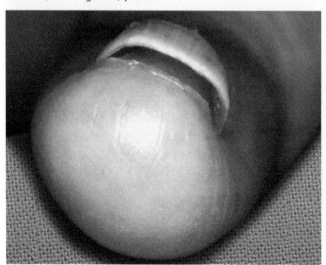

Onycholysis, due to tinea unguium.

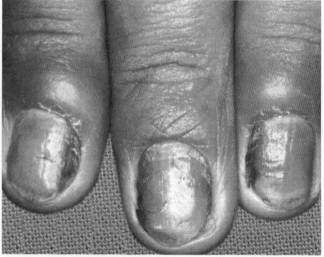

Nail changes due to cosmetics: paronychia and nail plate damage caused by nail polish and removers.

acquired, the latter often indicative of a systemic disease—cardiac disease, pulmonary suppuration or neoplasms. Generally bilateral. Finger nails more frequently involved. May resolve on treatment of primary condition.

Pitting

Uniform pitting of nail plates; multiple or all nails. Psoriasis, alopecia areata commonly responsible. Possibly caused by punctate parakeratosis of nail plate—parakeratotic portion dropping off. Pits may be uniform or confluent and ripple patterned.

- Psoriasis—Pits are more coarse, less In number and asymmetric.
- Alopecia areata—Pits are more fine, more numerous and symmetric.

Koilonychia

- Concave nails, i.e. depressed nail plate both longitudinally and horizontally.
- Nail plate thickness may or may not be altered.
- Most commonly associated with iron deficiency or hemochromatosis.
- Family history may be +.
- Occupational—Mechanics, hair dresses.

Beau's Lines

Transverse ridges or grooves on the nail plates. Indicate temporary cessation of nail plate formation. Result of severe systemic disease—from coronary artery disease to febrile illness or major physical accidents. Return to normalcy on recovery or convalescence. All finger and toe nails may be affected.

Onychogryphosis

Thickening, increase in length and curvature of nail plate. Great toe nails most frequently affected. Trauma, the most common factor. Psoriasis, pityriasis rubra pilaris, fungal infections responsible in some.

Treatment

Regular, careful clipping off of nails. Avulsion in some.

Pterygium Unguius (Dorsal)

Prolongation of the posterior nail fold onto the nail bed. Causes partial destruction of the nail plate. Most frequently seen in lichen planus.

Ventral Pterygium

Closure of space between hyponychium and free end of the nail plate. Occurs in systemic sclerosis, trauma, SLE.

Muehrcke's Nails/Paired White Bands

White bands parallel to the lunula, intervening pink area. Going across the full transverse diameter of the nail plate. Commonly seen in nutritional deficiencies, especially, hypalbuminemia. Nail changes reverse on correction of deficiency.

Half and Half Nails (Also, Lindsay's Nails)

Manifestation of chronic kidney disease, more so in patients on hemodialysis. Proximal half is white and distal half is pink/red/brown, with sharp demarcation.

Apparent Leukonychia

Due to pallour of the nail bed, nail appears white. Occurs in anemia, edema and vascular compromise.

Longitudinal Melanonychia (Pigmented Bands of Nails)

Common in blacks, infrequent in Caucasoids. Secondary to presence of active melanocytes in the nail matrix. A variant—may indicate a nevus in nail matrix.

Onycholysis

Separation of nail plate from nail bed. Idiopathic, due to psoriasis or onychomycosis. Photo-onycholysis (PUVA or PUVA sol), tetracyclines.

Trachyonychia

- Rough surface of up to all 20 nails (20 nail dystrophy).
- As known as 'Sand blasted nails'.

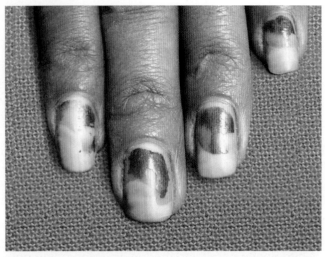

Housewife onycholysis: distal and lateral onycholysis of finger nails of dominant hand in a housewife.

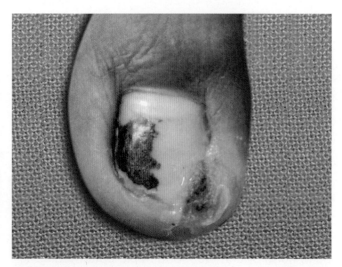

Ingrowing toe nail: lateral nail fold of great toe is swollen, with purulant discharge and excess granulation overlapping the nail plate.

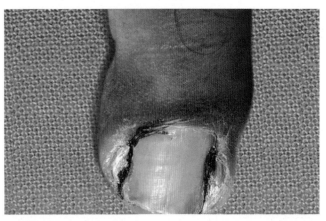

Ingrowing toe nail: bilateral lateral nail folds of great toe are swollen, with excess granulation.

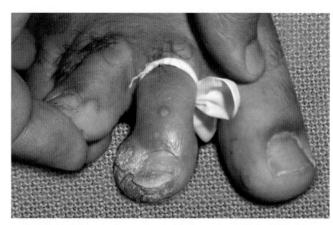

Periungual wart: huge wart involving the lateral fold, tip and nail bed of the great toe nail. Note distal and lateral onycholysis of the involved nail.

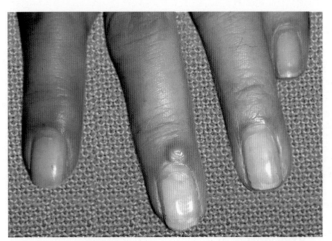

Myxoid cyst, middle finger: solitary cyst over the proximal nail fold and adjoining longitudinal gutter in the nail plate.

Courtesy: Dr Shanta Passi, Dermatologist, ESIC Hospital, Faridabad.

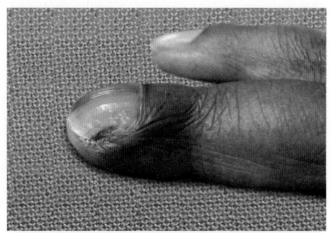

Nail bed glomus tumor: localized bluish discoloration visible in the lateral part of nail bed and adjoining lateral nail fold.

- More common in children.
- Associated with yellowish or greyish discoloration of nails.
- Self limiting in children, usually chronic in adults.

Cause

Psoriasis, alopecia areata, lichen planus, idiopathic.

Treatment

Topical steroid may provide temporal relief as with locally injected steroids. Topical 5-FU can be tried.

Nail Disorders and Cosmetics

Common. Females, of course, but not always. Nail cosmetics cause injury to nail plate, nail folds or skin at distant sites. Nail polish, polish removers or cuticle removers often responsible. Damage to or friability of nail plate. Allergic contact dermatitis of the nail fold or paronychia may be seen.

Ingrowing Nail (Onychocryptosis)

Most commonly the great toe nails. Usually nail plate impinges over the lateral nail fold in adults; in children usually it impinges distally. Major factor ill fitting footwear, others include sports with excess pressure on toes (kicking, football), anatomical defects (long toes, prominent lateral nail folds). Start with mild swelling and pain, followed by purulent discharge and exuberant granulation tissue. Conservative approach usually heals-topical steroid-antibiotic combinations, analgesics for pain relief, corrected footwear, avoiding repeated trauma. Surgery if no relief-lateral nail splinting, lateral nail spicule excision followed by chemical/surgical lateral matricetomy.

Idiopathic Housewife Onycholysis

Detachment of nail plate from the nail bed. Occupational dermatosis. More commonly distal and distal-lateral. Due to repeated mechanical friction, exposure to wet work involving detergents and possibly secondary colonization. Normal nail texture, no evident nail disease other than onycholysis.

Nail or Nail Fold Tumors

Periungual Warts

Warts more commonly involve the nail fold. Uncommonly the digital tip and the nail bed. Nail fold lesions cause nail plate ridging and bed lesions cause onycholysis. Treatment of choice is intralesional bleomycin injection 1 μ/mL 3 weekly for 3 doses. Other options include topical 5-fluorouracil cream, destructive therapies (radiofrequency, cryotherapy, laser), surgery (nail plate avulsion followed by radiofrequency).

Myxoid Cyst (Also, Mucoid Pseudocyst)

Known as pseudocyst because the wall is often not demonstrable. Classically located over the proximal nail fold, intermittently yields clear discharge and reduces in size only to refill. The adjoining nail plate shows a longitudinal gutter having transverse ridges inside it, corresponding to intermittent reduced pressure on nail matrix. Often found to have communication with distal interphalangeal joint. Treatment includes incision and drainage, locally destructive therapies (cryotherapy, laser, scerosant injection). Surgical excision has lower recurrence than the above.

Glomus Tumor

Characteristic moderate to severe pain which is aggravated by cold exposure. Tumors compressing the nail matrix produce longitudinal ridging and tumors of nail bed produce bluish or reddish discoloration seen through the nail plate. Suspicion should be strong in case of severe finger pain without signs. MRI investigation of choice in order to detect tumors as small as 2–3 mm and in case of suspected recurrence post surgery. Treatment is complete surgical excision.

16 Genodermatoses

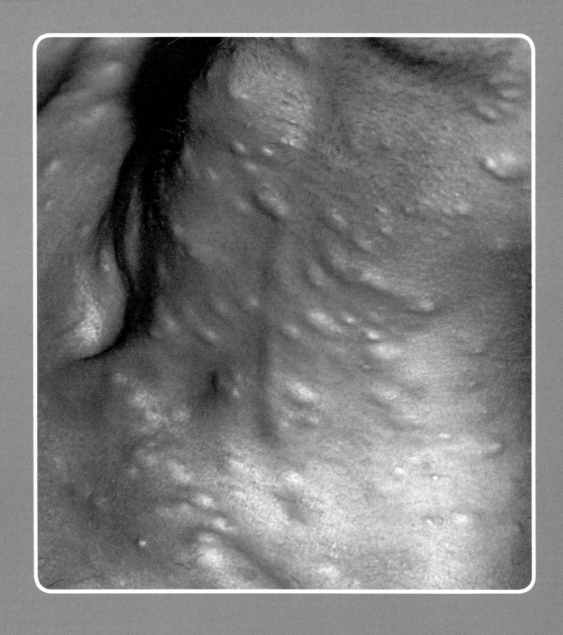

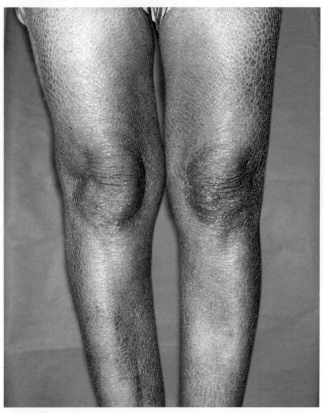

Ichthyosis vulgaris: fine scales on the extensors of lower limbs.

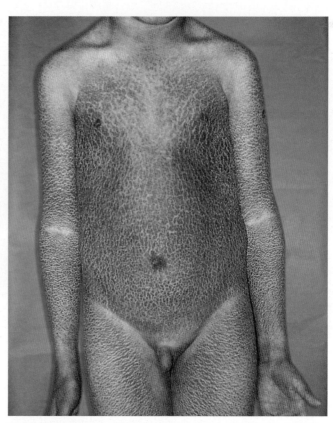

X-linked ichthyosis: black, pasted scales on the trunk and limbs. Flexures somewhat spared.

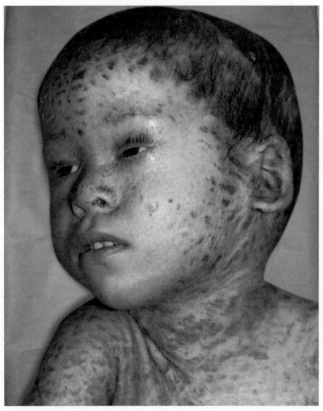

Lamellar ichthyosis: large, coarse scales. Note ectropion.

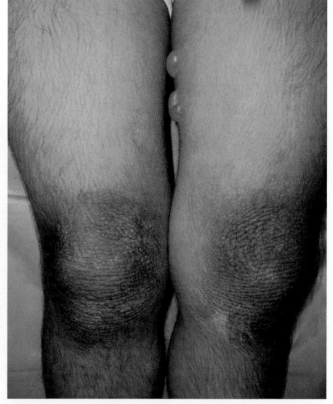

Epidermolytic ichthyosis: thick corrugated scales over both knees. Note blisters over the left inner thigh.

Dermatoses in which genetics plays a dominant, if not an exclusive, role. Environmental influences may modify clinical picture. Light, for instance, modifies manifestations in albinism, xeroderma pigmentosum and porphyrias; physical trauma in epidermolysis bullosa; heat in anhidrotic ectodermal dysplasia; dry climatic conditions exacerbate/precipitate ichthyosiform dermatoses. Dermatoses may manifest at birth or soon after, sometimes considerably later-around puberty or later.

Autosomal dominant inheritance, generally vertical (parents to offspring) and milder; autosomal recessive present amongst the siblings (horizontal). X-linked recessive confined to male members of the family, females being carriers.

KERATINIZING DISORDERS

Ichthyosiform Dermatoses

Common. Characterized by dry, fish-like scales (*ichthys* means fish). Several types. Rickets/vitamin D deficiency may be associated with any type.

Ichthyosis Vulgaris (Syn-Autosomal Dominant Ichthyosis)

Commonest variant. Autosomal dominant inheritance. Filaggrin gene mutation. Manifests in early childhood, *not* at birth. Small, white or light brown flaky scales fixed at one end. Extensors of extremities particularly involved, flexures

Ichthyosis, non-syndromic forms		
Disease	*Mode of inheritance*	*Common defective gene(s)*
Common ichthyoses		
Ichthyosis vulgaris	Autosomal semidominant	FLG
Recessive X-linked ichthyosis	X-linked recessive	STS
Autosomal recessive congenital ichthyosis		
Major variants		
Lamellar ichthyosis	Autosomal recessive	TGM1/NIPAL4z/ALOX12B
Congenital ichthyosiform erythroderma		ALOXE3/ALOX12B/ABCA12
Harlequin ichthyosis		ABCA12
Minor variants		
Self-healing collodion baby	Autosomal recessive	TGM1, ALOX12B, ALOXE3
Acral self-healing collodion baby		TGM1
Bathing suit ichthyosis		TGM1
Keratinopathic ichthyosis		
Major variants		
Superficial epidermolytic ichthyosis	Autosomal dominant	KRT2
Epidermolytic ichthyosis	Autosomal dominant	KRT1/KRT10
Minor variants		
Ichthyosis Curth-Macklin	Autosomal dominant	KRT1
Autosomal recessive epidermolytic ichthyosis	Autosomal recessive	KRT10
Annular epidermolytic ichthyosis	Autosomal dominant	KRT1/KRT10
Epidermolytic nevi	Somatic mutations	KRT1/KRT10
Other forms		
Loricrin keratoderma	Autosomal dominant	LOR
Erythrokeratodermia variabilis	Autosomal dominant	GJB3/GJB4
Peeling skin disease	Autosomal recessive	Unknown

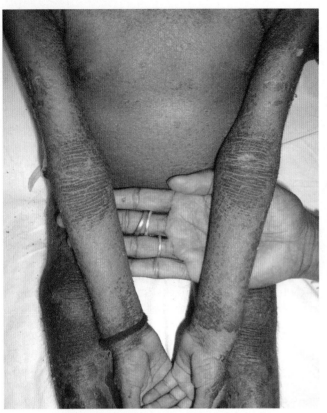

Epidermolytic hyperkeratosis: generalized erythema and scaling, corrugated scaling over joints. Note bilateral wrist widening suggestive of rickets.

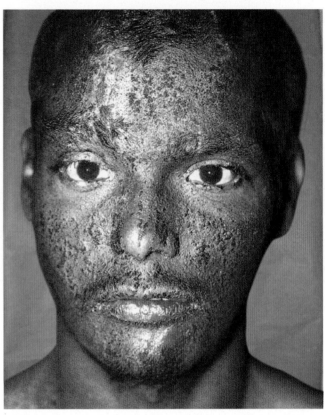

Epidermolytic hyperkeratosis: localized erythema and verrucous scales.

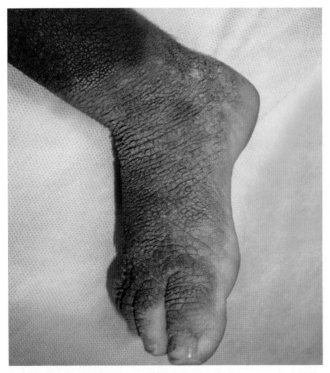

Ichthyosis hysterix generalized type: thick verrucous scales over dorsum of foot.

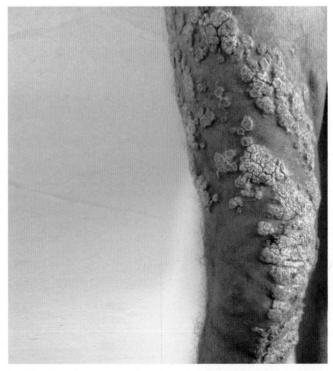

Ichthyosis hysterix nevoid type: Hyperkeratotic plaques arranged linearly on right thigh and leg.

conspicuously spared. Pronounced in cold dry weather. May completely remit in hot and humid season. Palmar creases accentuated with minimal or moderate hyperkeratosis. Heels dry and fissured. Significant association with atopy and keratosis pilaris.

X-linked Ichthyosis (Syn–Ichthyosis Nigra)

Relatively uncommon. X-linked recessive inheritance. Steroid sulfatase gene mutation. Only males affected. Manifests in infancy or early childhood. Large, brown to black (hence nigra), flat, adherent scales. Trunk, extremities, neck, sides of face, buttocks affected. Flexures not necessarily spared. Palmo-plantar keratoderma minimal. Heat and humidity help in relieving the condition. Extracutaneous associations include crypto-orchidism, non-blinding corneal opacities, male pattern baldness etc.

Lamellar Ichthyosis

Uncommon. Variable clinical severity but usually more extensive than IV and XLRI. Now classified under ARCI (autosomal recessive congenital ichthyosis). Autosomal recessive inheritance; consanguinous parents. Mutation in transglutaminase 1 gene. Present at birth. A parchment like membrane enveloping the whole body—*Collodion baby*. Membrane sheds off in a few days; generalized erythema (less than non-bullous ichthyosiform erythroderma, NBIE). Later, generalized coarse, large scales fixed in the center. Facial skin rigid and taut with ectropion and eclabion (eversion of lips). Offensive body odor. Blockage of sweat glands and heat intolerance. Marked keratoderma and fissuring of palms and soles. Deep fissures on flexures and joint surfaces. Flexion contractures, sclerodactyly may occur.

Epidermolytic Ichthyosis (Old Name Epidermolytic Hyperkeratosis)

Classified under keratinopathic ichthyosis since caused by mutation in keratin 1 and 10 genes. Rare. Autosomal dominant inheritance. Present at birth. Moist, superficially denuded skin. Soon, universal dry scaling on an erythematous background. Superficial vesicles that erode easily. Later, thick hyperkeratotic and verrucous corrugated scales particularly pronounced in the flexures. Offensive body odour. Heat intolerance. Variable palmo-plantar keratoderma. Localized epidermolytic hyperkeratosis resembles epidermal naevi.

Ichthyosis Hysterix

Spiny hyperkeratotic scales in localized, nevoid or generalized distribution. Localized more common. Autosomal dominant inheritance. Associated striate or diffuse paloplantar keratoderma. Erythema and blistering minimal.

Herlequin Ichthyosis

Severe erythrodermic variant. Autosomal recessive, sporadic. ABCA12 mutation. 'coat of armour' like appearance and distorted facies and extremities. Deep fissures, thick adherent skin. High mortality rate in first few weeks of life, improves with ICU care. Main concerns being fluid, electrolyte, feeding and temperature management.

Netherton Syndrome

Ichthyosiform syndrome. Autosomal recessive. SPINK5 mutation. Triad of erythroderma (ichthyosis linearis circumflexa), atopic dermatitis and hair shaft defect (trichorrhexis invaginata).

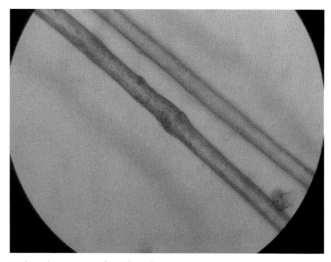

Hair microsopy of trichorrhexis invaginata: A case of netherton syndrome. Single node in hair shaft, the upper portion is tending to protrude into the lower portion which is tending to form a cup (10x).

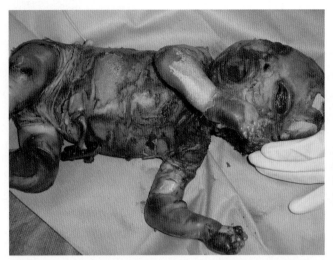

Herlequin ichthyosis: Deeply fissured thickened skin with ectropion, eclabium and mutilating deformity of hands and feet.

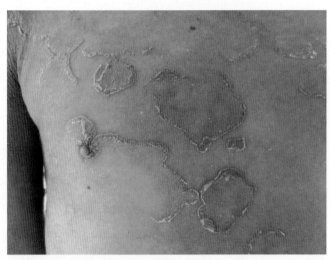

Netherton syndrome: Ichthyosis linearis circumflexa (plaques with double rimmed scales).

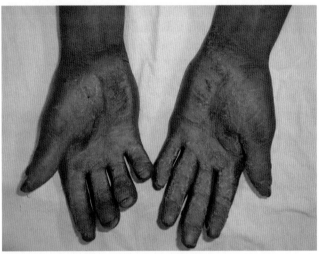

Unna Thost PPK: Diffuse yellowish thickening of palms with erythematous border.

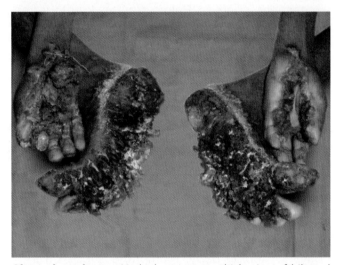

Olmsted syndrome: Marked verrucuous thickening of bilateral palms and soles causing functional disability.

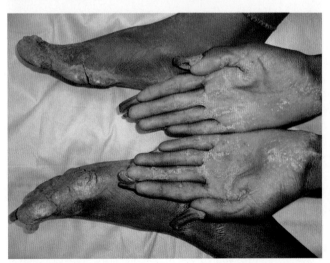

Pachyonychia congenita: Focal PPK of both palms and diffuse PPK of both soles. Marked tubular thickening of nails.

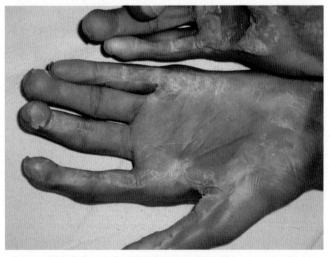

Striate palmoplantar keratoderma: Linearly arranged yellowish plaques involving the palms and fingers.

Treatment of Ichthyoses

Dependson severity. Mild to moderate cases, no therapy required in hot, humid climates. Winters, mild emollients—vaseline, lanolin, glycerine with water (equal parts) or 40–60% propylene glycol in water.

For more severe, particularly lamellar ichthyosis use keratolytics like 5–10% salicylic acid ointment or 20–40% urea in cream base: 0.025–0.05% retinoic acid may be helpful. Avoid in flexures. Severe cases need systemic retinoids (acitretin) 0.5–1.0 mg/kg per/day for coveral weeks—even life long! Oral retinoids avoided in epidermolytic ichthyosis since it can exacerbate blistering. Another method is to give intermittent retinoid therapy in winters when icthyosis is more severe.

Palmo-Plantar Keratodermas

Group of rare keratinizing disorders. More commonly autosomal dominant but recessive variants known. Classification as below (in attached power point). Diffuse PPK usually of earlier onset than focal/punctate variants. Mutilation occurs in Olmsted, Vohwinkel, Loricrin, Mal de Meleda and Sybert forms.

Because of thickness of keratin, hyperhydrosis malodour and secondary infection can occur. Erythema prominent in palms and soles in Mal de Meleda. Fissuring seen in Vorner. Transgradiens means extension to adjoining areas (example onto wrist/dorsae of hands and feet and achilles area) and progradiens means extension to distant areas (example elbows, knee, etc).

Unna Thost PPK

Diffuse non epidermolytic PPK. Early onset. Uniform yellowish thickening of palms and soles with sharp cut off at edges with erythema at the border. Hyperhydrosis and dermtophytic infection tendency.

Olmsted's Syndrome (Mutilating Palmoplantar Keratoderma with Periorificial Keratotic Plaques)

Autosomal dominant. Early onset, symmetric massive palmoplantar keratoderma leading to

Simple palmoplantar keratodermas	
Diffuse	
Non-transgradient	Epidermolytic (Vorner)
	Non-epidermolytic (Unna Thost)
	Huriez
	Olmsted
Transgradient	Loricrin
	Greither's
	Sybert
	Mal de Meleda
Focal/Areate	Focal
	Striate
	Pachyonychia congenita types 1 and 2
	Hidrotic ectodermal dysplasia
Punctate	Punctate
	Punctate keratosis of palmar creases
	Marginal papular keratoderma (acrokeratoelastoides, focal acral hyperkeratosis, degenerative collagenous plaques)

Complex/syndromic palmoplantar keratodermas	
Features	**Name of syndrome**
PPK with esophageal carcinoma	Howel Evans syndrome
Cicatrizing PPK with deafness	Vohwinkel syndrome
PPK with periodontitis and pyodermas	Papillon Lefevre syndrome
Oculocutaneous tyrosinemia	Richner Hanhart syndrome
PPK with eyelid cysts	Schopf Shulz Passarge syndrome
Striate PPK, woolly hair, cardiomyopathy	Naxos syndrome, Carvajal syndrome

flexion deformities and spontaneous amputation. Perioral, perianal and perineal keratosis, onychodystrophy and leukokeratosis.

Pachyonychia Congenita

Autosomal dominant. Mutations in keratin genes. Four types, recognized Type I (Jadassohn-Lewandowsky syndrome): Mutation in keratin 6

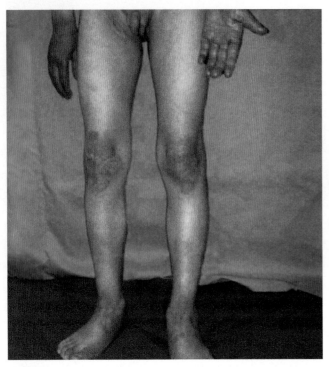

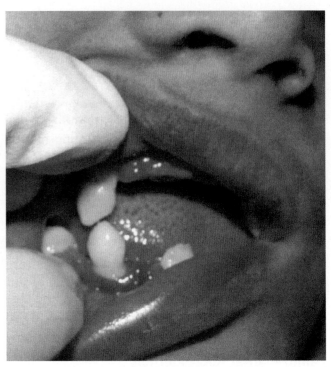

Papillon-Lefevre syndrome: symmetrical transgradient palmoplantar keratoderma; note scar in inguinal area of subsided abscess.

Papillon-Lefevre syndrome: periodontitis leading to loss of teeth.

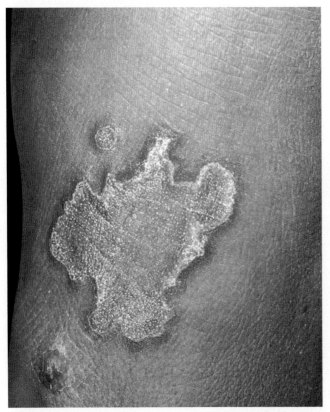

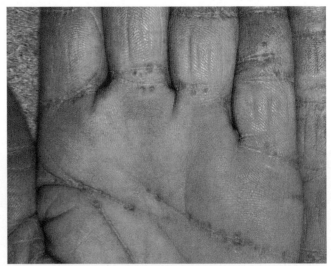

Punctate keratoderma of palmar creases: Punctate pits in the palmar and finger creases.

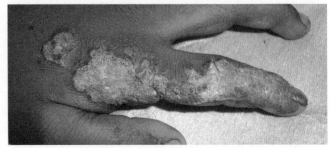

Parokeratosis of Mibelli: large irregular and small rounded plaques. Characteristic furrowed, hyperkeratotic border.

Linear porokeratosis: Linear Plaques with 'wiry' edge over the index finger and dorsum of hand.

or 16 gene. Thick and tented nails (fingers and toes) with onycholysis. Paronychia frequent. Follicular keratosis (elbows and knees) and palmoplantar hyperkeratosis. Oral cavity-leukokeratosis. Hoarseness, if larynx involved. Type II (Jackson-Lawler syndrome): Mutation in keratin 17 gene. Features of type I with natal teeth and steatocystoma multiplex. Type III (Schafer-Branauer syndrome): Features of type I with leukokeratosis of cornea. Type IV (pachyonychia congenita tarda): Late-onset in second or third decade.

Striate PPK

Linear thickening over palms, palmar aspect of fingers and soles. More focal/diffuse over soles. To look for woolly hair for syndromes.

Punctate Keratoderma of Palmar Creases

Keratotic papules involving the palmar creases, fall of leaving punctate pits at the places.

Papillon-Lefevre Syndrome

Autosomal recessive. Mutation in cathepsin C gene. Triad of symmetrical transgradient palmoplantar keratoderma, juvenile aggressive periodontitis and recurrent pyogenic infections of skin and internal organs, especially liver. Mental retardation, intracranial calcifications can occur.

Treatment of Palmo-plantar Keratodermas

Keratolytics mainstay of therapy. Salicylic acid (5–20%) ointment, retinoic acid (0.05–0.1%), propylene glycol (40–70%) in water. Systemic retinoids in patients with severe disease. Or mutilating variants—may prevent or delay mutilation. Oral retinoids may also improve periodontitis in papillon-lefevre syndrome.

Porokeratotic Disorders

Porokeratosis of Mibelli

Uncommon. Autosomal dominant inheritance, genetic basis unknown. Annular plaques with central, sometimes atrophic, depression. Characteristic edge: greyish, keratotic; often with a central furrow. Centrifugal spread. Limbs, trunk, face may be affected.

Linear Porokeratosis

Linear plaques along the lines of blaschko. Congenital or childhood onset, genetic basis unknown but aberration on chromosomes 12, 15 or 18 postulated as for disseminated superficial actinic porokeratosis. Morphology and histology similar to classic porokeratosis.

Histopathology of Porokeratotic Disorders

Parakeratotic plug (*cornoid lamella*) in the hyperkeratotic epidermis. Granular cell layer absent beneath the cornoid lamella.

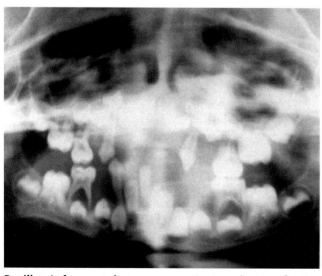

Papillon Lefevre syndrome: panoramic view, showing 'floating in air' appearance of teeth.

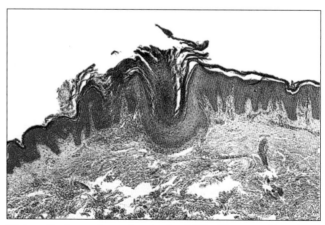

Histopathology of porokeratosis of Mibelli: cornoid lamella—a parakeratotic plug.

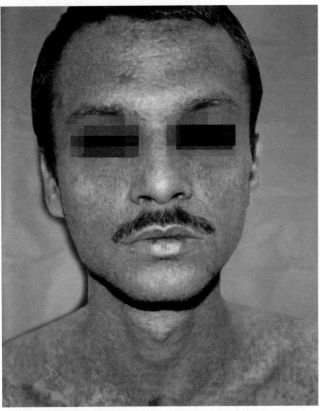

Darier's disease: scaly, discrete and confluent greasy papules in seborrhoeic sites.

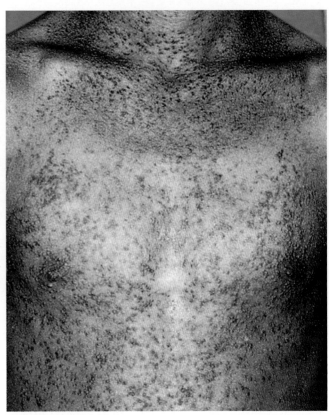

Darier's disease: characteristic greasy papules in a seborrhoeic distribution.

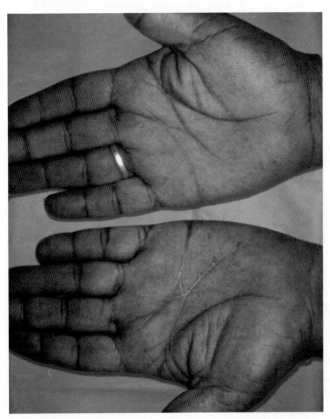

Darier's disease: characteristic pits on palms.

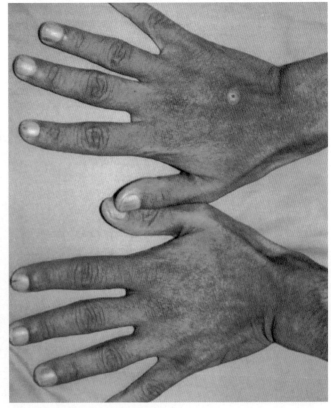

Darier's disease: acral lesions with angular nicks in the nails.

Treatment

Topical steroids and tretinoin help. Topical 5-flurouracil, imiquimod, oral acitretin (if extensive) also useful.

Darier's Disease (Keratosis Follicularis)

Uncommon disorder of keratinization. Autosomal dominant inheritance, variable penetrance. Mutation in ATP2A2 gene at chromosome 12q 24.1 that encodes for sarco- and endoplasmic reticulum calcium ATPase type 2, which maintain high calcium concentration in endoplasmic reticulum.

Begins at adolescence or early adult life. Asymptomatic. Discrete or confluent, brown or skin colored, firm, 'greasy', crusted, 'dirtylooking'

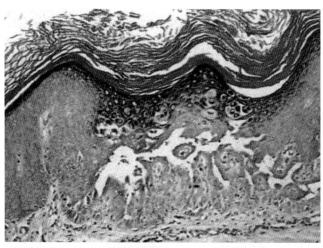

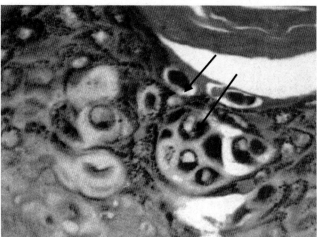

Histopathology of darier's disease: intra-epidermal split. Note dyskeratotic cells (corps ronds) in upper epidermal layers; top (10x), bottom (40x).

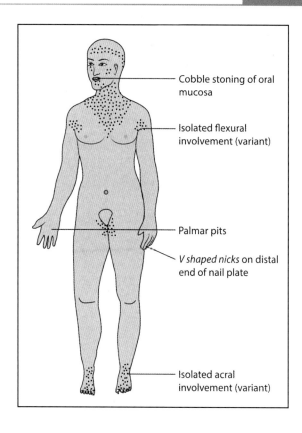

Cobble stoning of oral mucosa

Isolated flexural involvement (variant)

Palmar pits

V shaped nicks on distal end of nail plate

Isolated acral involvement (variant)

and foul-smelling papules or plaques. Seborrhoeic sites—scalp, face, nasolabial folds, chest, back, axillae and groins—preferentially affected. Palms and soles show minute pits. Dorsa of hands: small, flat, discrete papules (acrokeratosis verruciformis). 'Cobblestone' papules on the palate. Alternating longitudinal leuco- and erythronychia. Angular nicks in the nails. Runs a chronic course with exacerbations in summer and relative remissions in winter. Many variants described—comedonal, erosive, bullous, hypopigmented, keratoderma.

Histopathology

Moderate to marked hyperkeratosis, papillomatosis. Suprabasal split with villi, acantholysis and dyskeratotic cells in upper malpighian layers (corp ronds and grains).

Treatment

Treatment difficult and unsatisfactory. Mild cases, topical retinoic acid. Severe cases need systemic retinoids (acitretin, 0.5–1 mg/kg/day). Relapses occur on discontinuation of therapy.

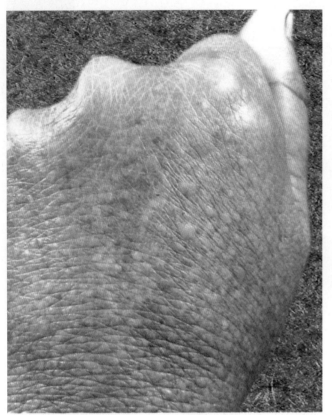

Acrokeratosis Verruciformis of Hopf: skin coloured plane topped papules over dorsum of left hand.

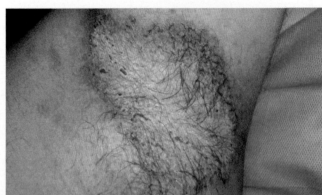

Hailey hailey disease: macerated plaque in axilla with linear fissures.

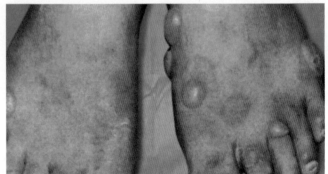

Epidermolysis bullosa simplex: intact blisters; healing with hyperpigmented macules.

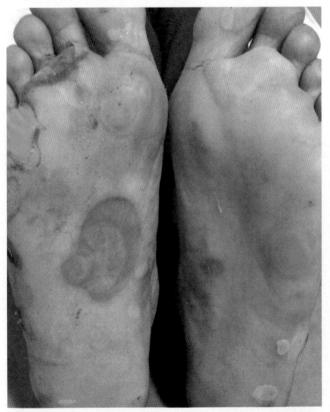

Epidermolysis bullosa simplex (Weber cockayne variant): Tense and flaccid bullae restricted to soles.

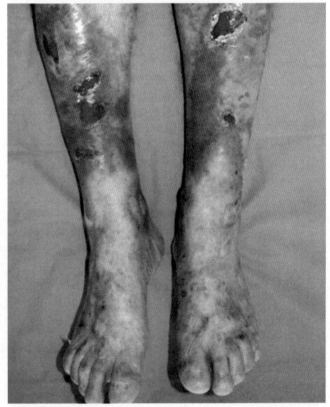

Epidermolysis bullosa, junctional, non-lethal: atrophy, hemorrhagic bullae, loss of nails.

Acrokeratosis Verruciformis of Hopf

Autosomal dominant. Relationship with Darier disease controversial, probably different phenotypes of a common gene defect in ATP2A2 gene. Skin-colored, plain topped papules. Symmetrically on dorsa of hands and feet. Punctate keratoses and interruptions of dermal ridges on palms and soles.

Histopathology

Hyperkeratosis, acanthosis and papillomatosis in 'church spire' pattern.

Treatment

Topical retinoids. Or ablation with radiofrequency, lasers or cryotherapy.

Benign Familial Chronic Pemphigus (Hailey-Hailey Disease)

Rare. Autosomal dominant inheritance with incomplete penetrance. Defect in gene ATP2C1 on 3q21. Onset: adolescence or later. Asymptomatic grouped vesicles. Rupture to form characteristic, almost diagnostic, irregular *fissures* or *cracks* in the skin. Axillae, groins, inframammary folds affected. Aggravation in summer, spontaneous remission in winter. Mucosal involvement rare. Longitudinal white lines in nails. Intra-epidermal irregular clefts.

Histopathology

Acantholytic dyskeratosis with extensive, acantholysis giving the so-called 'dilapidated' brick wall appearance. Occasional dyskeratotic cells.

Treatment

Treatment usually unsatisfactory. Topical antibacterial or anticandidal agents to get rid of secondary infections. Potent topical corticosteroids generally adequate. Occasionally systemic steroids needed. Tendency to recur if treatment discontinued. Locally destructive therapies like Cryosurgery, radio-surgery and laser ablation provide longer relief.

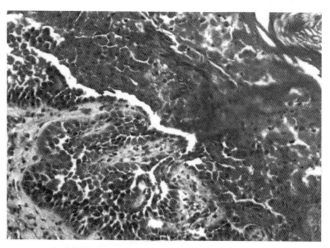

Histopathology of benign familial chronic pemphigus: irregular intraepidermal clefts with acantholytic cells. Note dyskeratotic cells in upper layers.

EPIDERMOLYSIS BULLOSA (EB)

Uncommon genodermatoses. Increased fragility of the skin. Blistering and peeling off—on minor trauma, hence also labelled *mechanobullous dermatoses*. Heterogeneous group. Dominantly inherited forms—mild. Recessively inherited variants— severe, serious or fatal. 'Spontaneous' blistering, mucosal involvement, and nail involvement in severe forms. *Simplex, junctional* and *dystrophic* forms. Split in simplex form truly epidermal (basal cell layer); in junctional forms in the lamina lucida and in the dystrophic forms in upper dermis.

Epidermolysis Bullosa Simplex

Commonest form. Generalized or localized. Autosomal dominant inheritance. Bullae caused by disintegration of basal and suprabasal epidermal cells. Blisters, generally in the first year of life, caused by trauma of crawling or walking. Some patients improve at puberty. Worse in warm weather. Clear blisters on the hands, feet, legs and arms. Heal without scarring. No mucosal or nail involvement.

Localized (Weber-Cockayne) form: onset in childhood or adulthood. Localized to feet, less frequently to hands. Worse in summer. Precipitated by use of heavy boots or in individuals on long marches.

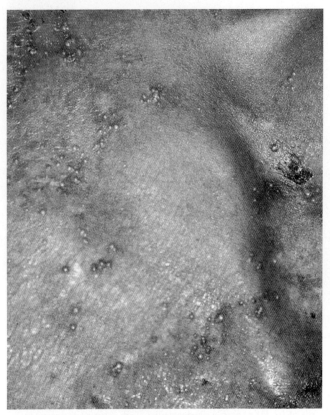

Epidermolysis bullosa dominant dystrophic: note milia and scarring.

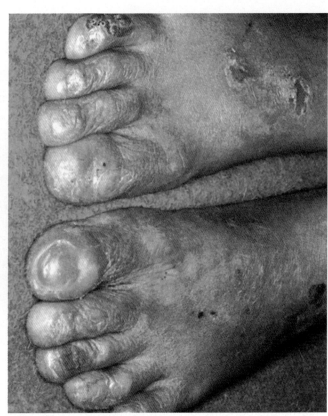

Epidermolysis bullosa dominant dystrophic: atrophic scars, milia and partial loss of nails.

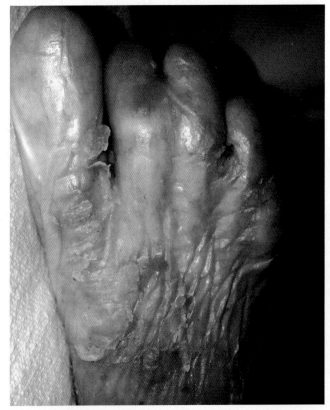

Recessive dystrophic EB: 'Mitten like' appearance of toes.

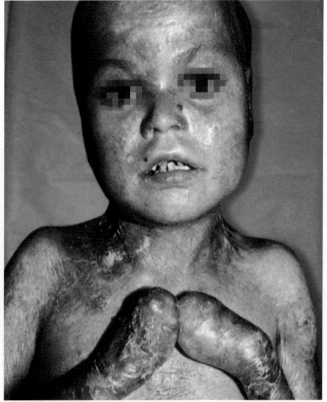

Epidermolysis bullosa, recessive dystrophic: mitten-like hands, poor dentition and cicatricial alopecia.

Level of blister	EB type	EB subtypes	Defective protein(s)
Intraepidermal	EB Simplex	Suprabasal EBS	Transglutaminase 5; plakophilin 1; desmoplakin; plakoglobin
		Basal EBS	Keratins 5 and 14; plectin; bullous pemphigoid antigen 1
Intralamina lucida	Junctional EB	Localized JEB	Collagen 17; laminin-332; α6β4 integrin
		Generalized JEB	Lamin-332; collagen 17; α6β4 integrin
Sublamina densa	Dystrophic EB	Dominant DEB	Collagen 7
		Recessive DEB	Collagen 7
Mixed	Kindler syndrome	—	Kindlln-1

Major types of epidermolysis bullosa

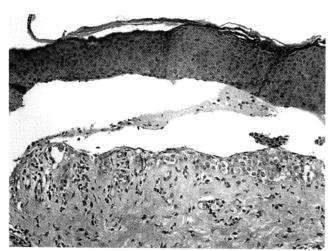

Histopathology of epidermolysis bullosa simplex: intra-epidermal split.

Junctional Epidermolysis Bullosa

Autosomal recessive inheritance; split in the lamina lucida. One variant lethal (Herlitz). Bullous lesions and peeling off of the skin, at birth or soon after. May be generalized. Healing with atrophy. No scarring or milia. Mucosal involvement present. Death generally in infancy due to infection in the *lethal (Herlitz)* form. Nail and teeth involved in the non-lethal variant.

Dominant Dystrophic Epidermolysis Bullosa

Uncommon. Autosomal dominant inheritance. Dermo—epidermal split beneath the lamina densa due to damage to anchoring fibrils. Onset: early infancy. Blisters at sites of trauma; heal with hypertrophic scarring and milia. Mucous membranes and nails involved but less frequently and less severely than in the recessive form.

Pretibial localization seen in some families (pretibial variant). White, perifollicular papules on lumbo-sacral region in some others (*albopapuloid* variant of Pasini); not associated with blistering.

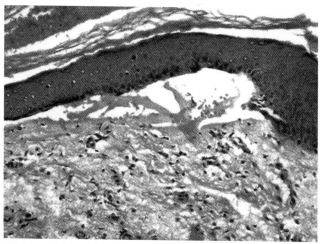

Histopathology of epidermolysis bullosa dystrophica: subepidermal split.

EB Pruriginosa

Very itchy linearly arranged vesicles and papulonodular lesions over the shins. Onset in infancy or childhood, may occur later. Commonly sporadic. Scarring, milia, nail dystrophy.

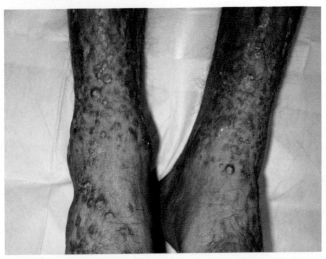

EB pruriginosa: Excoriated nodules and vesicles over the legs and feet.

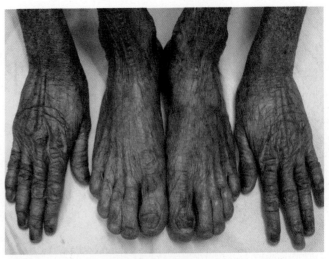

Kindler syndrome: generalized wrinkling on dorsae of hands and feet, atrophic scars on knuckles and fingers and nail dystrophy.

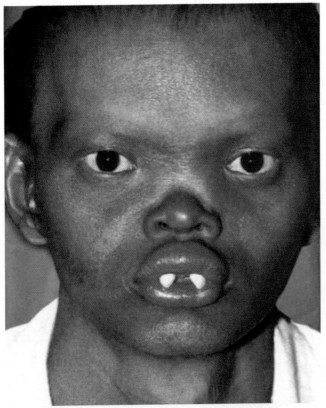

Anhidrotic ectodermal dysplasia: typical facies with saddle-shaped nose, thick everted-lips and peg-shaped teeth.

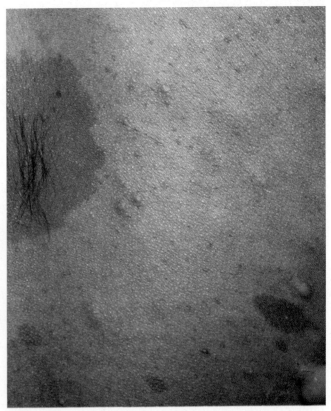

Neurofibromatosis: irregular, uniformly light brown, cafe-au-fait macules.

Recessive Dystrophic Epidermolysis Bullosa

Rare. Severe form. Blisters in the upper dermis. Onset at birth or early infancy. Spontaneous blistering. Large, flaccid, hemorrhagic bullae that heal with atrophic scarring and milia. Scarring may join fingers to give a 'mitten-like' appearance. Mucosal involvement common; buccal lesions may cause difficulty in feeding. Esophageal strictures may develop.

Treatment of Epidermolysis Bullosa

Genetic counselling important. No treatment effective yet: pivots around prevention of trauma. Oral steroid and dapsone tried in progressive disease with some benefit. Issues to be addressed wound healing, infection control, care of oral, anal and upper airway mucosa, and early detection and treatment of malignancies. Experimental therapies include—wound dressing with honey, gene therapy (currently underway on laminin 5 and collagen 7).

Kindler Syndrome

Rare autosomal recessive disorder characterized by poikiloderma, trauma-induced blisters and variable photosensitivity. Defect in KIND1 gene which encodes kindlin-1 protein involved in actin cytoskeleton. Blistering and photosensitivity start infancy or early childhood, poikiloderma appears later and is progressive. Blisters mainly over injury prone areas like hands and feet, less commonly over elbows, kneel and buttocks. These heal with atrophic scars, wrinkling and nail dystrophy/loss. Mucosal blisters heal with scaring (oral, conjunctival etc.) and strictures (urethral, anal etc.). Photsensitivity variable, actinic keratoses may develop.

Treatment

Mainly symptomatic-sun protection and wound care.

ECTODERMAL DYSPLASIAS

A large heterogeneous group. Primary defect in sweat glands, teeth, hair and nails.

Anhidrotic (Hypohidrotic) Ectodermal Dysplasia

Uncommon. X-linked inheritance; occasionally autosomal recessive. Complete syndrome in boys. Female carriers may have incomplete syndrome. Poor or absent sweating, sparse hair and poor dentition. *Characteristic facies*: saddle nose, frontal bossing, prominent supraorbital ridge, peg-shaped teeth, thick everted lips. Most patients look strikingly similar. *Hair:* scanty, fine, dry, light colored. Absent or sparse scalp hair, eyebrows and eyelashes. Axillary and pubic hair and beard—poor growth. *Teeth:* conical and spaced; occasional anodontia. *Glandular development:* poor development of salivary, lacrimal and mucous glands. Patients develop increased body temperature in hot weather due to absent or poor sweating. Also hyperthermia during febrile episodes. Intelligence generally normal.

INHERITED TUMORS AND TUMOR SYNDROMES

Neurofibromatoses

Common. Autosomal dominant inheritance, variable expression. Several distinct genetic disorders (including NF1, NF2, segmental NF1, familial

Diagnostic criteria for NF-1 (two or more required for diagnosis)
1. Six or more cafe-au-lait macules over 5 mm in greatest diameter in prepubertal individuals, and over 15 mm in postpubertal individuals
2. Two or more neurofibromas of any type or more plexiform neurofibroma
3. Freckling in the axillary or inguinal regions
4. Optic glioma
5. Two or more irris Lisch nodules
6. A distinctive osseous lesion such as sphenoid dysplasia or thinning of long bone cortex with or without pseudarthrosis
7. A first-degree relative (parent, sibling, or offspring) with NF-1 by the above criteria

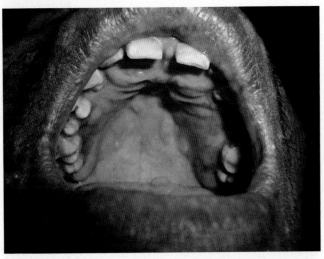

Neurofibromatosis 1: Mucosal neuromas over palate and dorsum of tongue.

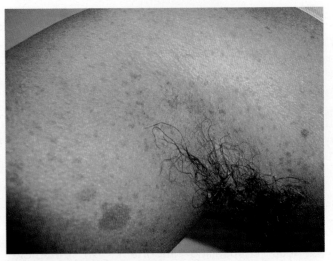

Neurofibromatosis 1: Crowe sign (axillary freckling).

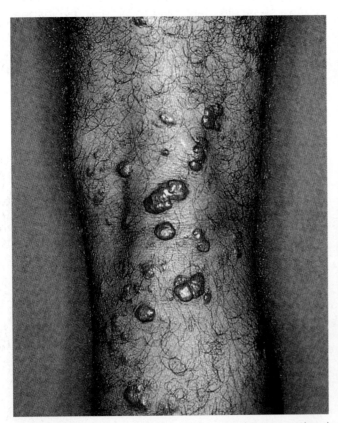

Neurofibromatosis: multiple soft skin-brown colored neurofibromas.

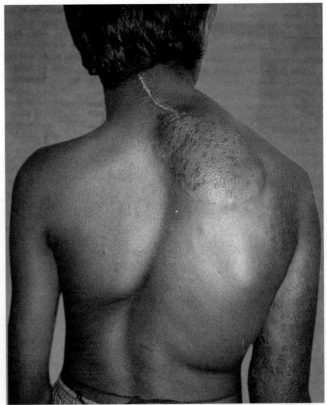

Mosaic/segmental neurofibromatosis type 1: Plexiform NF over the right upper back and involving the right upper limb with CALMs, soft tissue hypertrophy of limb and kyphoscoliosis.

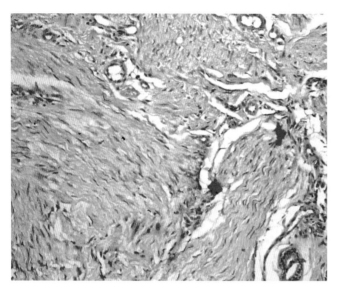

Histopathology of neurofibroma: numerous spindal cell fascicles seen with nuclear buckling and wavy nerve fibers.

cafe-au-lait macules & schwannomatosis). One type chiefly skin related (NF1/*von Recklinghausen's disease*) and the other related to nervous system (NF2).

Etiology of NF1

Mutation of NF1 gene on chromosome 17, reduced production of neurofibromin protein.

Clinical Manifestations

Cutaneous neuromas, cafe-au-lait macules and freckling. Cutaneous neuromas (molluscum fibrosum): soft, skin or brown colored, dome-shaped, sessile or pedunculated cutaneous or subcutaneous tumors. Vary in number and size. Plexiform neurofibromas—large, with a 'worms-in-a-bag' feel. Asymptomatic. Cafe-au-lait macules: sharply defined, uniformly light brown macules of varying sizes; margin irregular. Often the first manifestation of the disease; increase in number and size during the first decade. Axillary freckling (Crowe sign) and palmar freckling (Premlata Yesudian or 'PY' sign) are diagnostic. Neural fibromas occur along the cranial or peripheral nerves or in spinal cord. Acoustic and optic nerve

neuromas fairly common. Malignant peripheral nerve sheath tumor in plexiform NF (uncommon).

Histology: Dermis based non-encapsulated tumors. Thin neural fascicles with wavy nuclei lying singly in the loose connective tissue matrix. Mucin +/–. In plexiform NF, large nerve fascicles, loose but cellular matrix, abundant mucin, primarily deep dermal and subcutaneous but extension dermal extension in huge masses.

Segmental NF

Mosaic localized NF1 better term. Usually somatic mosaicism. Conadal mosaicism possible. Involvement of a part of body with CALMs and neurofibromas.

Treatment

Multiplicity of lesions makes treatment difficult. Excise large or unsightly tumors or ones suspicious of a malignant change. Offer genetic counseling. Surgical management of systemic conditions likeoptic nerve tumors, kyphoscoliosis. Experimental treatments for plexiform NFs include sirolimus, imatinib, pegylated interferon alpha etc.

Tuberous Sclerosis (Epiloia)

Uncommon. Autosomal dominant inheritance. Mutation in either TSC1 or TSC2 genes. Varied cutaneous and neurological manifestations. *Skin lesions:* depigmented macules: oval, well-defined, depigmentation on the back or trunk—ash–*leaf macules* may be the *first manifestation*.

Angiofibromas (adenoma sebaceum, a misnomer): small, firm, skin colored or pink papules or nodules present in the central part of the face particularly in the naso-labial folds. Also pale-yellow, or skin colored, slightly elevated, plaques—*shagreen* patches. Periungual fibromata —*Koenen's tumors*—firm, skin colored 'clove-like' projections from the nail folds.

Neurological manifestations: variable—mental deficiency, epileptiform seizures; cortical calcifications. Rarely renal, cardiac or pulmonary hamartomas.

Course: unpredictable but not unfavorable except in full blown cases.

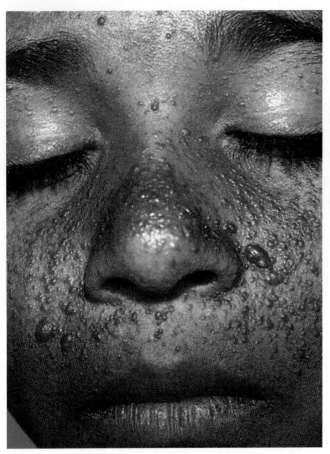

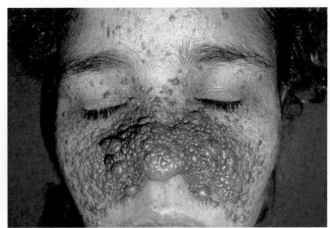

Tuberous sclerosis: angiofibromas coalescing over the centro-facial area to form of plaque.

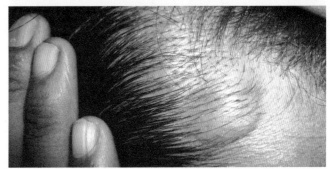

Tuberous sclerosis: angiofibromas on the nose and cheeks.

Tuberous sclerosis: collagenoma on the forehead('fibrous fore-head plaque').

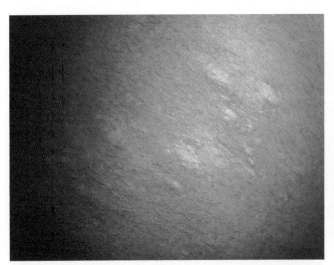

Tuberous sclerosis, shagreen patch: skin colored grouped papules and plaques over trunk.

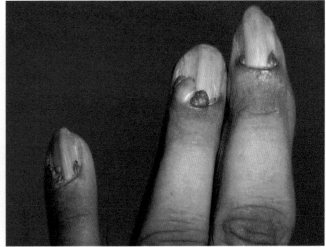

Tuberous sclerosis, periungual fibromas: fleshy papules and nodules arising from the nail folds producing guttering of the nail plate.

Tuberous sclerosis: multi-system clinical manifestations

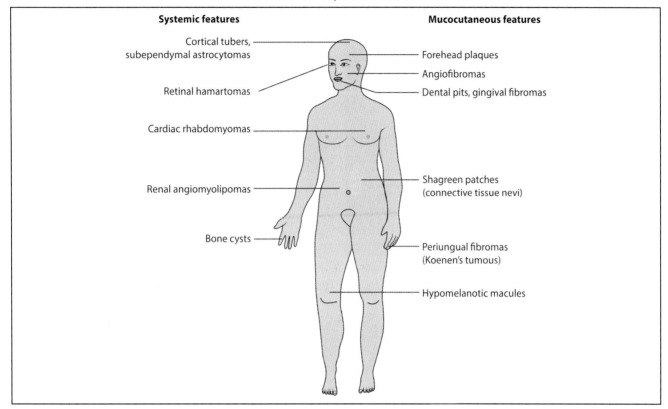

Systemic features	Mucocutaneous features
Cortical tubers, subependymal astrocytomas	Forehead plaques
	Angiofibromas
Retinal hamartomas	Dental pits, gingival fibromas
Cardiac rhabdomyomas	
Renal angiomyolipomas	Shagreen patches (connective tissue nevi)
Bone cysts	Periungual fibromas (Koenen's tumous)
	Hypomelanotic macules

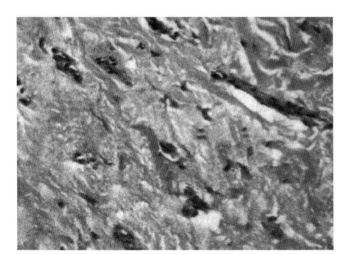

Histopathology of angiofibroma: dense dermal collagen and multiple blood vessels.

Treatment

Electrofulguration or laser ablation. Symptomatic treatment of seizures.

Trichoepithelioma

Uncommon. Hamartoma of pilosebaceous apparatus. Multiple familial trichoepitheliomas has autosomal dominant inheritance. Gene for multiple trichoepitheliomas mapped to chromosome 9.

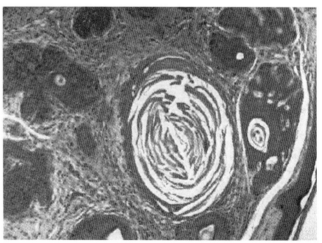

Histopathology of trichoepithelioma: focal collection of basaloid cells; hairshaft like structures in the center.

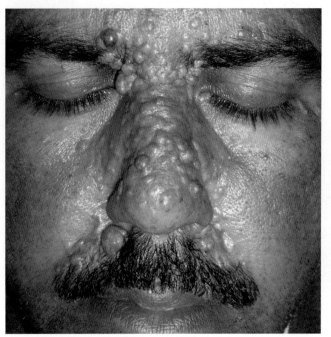

Trichoepitheliomas: multiple skin colored to few yellowish papules and nodules over centrofacial area.

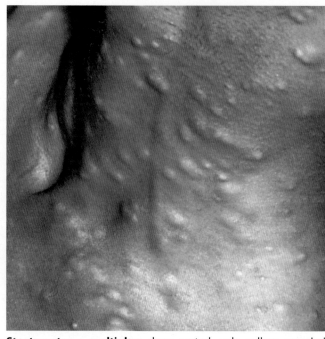

Steatocystoma multiplex: deep seated, pale yellow rounded and oval nodules.

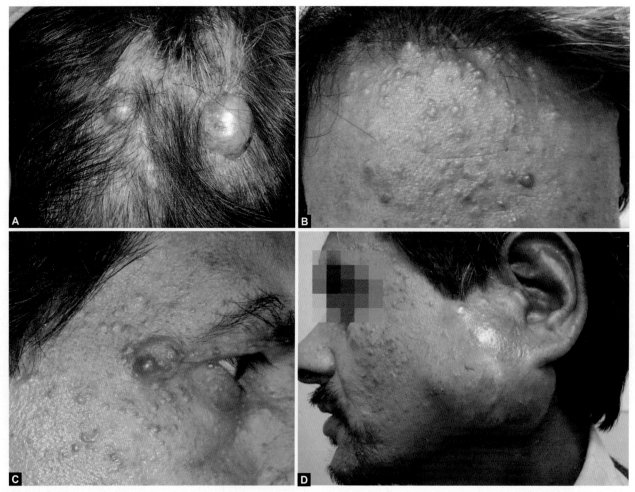

Brooke spiegler syndrome: composite image (A) scalp cylindromas; (B) forehead trichoepithelomas; (C) eccrine spiradenoma near outer canthus; (D) parotid tumor.

Non-familial or sporadic cases more common. Appearance at puberty or young adults. Solitary lesions as smooth nodules on face. Multiple, lesions as pale-yellow, dome shaped papules or nodules over centrofacial area-nose, philtrum area, nasolabial folds, eyelids. Symmetrical. May increase in number. Rare transformation to basal cell carcinoma.

Brooke-Spiegler Syndrome

Rare. Autosomal dominant inheritance. CYLD gene mutation, chromosome 16q. Characterized by multiple trichoepitheliomas and cylindromas, with or without spiradenomas. Several rarer benign appendageal tumors reported, along with composite tumors (e.g. spiradenocylindroma, etc.). Few associated with parotid basal cell adenoma/carcinoma. No specific treatment. Palliative-excision (blade, radiofrequency, Moh's, CO_2 laser). Topical salicylate tried for cylindromas.

Steatocystoma Multiplex

Rare. Autosomal dominant inheritance in many cases which have keratin 17 mutation. Multiple, asymptomatic, smooth, firm or soft, yellowish dermal cysts on neck, chest, proximal parts of upper extremities. Variable sized—a few millimetres to larger. No punctum. Cheesy material or oily fluid extrudes on puncturing. No definitive treatment. Radio-frequency induced puncture and expression helps.

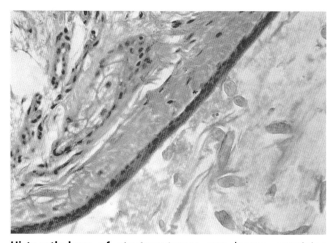

Histopathology of steatocystoma: cyst lumen containing numerous vellous follicles, wall showing eosinophilic cuticle and a sebaceous gland lobule.

Cowden Disease

Mutation in PTEN1 or TGF beta receptor. Skin colored papules around eyes and mouth, papillomatosis of labial and buccal mucosa, punctate keratosis of palms & soles. Craniomegaly. Association with carcinomas breast, thyroid.

DISORDERS OF CONNECTIVE TISSUE

Pseudoxanthoma Elasticum (PXE)

Uncommon. Mutation in ATP binding cassette (ABCC6). Autosomal recessive disorder, thought of as primarily metabolic disease with elastic tissue involvement. Complete syndrome skin changes (pseudoxanthoma elasticum), ocular lesions (angioid streaks) and vascular disturbances (hypertension, gastrointestinal hemorrhages and ischemic heart disease). *Skin lesions:* Yellowish (pseudoxanthomatous) discrete to confluent papules in skin folds (neck, axillae, cubitals, periumblical, groins etc) giving 'chicken skin', 'Moroccon leather' or cobblestone appearance. Reticulate or linear configuration. Skin: soft, lax and finely wrinkled. Lesions persistent and unaltered. Sites at predilection: sides of neck, axillae, groins and abdomen. Ocular changes: angioid streaks-radiating greyish streaks on the retina. *Vascular changes:* death from coronary occlusive disease or gastrointestinal hemorrhages.

Histopathology

Fragmented basophilic staining elastic fibers in the mid dermis.

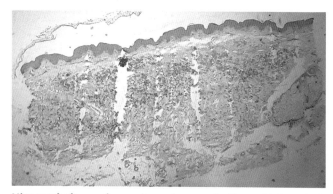

Histopathology of pseudoxanthoma elasticum histopathology: Deep pink, fragmented and calcium laden elastic tissue in mid dermis (Haematoxylin and Eosin, 4x)

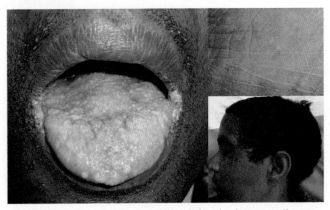

Cowden disease: Composite photo; left side shows papilomatosis over angles of mouth and tongue, right upper shows palmar keratosis, right lower shows craniomegaly.

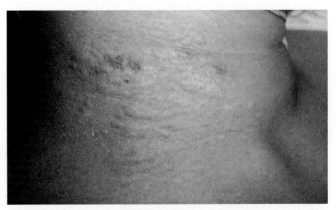

Pseudoxanthoma elasticum: Yellowish confluent papules over the side of neck, producing 'cobblestone' appearance.

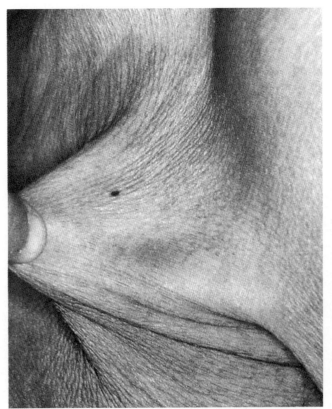

Ehlers-Danlos syndrome: hyperextensible skin.

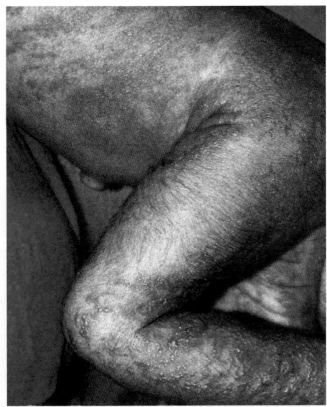

Incontinentia pigmenti: vesicular and verrucous lesions, lower limbs and trunk.

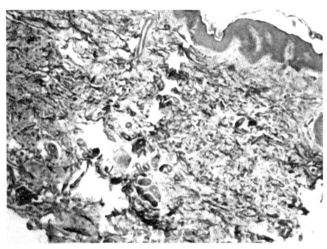

Histopathology of pseudoxanthoma elasticum: fragmented elastic fibers (black fibers), mid dermis (Verhoeff-van Gieson stain, 10x).

Treatment

Chiefly directed at preventing and combating vascular complications. Skin lesions only cosmetically objectionable.

Ehlers-Danlos Syndrome (Cutis Hyperelastica)

Rare. Genetic defects variable and not known in many variants; mutations in collagens 1, 3 and 5, fibronectin etc. Several variants: autosomal dominant. Or recessive. Or X-linked recessive inheritance. *Skin:* soft, smooth, hyperextensible (not lax atrophic scars, molluscoid pseudotumors, easy bruisability etc.). *Others:* hypermobile joints, fragile blood vessels, risk of bowel rupture, bony deformities, kyphoscoliosis etc.

Course: severity and prognosis variable.

PIGMENTARY DISORDERS

Incontinentia Pigmenti (Bloch-Sulzberger Syndrome)

Rare. X-linked dominant inheritance. Lethal in males, so patients always females barring anecdotal cases of gonadal mosaicism. NEMO (nuclear factor kappa B essential modulator) gene mutation on X chromosome. Three independent or overlapping phases: *vesiculobullous, verrucous*

and *pigmentary.* Onset, *in utero* or soon after birth. *Vesiculobullous* phase: localized or generalised crops of clear, tense, grouped bullae. Limbs often affected. Recur for days or weeks. *Verrucous phase:* irregular linearly distributed warty papules on the limbs or trunk. Sites, those affected by vesiculo-bullous lesions or independent. *Pigmentary phase:* characteristic, slate-grey or brown, bizzarre, *whorled* or splashed pigmentation. May persist or gradually fade. *Associated:* cicatricial alopecia, dental, ocular and neurological abnormalities (mental retardation, epileptiform seizures. Eosinophilia common.

Histopathology

Intraepidermal spongiotic vesicle containing eosinophils in the vesicular stage. Verrucous phase: hyperkeratosis and irregular acanthosis. Incontinence of pigment in the pigmentary stage conspicuous.

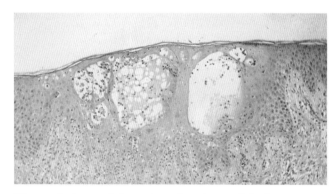

Histopathology of incontinentia pigmenti bullous stage: Intra-epidermal spongiotic vesicles containing eosinophils.

Treatment

No treatment available, topical steroids and tacrolimus may help reducing pruritus in vesicular/ verrucous stage.

Linear and Whorled Nevoid Hypermelanosis

Disorder of chromosomal mosaicism. Hyperpigmentation in linear and whorled configuration over the trunk and limbs, sparing face, palms and soles. Extracutaneous features include developmental and growth retardation, body asymmetry. No treatment available.

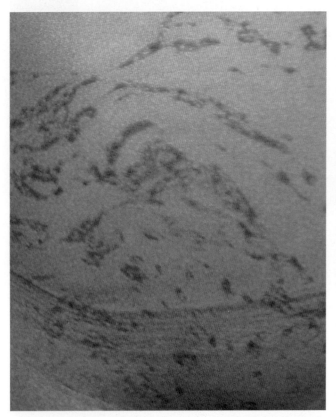

Incontinentia pigmenti stage 3: Streaky whorled hyperpigmentation over trunk in a child.

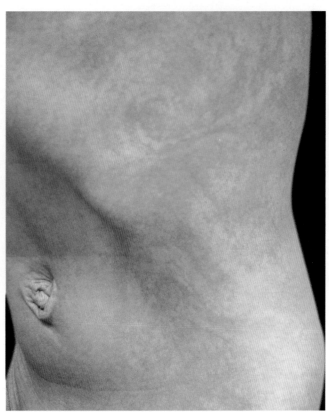

Linear and whorled hypermelanosis: Fine hyperpigmented lines in blaschoid pattern over trunk.

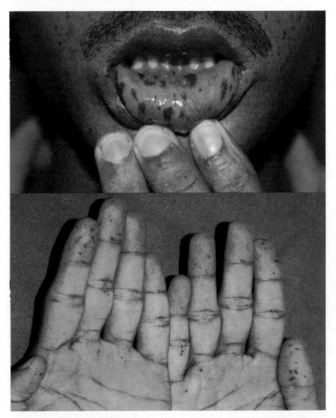

Peutz Jegher syndrome: brown-black lentigines involving perioral area, lip mucosa and fingers.

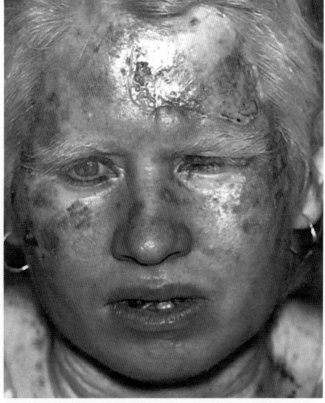

Oculo-cutaneous albinism: tyrosinase negative type. Pink irides, white hair and actinic keratosis—a total lack of pigmentation.

Peutz-Jeghers Syndrome (Periorificial Lentiginosis)

Rare. Autosomal dominant inheritance. Inactivating mutations in serine threonine kinase gene LKB1. A combination of mucocutaneous pigmentation and gastrointestinal polyps. Onset at birth or early childhood. Oval, circular or irregular, brown black to black macules. Mucosa consistently involved. The lips, gums or buccal mucosa and perioral area affected. Face, hands and feet. Polyposis generally in small intestine. Abdominal pain, vomiting, bleeding per rectum or hematemesis. Increased risk of malignancies in several organs. Pigmentation without polyposis may occur.

Treatment

Surgical removal of polyps. Lasers tried with success for mucocutaneous pigmentation.

Albinism (Oculo-Cutaneous Albinism)

Widely varying prevalence. Autosomal recessive inheritance. Failure to form melanin in the skin and the eyes. Two types: *tyrosinase positive* and *tyrosinase negative*, the latter less common, but more severe. Dead white skin that sunburns easily. Pink irides, photophobia, nystagmus and impaired visual acuity. Progressive solar damage of light exposed skin: solar elastosis, actinic keratoses and squamous cell carcinomas.

Tyrosinase positive albinism: some pigment present in the skin, hair and irides. Freckling and irregular pigment formation in light exposed skin. Patients improve with age.

Treatment

Total protection from sunlight. Nocturnal living. *Surveillance for neoplasms:* treat solar keratoses with 5-fluorouracil; excise squamous cell carcinomas.

Piebaldism

Autosomal dominant. Mutated c-kit protooncogene on chromosome 4q12, causes defective migration and differentiation of melanoblasts from neural crest. Depigmented macules; characteristic islands of hyperpigmentation occur within these macules.

Mid-forehead, central eyebrows, neck, anterior trunk, mid extremities, feet, back, shoulders, and hips. White forelock seen in 80–90%.

Treatment

Camouflage. Autologous, cultured epithelial grafts help.

Waardenburg Syndrome

Autosomal dominant syndrome of hypopigmented patches, dystopia canthorum, white forelock, sensorineural deafness.

DISORDERS OF GENOMIC INSTABILITY

Xeroderma Pigmentosum

Etiology

Autosomal recessive inheritance. Genetically heterogeneous subtypes, called *complementation* groups A-G. And *XP variant*. XP complementation groups with corresponding mutations in genes XP-A to XP-G, XP variant with mutation in a subtype of DNA polymerase.

Cells have a defective endonuclease activity, thus lack the ability to normally repair the UV light induced damage to DNA. Rare group of disorders characterized by photosensitivity, predisposed to develop cutaneous and internal malignancies. Occasional neurological involvement.

Clinical Manifestations

Manifestations confined to or predominant in light exposed parts of the skin. Onset: infancy or early childhood, rarely adulthood. Skin: easy sunburning, often the initial manifestation. Hallmark is skin dryness (xerosis), mottled hyper – and hypopigmentation and background telangiectasias. Freckling, rough hyperkeratotic papules (actinic keratoses), angiomata, superficial ulcerations and atrophic, white spots follow. Patients have 10,000 fold increased risk of skin cancer and 10–20 fold risk of developing internal malignancy. Cutaneous malignancies frequent and early. Commonly, basal or squamous cell carcinomas and malignant melanomas. Multiple metastases cause early death, generally before adolescence. *Ocular manifestations:*

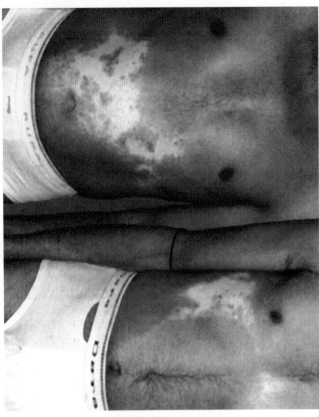

Piebaldism: depigmented macules on the ventral aspect of trunk with islands of hyperpigmentation.

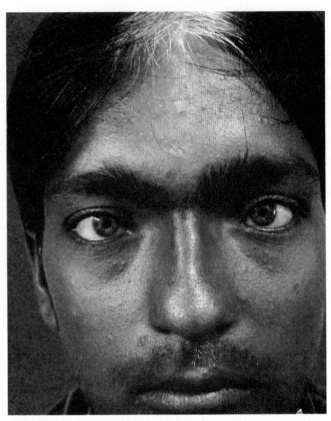

Waardenburg syndrome: White forelock, dystopia canthorum, blue iridis.

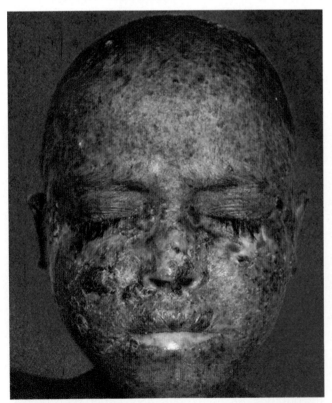

Xeroderma pigmentosum: mottled hypo- and hyperpigmentation on sun exposed areas, dry skin and multiple basal and squamous cell carcinomas.

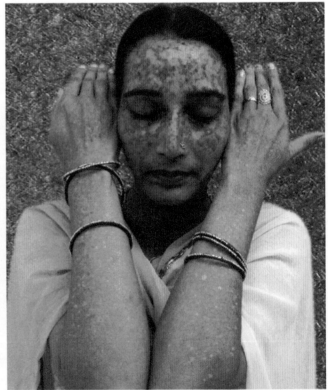

Xeroderma pigmentosum variant(pigmented xerodermoid): mottled hypo- and hyperpigmentation over face and sun exposed areas of upper limbs.

common—photophobia, corneal opacities, ectropion. Occasionally *neurological manifestations:* severe mental retardation, microcephaly. As also hypogonadism, dwarfism and deafness all seen in *xerodermic idiocy* or *De Sanctis—Cacchione syndrome.* XP variant or *pigmented xerodermoid*: Late onset. Mild photosensitivity.

Course

Progressively downhill. Life expectancy severely compromised.

Treatment

Strict and complete protection from sunlight. Mainly protection required from UVB but broad spectrum sun screens preferred. Prenatal diagnosis possible; termination of pregnancy if desired and legally permissible. Oral retinoids (isotretinoin at 0.5 mg/kg) helpful in prophylaxis of cutaneous malignancies. Topically applied bacterial endonuclease named denV T4 endonulease may be promising for future. Facial skin changes shown to respond to topical imiquimod.

Bloom Syndrome

Autosomal recessive. Mutant gene, BLM, on 15q26.1, controls DNA helicase activity and maintains genomic stability. Boys. Telangiectatic erythema in butterfly distribution, bird-like facies, short stature, long limbs high-pitched voice. Increased susceptibility to infections (respiratory and gastrointestinal tract) and malignancies (leukemia, lymphoma and gastrointestinal adenocarcinoma).

POIKILODERMATOUS DISORDERS

Dyskeratosis Congenita

X-linked recessive. Mutant gene, DKC1, encodes protein dyskerin. *Triad:* reticulate or mottled pigmentation, nail dystrophy and premalignant leukoplakia. *Other features:* palmo-plantar hyperkeratosis and adermatoglyphia (absent dermal ridges on fingers and toes). Progressive pancytopenia in most patients—principal cause of mortality.

Rothmund-Thomson Syndrome

Rare. Autosomal recessive inheritance; mostly affects females. Mutation in DNA helicase gene, RECQL4. Begins in infancy or early childhood. Poikilodermatous changes—atrophy, telangiectasia, pigmentation, particularly on the cheeks and later other light exposed areas. Skin lesions unaltered. Solar keratoses or squamous cell carcinoma may develop around puberty.

SYNDROMES WITH SILVER HAIR

Griscelli Syndrome

Autosomal recessive. Silver grey hair. Associated with neurological abnormalities (type 1; myosin SA gene mutation), immunodeficiency (type 2; RAB27 A gene mutation) or no abnormality (type 3; melanophilin gene mutation). Giant granules in granulocytes absent (c.t. Chediak Higashi syndrome).

Hair Microscopy

Characteristic; large clumps of pigment distributed irregularly along the hair shaft.

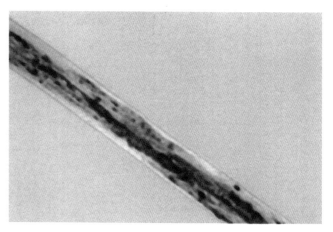

Griscelli syndrome: light microscopy of hair shows large clumps of pigment distributed irregularly along the shaft.

Histopathology

Enlarged hyperpigmented basal melanocytes with sparse pigmentation of adjacent keratinocytes.

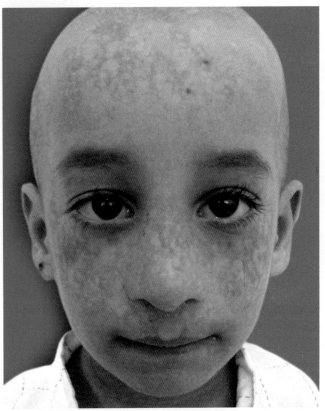

Bloom syndrome: erythematous/telangiectatic macules on face, prominent nose and malar hypoplasia.

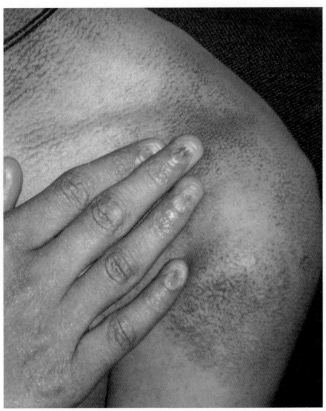

Dyskeratosis congenita: reticulate pigmentation (poikiloderma), multiple nails dystrophic.

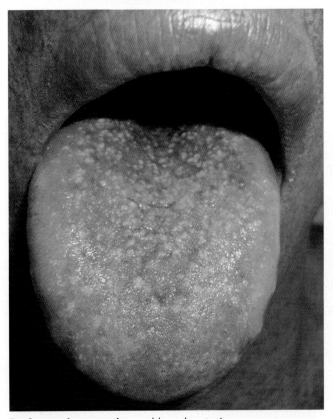

Dyskeratosis congenita: oral leucokeratosis.

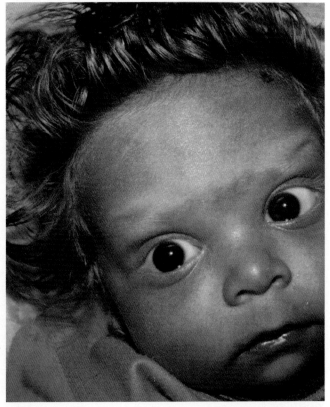

Griscelli syndrome: silvery grey hair, hypopigmentation and normal eyes.

Treatment

Genetic counselling. Also seizure control (Type 1). Bone marrow transplantation (Type 2), systemic steroids and immunosuppressives, palliative.

Elejalde Syndrome (Neuroectodermal Melano-lysosomal Syndrome)

Genetic linkage not known. Silver grey hair, photosensitivity and profound neurological dysfunction. Immune system normal. Hair microscopy and skin histology: similar to Griscelli syndrome.

Treatment

Supportive.

Chediak Higashi Syndrome

Autosomal recessive: mutation in lysosomal trafficking regulator gene on chromosome 1 q42.1. Silver grey hair, photophobia, nystagmus, neutropenia; susceptibility to infection and lymphoma. Granulocytes show giant granules.

Hair Microscopy

Small clumps of pigment distributed uniformly along the hair shaft.

Treatment

Supportive: control infections and seizures. Definitive: bone marrow transplantation. Palliative: systemic steroids and immunosuppressives.

OTHER GENODERMATOSES

Monilethrix

Rare, autosomal dominant hair shaft disorder. Mutation in genes encoding for human hair keratins hHb1 and hHb6.
Hair shaft is beaded at regular intervals (nodes and internodes), breaks easily at the internodes. Variable clinical severity. Hair loss and breaking off associated with follicular keratosis, mostly over the nape of neck and occiput. Eyebrows, eyelashes, axillary and pubic hair may also be affected.

Treatment

Spontaneous improvement known in some cases. Oral retinoids gave relief, probably in follicular keratosis. Topical minoxidil may give some relief.

Acrodermatitis Enteropathica

Rare. Inheritance, probably autosomal recessive. Basically a defect in zinc absorption. Gene defect in SLC39A4 encoding intestinal zinc transporter. Onset in infancy—within a few weeks of weaning off breast feeds. Steatorrhea or diarrhea. Loss of weight. Stunted physical growth. Behavioral disturbances. *Skin:* bullous, psoriasiform or eczematous erosive lesions around the orifices and acral parts of extremities. Candidal, bacterial or other infections (either cutaneous or systemic). Hair: Brittle, diffuse alopecia, light and dark bands on polarizing. Untreated, patients die in early childhood. Raised serum alkaline phosphatase levels helpful but low serum levels of zinc diagnostic.

Treatment

Zinc sulfate with elemental zinc at 2–3 mg/ kg/day brings about a fairly dramatic response. Continue therapy till adulthood to prevent relapse.

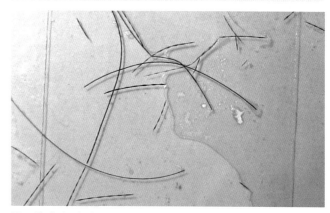

Monilethrix, hair mount: Hair shafts beaded at regular intervals seen on naked eye examination itself.

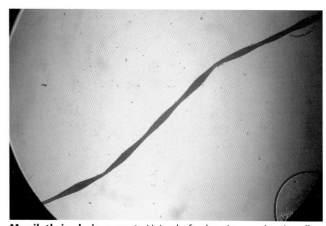

Monilethrix, hair mount: Hair shaft showing nodes (swollen areas) and internodes (constricted areas) at regular intervals.

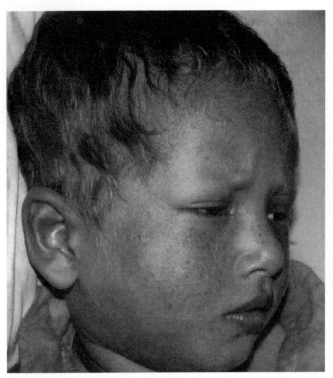

Elejalde syndrome: silver-grey hair, photophobia and photosensitivity giving bronze colored skin.

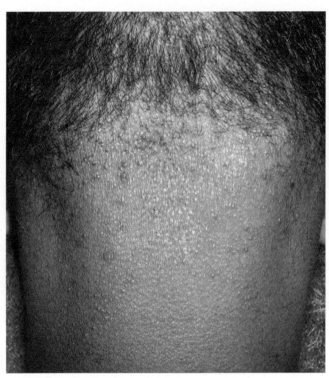

Monilethrix: keratotic papules over nape of neck. Note: hair loss involving the occipital scalp.

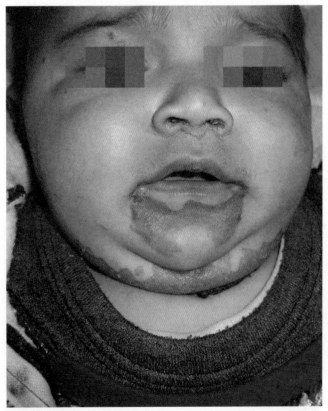

Acrodermatitis enteropathica: scaly psoriasiform plaques involving perinasal, perioral and neck regions.

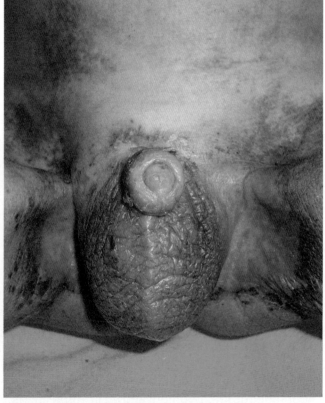

Acrodermatitis enteropathica: erosive eczematous plaques involving genitalia and groins.

Pachydermoperiostosis

Primary also known as Touraine-Solente-Gole syndrome. Or secondary—often associated with pulmonary malignancy, endocrinopathies or suppuration.

Primary: Rare. Autosomal dominant or recessive inheritance. Some cases have defect in hydroxy-progesterone dehydrogenase gene. Onset around puberty. Thickened and folded skin of the face, forehead and scalp (*cutis verticis gyrata*). Increased sebaceous gland activity on the face. Palmo-plantar hyperhidrosis. Thickened phalanges and ends of long bones. Clubbing of finger and toe nails. Painful polyarthropathies. Course, unpredictable, generally not unfavorable. Life span may be lowered. Medical therapy mainly for polyarthropathies (NSAIDs, steroids, colchicine). For forehead wrinkling, ptosis and hyperhydrosis, botulinum toxin may help.

Epidermodysplasia Verruciformis

Autosomal recessive. Specific defect of cellmediated immune response to human 'papilloma virus' resulting in widespread persistent infection. Polymorphic macules resembling pityriasis versicolor and warty flattopped papules resembling verruca plana or flat warts. Papules coalesce to form large plaques. Malignant transformation common, usually in sun-exposed areas.

Histopathology

Clear cells in granular and spinous layers with enlarged hyperchromatic, atypical nuclei.

Treatment

Sunscreens. Systemic acitretin (retinoid) and interferons may help. Regular follow-up needed for early detection of malignancies.

Hyper IgE Syndrome (Syn—Job Syndrome, Buckley Syndrome)

Rare. Most cases sporadic or autosomal dominant with variable penetrance. Autosomal recessive uncommon.

Different gene defects known but most common in STAT3 (signal transducer and activator of transcription). Absent Th17 type of T cells, making patient prone to recurrent bacterial and fungal infections.

Clinical Manifestations

Classic triad of recurrent staphylococcal abscesses on skin, pneumonia with pneumatoceles and high serum IgE levels. Atopic dermatitis develops in childhood. Mucocutaneous candidiasis also common. Facial and skeletal abnormalities—coarse facial features, dental anomalies, scoliosis, hyper-extensible joints.

Treatment

Anti-staphylococcal antibiotics and atifungals for candidal infections effective episodically and prophylactically. Intravenous immunoglobulin is most effective. Vitamin C and cimetidine also used with good effect in some. Bone marrow transplant not yet effective.

Fabry's Disease

Rare X-linked lysosomal storage disorder. Males show high penetration, milder/variable disease expression. Defect in GLA gene for α-galactsidase-A enzyme, leading to depositon of sphingolipids in lysosomes in various tissues and fluids. Onset in early childhood. Skin lesion in form of timing red papules all over the body (angiokeratoma corporis diffusum, ACD), more in number over trunk (concentrate between umblicus and knees). Also, these lesions involve oral and conjunctival mucosa. Other features—hypohidrosis, Raynaud's phenomenon, acro-paraesthesias, corneal opacities, and GI, renal, CNS and cardiac disease. Latter two responsible for morbidity and shortening of life span.

Histpathology

Biopsy of ACD shows finding same as other angiokeratomas—dilated capillaries abutting and expanding the dermal papillae.

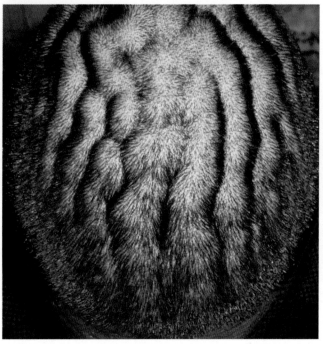

Pachydermoperiostosis: cutis verticis gyrata (cerebriform folds) of the scalp.

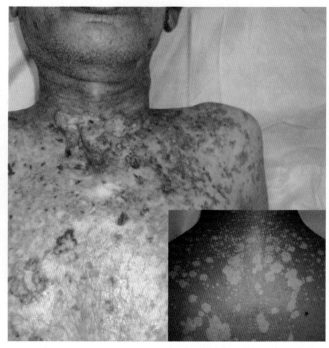

Epidermodysplasia verruciformis: different types of lesions—hyperpigmented macules and barely elevated papules, seorrheic keratosis like lesions, few plaques of bowen's disease and basal cell carcinoma. Inset shows pityriasis versicolor like lesions on back.

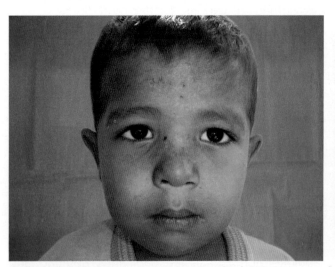

Hyper IgE syndrome: coarse facial features—wide nasal root, broad nasal tip, prominent forehead. Scaly papules (few excoriated) over face suggestive of atopic dermatitis.

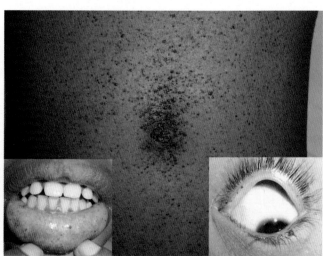

Fabry's disease: red papules on abdomen, most concentrated around umblicus. Inset shows similar lesions over lip mucosa and conjunctiva.

Treatment

Enzyme repacement therapy—Fabrazyme (α-galactsidase type B enzyme), Replagel (α-galactsidase type A enzye) only definitive treatment. Symptomatic treatment as per clinical manifestations.

Summary of common inheritance pattern in genodermatoses

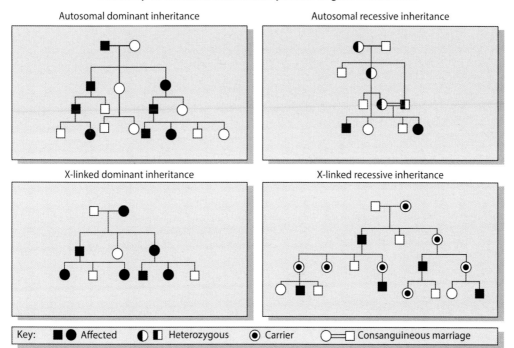

17

Nevoid Conditions

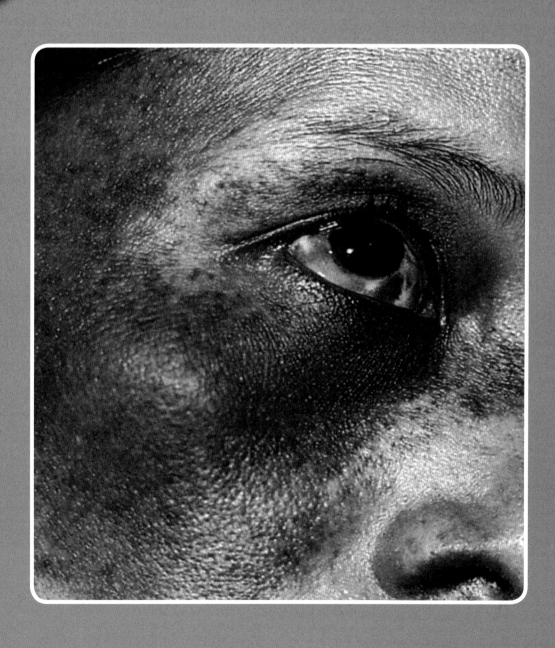

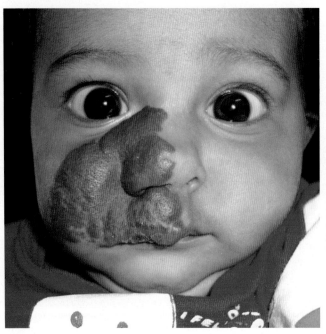

Infantile hemangioma, superficial type: large plaque with sharp midline demarcation, with focal atrophy and upper lip ulceration.

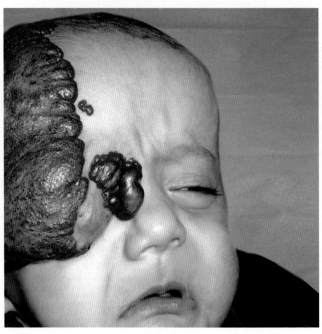

Infantile hemangioma, proliferative phase: massive, confluent, hypertrophic plaque involving the right side of face and causing visual obstruction (certain indication for systemic therapy).

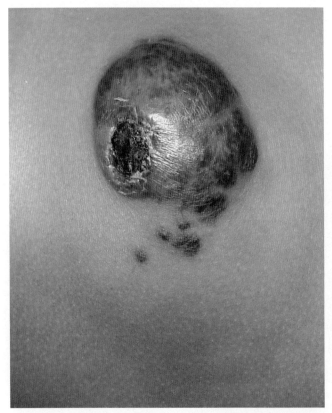

Infantile hemangioma, mixed type: superficial ulcerated hemangioma overlying a faint green swelling suggestive of deep component.

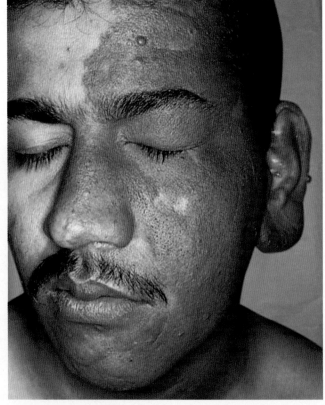

Capillary malformation, port wine stain type: unilateral vascular malformation confined to trigeminal distribution. Patient also had seizures (Sturge-Weber syndrome).

Developmental anomalies or *hamartomas* (abnormal quantity of normal tissues present in the skin). Common. Present at birth. Or appear in early childhood, occasionally later. Caused possibly by interactions between environmental and genetic factors. The term 'nevus' is prefixed by a term depicting the tissue affected; vascular nevi, connective tissue nevi, melanocytic nevi, etc. Other nevoid conditions may involve connective tissue, epidermis or adnexa such as hair, sebaceous and sweat glands. Malformations are anatomical defects resulting from abnormal tissue or organ development.

VASCULAR NEVI

Two types of lesions recognized: vascular malformations and hemangiomas.

Superficial Hemangioma (Older Term– Strawberry Hemangioma)

Common. Present at birth/appears in infancy. Frequent in premature children. Enlarges for few months to a year. Face, trunk frequently affected. Often single, occasionally multiple. Smooth or lobulated plaque or dome shaped nodule. Strawberry colored-as also stippled. May bleed, ulcerate/get infected. Spontaneous resolution in 5–7 years, universal. Multiple angiomatous nevi complicated by thrombocytopenia due to sequestration of thrombocytes.

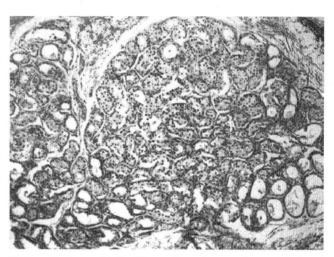

Histopathology of infantile capillary hemangioma: lobulated aggregate of capillaries, many showing proliferative changes.

Classification of vascular anomalies/nevi	
Vascular tumors	*Vascular malformations*
• Infantile hemangiomas	Slow-flow vascular malformations:
• Congenital hemangiomas (RICH and NICH)	• Capillary malformation (CM) Port wine stain Telangiectasia Angiokeratoma
• Tufted angioma (with or without Kasabach–Merritt syndrome)	• Venous malformation (VM) Common sporadic VM Bean syndrome Familial cutaneous and mucosal-glomangioma/ Glomuvenous malformation (GVM) Maffucci syndrome
• Kaposiform hemangioendothelioma (with or without Kasabach–Merritt syndrome)	• Lymphatic malformation (LM)
• Spindle cell hemangioendothelioma	Fast-flow vascular malformations:
• Other, rare hemangioendotheliomas	• Arterial malformation (AM)
• Dermatologic acquired vascular tumors (glomeruloid hemangioma, pyogenic granuloma, targetoid hemangioma, etc.)	• Arteriovenous fistula (AVF) • Arteriovenous malformation (AVM)
	Complex-combined vascular malformations:
	• CVM, CLM, LVM, CLVM, AVM-LM, CM-AVM

RICH: Rapidly involuting congenital hemangioma
NICH: Non-involuting congenital hemangioma

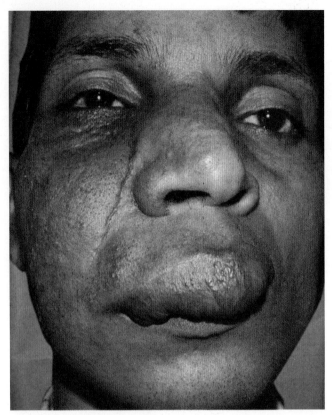

Hypertrophic port wine stain: hypertrophy of right side of face, especially upper lip. Capillary malformation is seen focally-over upper lip, right nasal ala and around the right eye.

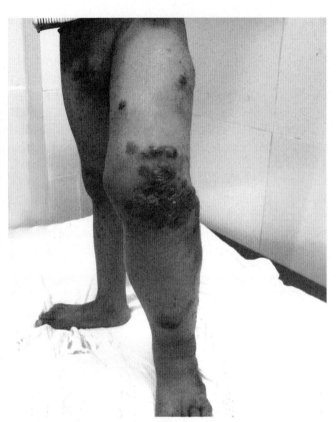

Klippel-Trénaunay syndrome: hypertrophic port wine stains, upper thigh venous dilatations (seen as faint green discoloration) and soft tissue hypertrophy of the left lower limb.

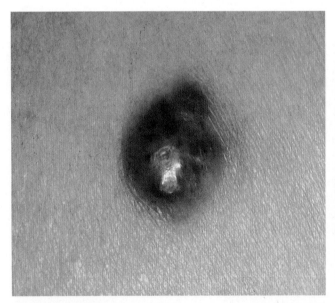

Blue rubber bleb nevus syndrome: deep blue nodule on trunk (tender on palpation).

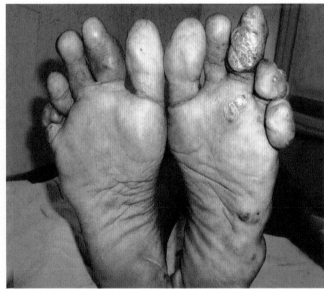

Maffucci syndrome: multiple blue nodules over the toes and soles. Enchondroma involving the right second toe.

Differences between infantile hemangiomas and vascular malformations		
	Infantile hemangioma	*Vascular malformations*
Age of occurence and course	Infancy and childhood	Everlasting if not treated
Course	Three stages: proliferating, involving, involuted	Commensurate growth or slow progression
Sex prevalence	3–9 girls/1 boy	1 girl/1 boy
Cellular	Increased endothelial cellular turnover Increased mastocytes Thick basement membrane	Normal cellular turnover. Normal number of mastocytes. Normal thin basement membrane
Factor causing flare	None (or unknown)	Trauma, hormonal changes
Pathology	Distinctive aspects of the three phases of the tumor. GLUT1+	CM, VM, LM, AVM, depending on the type. GLUT1–
Radiological aspects on MRI	Well-delineated tumor with flow voids	Hypersignal on T2-sequences with VM or LM. Flow voids without parenchymal staining with AVM
Treatment	Spontaneous involution, or pharmacological treatment, or surgery, lasers	Lasers, or surgery and/or embolization/sclerotherapy depending on the type

Treatment

Generally not required. Spontaneous resolution the rule with good cosmetic results—earlier the onset of resolution, better the results. Indication for treatment—disfiguring facial hemangiomas, involving vital structures, affecting vital functions, systemic involvement, ulceration in hemangioma. Currently, oral propranolol (dose 2–3 mg/kg/day) seems safest and best treatment option. Systemic steroids (dose 2–4 mg/kg/day) conventionally used but risk of side effects. Other modalities include topical timolol, imiquimod, etc.

Deep Hemangioma (Older Term-Cavernous Hemangioma)

Relatively uncommon. Present at birth. Large, ill defined, soft, bluish lobulated mass deep in the dermis or subcutis. 'Bag of worms' feel. Spontaneous resolution infrequent.

Telangiectatic Nevus Port Wine Stain (Nevus Flammeus)

Common. Ectatic superficial and deep dermal blood vessels. Present at birth. No increase in size. Face most often affected, unilaterally. Rarely acquired, more common over extremities. Sharp midline margination. Color varies from pink to purple. Long standing lesions become darker red and develop thickening and hyperkeratotic changes. Facial lesions may not respect trigeminal dermatomes, involving more than one dermatome partially. On limbs may lead to soft tissue hypertrophy and bony changes. Numerous lesions over the back may suggest underlying spinal dysraphism. Sturge-Weber syndrome a triad of triad of facial dermal capillary malformation, ipsilateral central nervous system (CNS) vascular malformation (leptomeningeal angiomatosis), and vascular malformation of the choroid of the eye associated with glaucoma. Incomplete forms known. Neurological symptoms include seizures, hemiplegia and mental retardation. CNS involvement more in port wine stains of V1 dermatome.

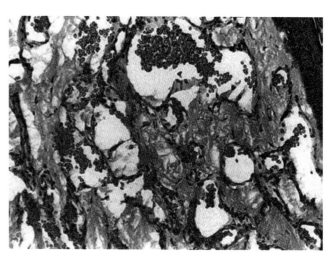

Histopathology of capillary malformation: collection of dilated capillaries in upper dermis.

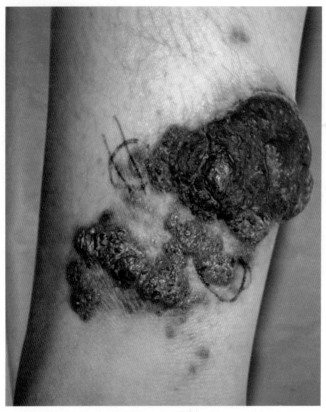

Angiokeratoma circumscriptum: localized keratotic plaque over capillary malformation, left leg.

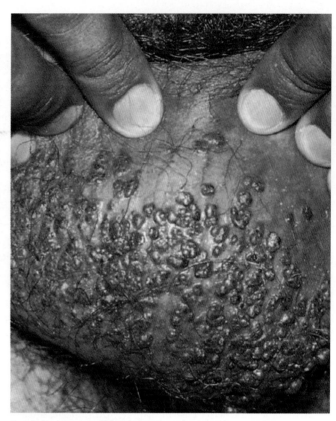

Angiokeratoma of fordyce: vascular papules, scrotum.

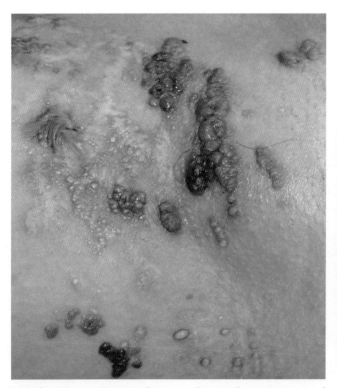

Lymphangioma circumscriptum, microcystic type: grouped vesicles, clear ('frog spawn' appearance) as well as hemorrhage.

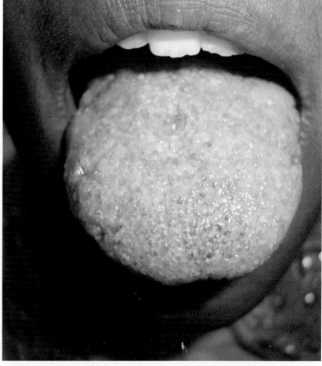

Lymphangioma circumscriptum, microcystic type: grouped vesicules causing macroglossia.

Treatment

Pulse dye lasers provide good relief. Centrofacial lesions and long standing/hypertrophic lesions show poor response. Best results achieved when laser done in childhood and on lateral face. Cosmetic camouflage. Surgery not helpful.

Klippel-Trenaunay Syndrome

Classically, capillary malformation of the skin with soft tissue and bony hypertrophy of the affected limb, and varicose veins with or without deep venous anomalies. Orthopedic consultation needed for limb length discrepancy. Recurrent thrombophlebitis and cellulitis may complicate the picture. Risk of deep venous thrombosis also there.

Blue Rubber Bleb Syndrome

Mostly sporadic. Few reports of familial cases. Cutaneous and gastrointestinal venous malformations. Most characteristic are blue compressible subcutaneous nodules on skin. Commonly on trunk and extremities. Gastrointestinal malformations cause for morbidity. Whole GI tract may be involved. Rectal occult bleeding or frank blood loss from upper or lower GI tract. Symptoms in childhood or adulthood. Malformation may involve CNS, orbit or genitourinary tract.

Maffucci Syndrome

Sporadic genetic disorder. Combination of enchondromas and vascular anomalies (superficial and deep venous malformations, hemangioendotheliomas, etc). Blue to purple soft nodules, may be tender. Usually on distal extremities, may involve internal viscera. Enchondromas involve phalanges and long bones.

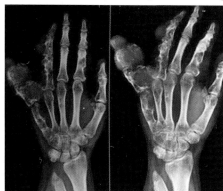

Maffucci syndrome: X-ray both hands showing multiple areas of bony destruction and lucencies in phalangial bones, suggestive of multiple enchondromas.

Angiokeratoma Circumscriptum

Localized capillary-lymphatic (mixed) malformation. Onset at birth, not inherited. Often on extremities. Pink to reddish blue raised hyperkeratotic plaques, may bleed on trauma. Separate capillary and lymphatic components may be seen.

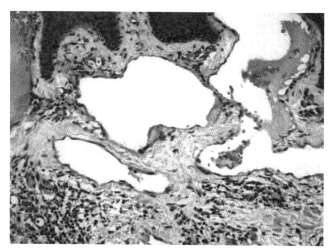

Histopathology of angiokeratoma: dilated blood vessels in papillary and mid dermis.

Angiokeratoma of Fordyce

Uncommon. Superficial ectatic blood vessels in superficial dermis. Elderly or adults. Deep red or purple, 1–5 mm, vascular papules on the scrotum, and infrequently on the glans penis. Usually asymptomatic. Occasionally bleed. Associated varicocele.

Treatment

Left alone or ablate with radiofrequency, cryotherapy or laser.

Lymphangioma Circumscriptum

Uncommon. Present at birth or appears during early childhood. Axillae, neck, upper trunk, proximal parts of extremities. Or mucosa affected. Multiple, closely-set, mulberry—like, clear or hemorrhagic vesicular lesions. Underlying deep seated subcutaneous lymphangioma. Associated hemangiomatous component may be present.

Treatment

Superficial lesions: destroyed with electric diathermy. Or radiofrequency ablation. Deep component poorly delineated and thus not easy to treat, even surgically.

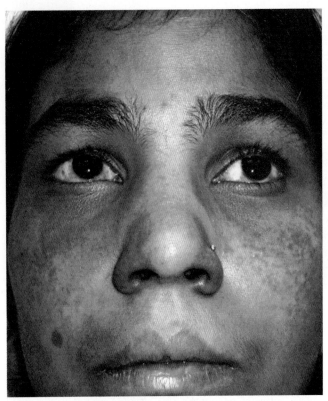

Phakomatosis pigmentovascularis type 2: combination of port wine stain (right half of face) and bilateral nevus of Ota (cheeks, nasal alae, periorbital and sclera).

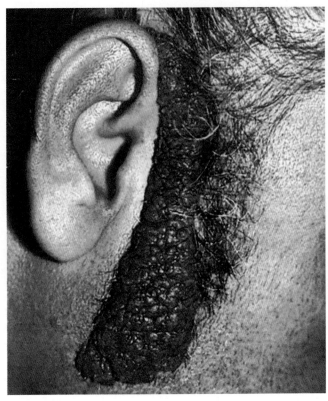

Verrucous epidermal nevus: a linear verrucous lesion.

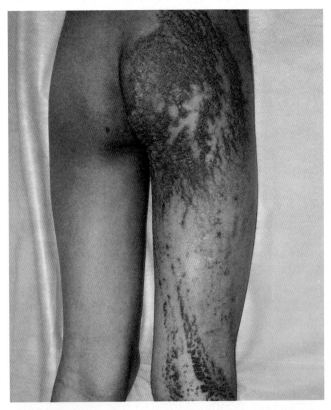

Verrucous epidermal nevus: nevus unius lateris (unilateral, widespread VEN).

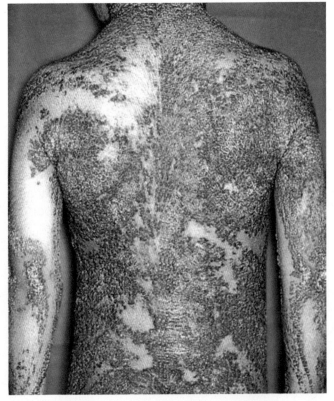

Verrucous epidermal nevus: systematized lesions.

Treatment of vascular nevi		
Modality	*Vascular tumors*	*Vascular malformations*
Pharmacological therapies (systemic steroids, propranolol, interferons-α 2a or 2b, vincristine, cyclophosphamide, bleomycin)	+++	+/–
Lasers PDL, Nd:YAG, diode, etc.	+	CM +++ VM and LM +
Surgical excision/resection (only for small localized lesions)	++	++
Sclerotherapy	–	VM and LM +++ AVM +
Arterial embolization	+/– (liver hemangiomas, hemangiomas with congestive cardiac failure)	AVM +++ VM +/–

Phakomatosis Pigmentovascularis

Rare, sporadic occurrence. Combination of different vascular, pigmented and epidermal nevi. Of several subtypes: type 1-port wine stain (PWS) with epidermal nevus; type 2-PWS and aberrant blue spot (mongolian or other dermal melanocytosis); type 3-PWS with nevus spilus, type 4-PWS with nevus spilus and aberrant blue spot; type 5-aberrant blue spot with cutis marmorata telangiectatica congenita.

EPIDERMAL NEVI

Hamartomas arising from ectodermal cells. Differentiate towards keratinocytes or epidermal appendages. Admixtures of varying proportions.

Verrucous Epidermal Nevus

Common. Present at birth, or appears during childhood. Skin colored or dark brown, localized, warty or flat, linear or irregular plaques. If widespread, called systematized nevi: present over most parts of the body. Widespread nevus involving 1 half of trunk/limb called nevus unius lateris. Follow lines of Blaschko. Vertical configuration along the limbs and horizontal, S-shaped on the trunk. Asymptomatic. May increase upto puberty and persist. Classified as either epidermolytic or non-epidermolytic type—based on clinical features and more on histology. Epidermolytic made out by variable height and verrucosity of the plaque, areas of verrucous plaque may shed of leaving hypopigmented areas.

Classification of nevi (excluding vascular and melanocytic)			
Epidermal nevi	*Example*	*Dermal and subcutaneous nevi*	*Example*
Keratinocyte nevi	Verrucous epidermal nevus	Connective tissue nevi	Collagenoma
Inflammatory epidermal nevi	Inflammatory verrucous epidermal nevus	Muscle nevi	Smooth muscle hamartoma
Epidermal nevus syndromes	Sebaceous nevus syndrome	Fat nevi	Nevus lipomatosus cutaneous superficialis
Sebaceous nevi	Nevus sebaceous		
Follicular nevi	Nevus comedonicus		
Apocrine nevi	Syringocystadenoma papilliferum		
Eccrine nevi	PEODDN		
Becker's nevus			

PEODDN: Porokeratotic eccrine osteal and dermal duct nevus

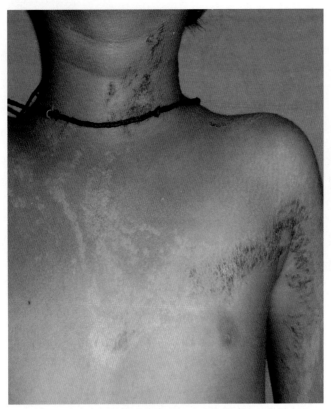

Epidermolytic verrucous epidermal nevus: most of the plaque has shed its raised part, leaving hypopigmented areas. Remaining VEN seen as hyperpigmented verrucous areas.

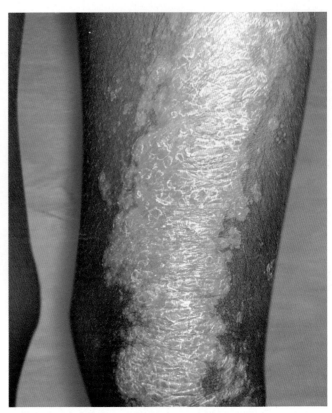

Inflammatory linear verrucous epidermal nevus: vertically alternating ortho- and parakeratotic hyperkeratosis.

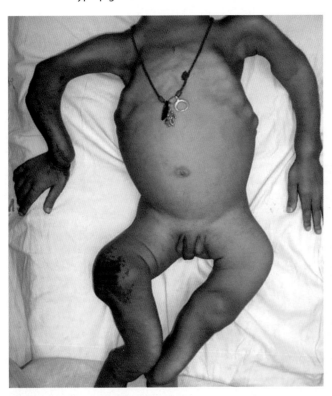

Epidermal nevus syndrome: unilateral VEN involving the right forearm and right lower limb. Severe, deforming hypophosphatemic rickets.

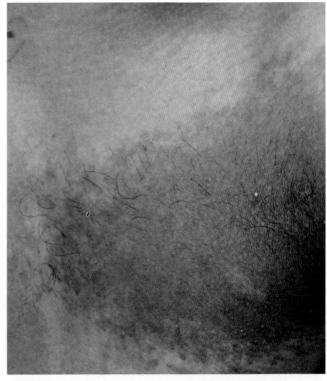

Becker's nevus: dark brown macules with 'splashed' appearance and overlying hypertrichosis. (Typical site- upper chest and proximal arm).

Histopathology

Two variants: epidermolytic and non-epidermolytic. Both show hyperkeratosis and acanthosis. Only minimal infiltrate indermis. Epidermolytic variant shows vacuolization of keratinocytes, begins in granular layer and may extend to basal layer. Within vacuolated keratinocytes, keratohyalin and trichohyalin granules seen.

Histopathology

Vertically alternating orth—and parakeratotic hyperkeratosis. Varying picture—dermatitic, psoriasiform or lichenoid. Infiltrate conspicuous.

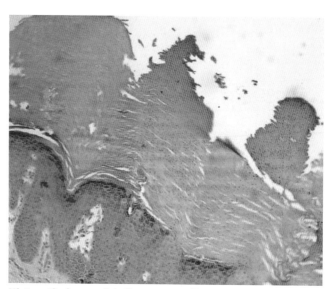

Histopathology of inflammatory linear verrucous epidermal nevus: vertically alternating ortho- and parakeratotic hyperkeratosis.

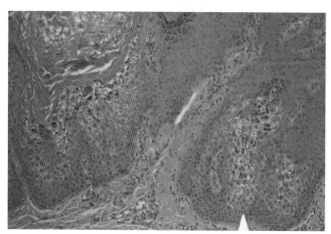

Histopathology of epidermolytic type of verrucous epidermal nevus: hyperkeratosis, acanthosis. Focal vacuolization of keratinocytes (one focus indicated by yellow arrow head) extending from top to basal layer of epidermis. Within the vacuolization, keratohyaline (deep purple dots) and trichohyaline (deep pink dots) granules seen.

Treatment

Topical retinoic acid 0.05–0.1% or tazarotene once daily may help some patients; caution in flexures—may cause irritation. Maintenance applications required. Shave off or dermabrade. Radiofrequency ablation or surgical excision, if lesion cosmetically objectionable. Systemic acitretin in systematized disease.

Inflammatory Linear Verrucous Epidermal Nevus (ILVEN)

Uncommon. Onset, infancy or childhood. Inflammatory—dermatitic. Or psoriasiform (psoriasiform epidermal nevus, or PEN). Or lichenoid. *Itchy*, linear band along the whole, often the lower, limb. May persist or spontaneously resolve.

Treatment

Unsatisfactory. Combination of potent steroids and salicylic acid may help. Cryotherapy or surgical excision.

Epidermal Nevus Syndrome

Umbrella term for systemic association with any form of epidermal nevus in form of various cutaneous, neurologic, skeletal, cardiovascular, ocular or urogenital developmental anomalies. Common epidermal nevi associated include verrucous epidermal nevus (VEN), sebaceous nevus, comedo nevus and becker's nevus. Nevus unius lateris more common among VEN.

Becker's Nevus (Pigmented Hairy Epidermal Nevus)

Common. An epidermal nevus with pigmented component. Appears around adolescence. Males more often affected. Shoulder region, front and back most frequently involved. Unilateral. Variegated

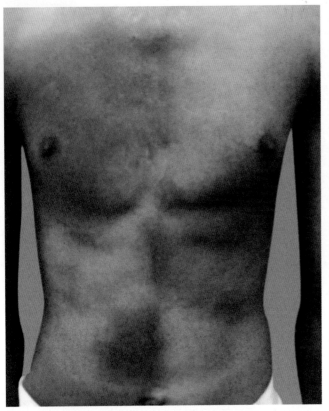

Becker's nevus: multiple becker's nevi in 'checker-board' (chessboard) pattern.

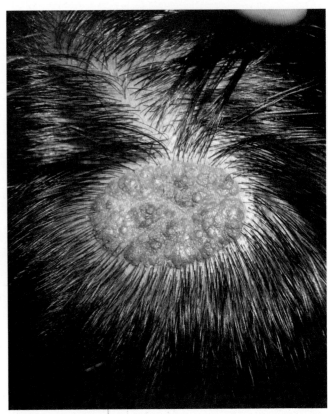

Nevus sebaceous: oval, yellow-brown, hairless waxy verrucous plaque on scalp.

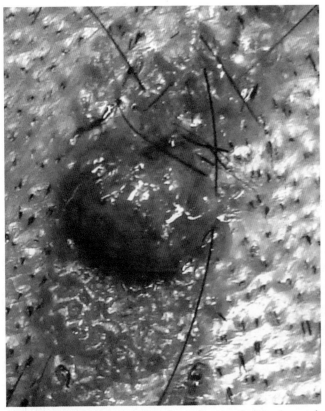

Syringocystadenoma papilliferum: solitary red glistening nodule over nevus sebaceous (scalp).

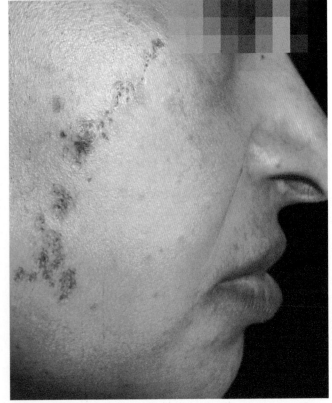

Nevus comedonicus: linearly arranged large open comedones over cheek arranged in linear fashion.

brown pigmented area, the size of a palm with small satellite pigmented macules—so called *splashed appearance*. Locally increased androgen receptors and their sensitivity my cause acneform eruption, comedones and hypertrichosis. Rare associations with other ipsilateral developmental anomalies like breast hypoplasia, supernumerary nipples, scoliosis, pectoralis major muscle aplasia, limb reduction and lipoatrophy.

Histopathology

No nevus cells. Variable epidermal changes like hyperkeratosis, mild acanthosis may be seen. Increased basal pigmentation and few dermal melanophages. Dermis may show thickened or increased smooth muscle fibers, suggestive of, smooth muscle hamartoma.

Treatment

Several pigmentary and hair reduction laser tried with variable and modest response. Q switched ruby laser and Er:YAG lasers shown best response.

Nevus Sebaceous

Sometimes called organoid nevus due to hamartomatous involvement of epidermis, pilosebaceous unit as well as other appendages. Uncommon usually solitary. Well demarcated, yellow-brown hyperpigmented oval, circular or irregular, plane topped to mildly verrucous, waxy plaque(s), most common on scalp but also occurs on face, chest. Scalp lesions have associated alopecia. Enlarge around puberty. Prone to develop benign tumors over time and rarely malignant. Commonest benign tumors: syringocystadenoma papilliferum and trichoblastoma. Others include leiomyoma, syringoma, spiradenoma, hidradenoma and keratoacanthoma. Malignant tumors may develop: basal cell carcinoma, apocrine carcinoma, squamous cell carcinoma and malignant eccrine poromas. Occasional malignant transformation to basal cell carcinoma.

Histopathology

Epidermis showing changes of hyperkeratosis, acanthosis, papillomatosis. Sebaceous glands present higher up in dermis. Mature sebaceous follicles—increased in number, increased size of lobules which are closely set, increased ducts.

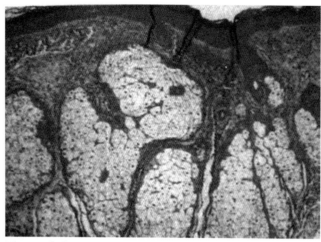

Histopathology of nevus sebaceous: hypertrophic sebaceous glands in upper dermis-increased size, close set lobules.

Syringocystadenoma Papilliferum

Rare. Usually over an underlying sebaceous nevus. Origin from apocrine gland, uncommonly from eccrine gland. Most common on scalp. Solitary or linearly arranged pink-brown nodules, friable/glistening surface. Enlarge around puberty. Rapid increase suggests basal cell carcinoma.

Histopathology

Multiple dilated ducts connecting epidermis to dermal cysts. Latter lined by twin layers of cuboidal or columnar cells, containing papillary projections and villi. The stroma shows moderately dense infiltration by plasma cells.

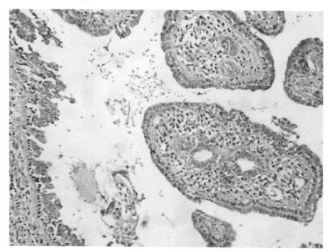

Histopathology of syringocystadenoma papilliferum: high power showing numerous villi in a cavity. Both villi and the cavity lined by twin layer of cuboidal cells and stroma showing plasma cell infiltrate. Many cells lining cavity show apical pinching off, suggestive of apocrine differentiation.

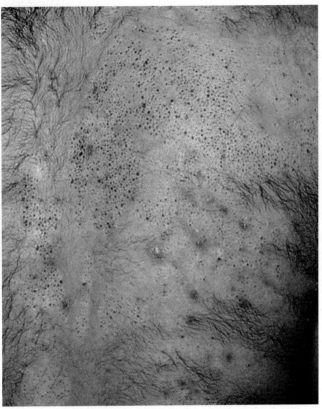

Nevus comedonicus: unilateral lesions of grouped comedones along lines of Blaschko.

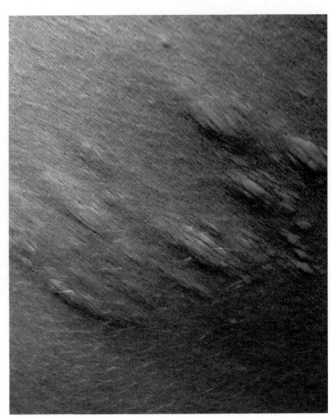

Shagreen patch: grouped, skin colored papules and nodules over trunk.

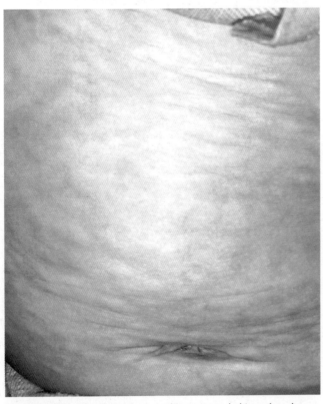

Buschke-Ollendorff syndrome: disseminated skin colored papules and plaques on trunk of an infant.

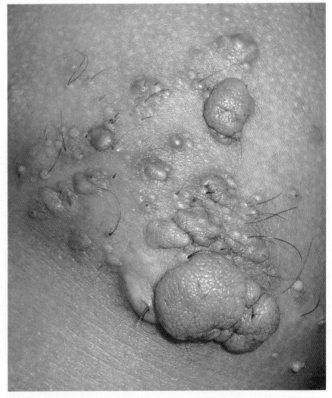

Nevus lipomatosus cutaneous superficialis: grouped skin colored papules and nodules over the right buttock, increased hair growth.

Treatment

Complete surgical excision.

Nevus Comedonicus

Hamartoma of pilosebaceous apparatus. Large grouped comedones and some inflammatory papules. Face, trunk, neck generally affected. Rarely be generalized or systematized. Recurrent secondary infection, abscess formation, foul smelling discharge may be a problem. Sometimes, acne may be interspersed over the lesion.

Treatment

Complete surgical excision. Deep excision may be required for complete removal of abnormal pilosebaceous units.

Shagreen Patch

It is a clinical form of collagenoma, one of the major criterias for tuberous sclerosis. Located as a skin colored plaque or coalescing papules and nodules over the trunk. Peaud' orange (orange peel) appearance may be there.

Histopathology

Dense sclerotic bundles of collagen in reticular dermis.

Juvenile Elastomas/Buschke-Ollendorff Syndrome

Association of connective tissue nevi and osteopoikilosis. Autosomal dominant. Two types of presentations. Asymmetric yellow nodules coalescing to form plaques. Less common is generalized eruption of waxy yellowish/lichenoid papules (dermatofibrosis lenticularis disseminata).

Histopathology

May appear normal on H&E staining, elastin stains show thick, interlacing elastin fibers between normal collagen bundles.

Nevus Lipomatosus Cutaneous Superficialis

Two types of presentations. Classic (Hoffman-Zurhelle), more common—since birth or early childhood, grouped, soft, fleshy, nodules over the lower trunk/buttocks/upper thigh. Occasionally hairy with open comedones. Other type presents as solitary skin colored papule in adults, on lower trunk and knees.

Histopathology

Mature adipocytes higher up in dermis amid collagen fibers, not connected to subcutaneous fat.

PIGMENTED LESIONS

Freckles

Common in whites, particularly red-haired or blondes with blue irides. Light brown, small macules with ill-defined edges. Present on the face and other light exposed parts of the body. Pigment accentuated on exposure to UV light! sunlight; become lighter on withdrawal.

Treatment

Protect from sunlight. Q switched Nd:YAG laser very effective but recurrence common if sun protection inadequate. If few lesions, may be ablated with radiofrequency or trichloroacetic acid touch.

Lentigines

Common. Dark brown macules anywhere on the body. Circular, oval or irregular, 2–3 mm sized macules. Uniform brown pigmentation, not related to sunlight exposure. Appear in childhood and increase upto adult life. May spontaneously fade away.

Treatment

Q switched Nd:YAG laser very effective. If few lesions, may be ablated with radiofrequency or trichloroacetic acid touch.

Freckles	Lentigines
Individuals are fair skinned, red haired/blondes with blue irides	Any skin color
Photoexposed parts only	Any part of skin; even mucosa
Lesions show variegation in color	Lesion show uniform color
Ill-defined edge	Better defined edge
Darken on sunexposure	No change in color on sunexposure

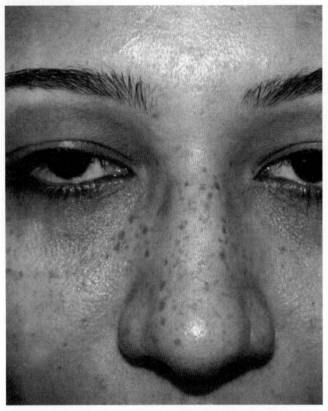

Freckles: dark brown macules, face–photoexposed part.

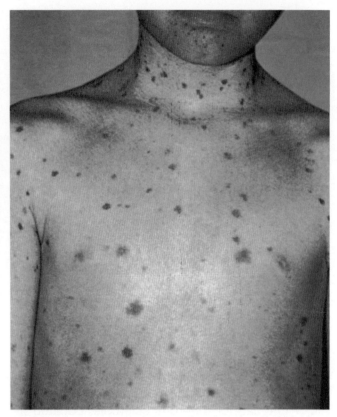

Lentiginosis: irregular dark brown macules all over trunk.

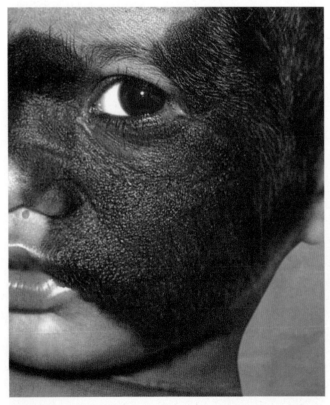

Giant melanocytic nevus on the face: dark brown to black with terminal hair.

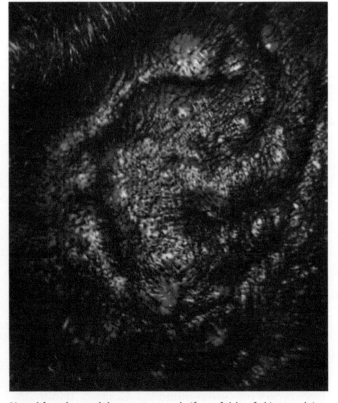

Nevoid cutis verticis gyrata: cerebriform folds of skin overlying a melanocytic nevus.

Melanocytic Nevi (Nevocellular Nevi)

Common. Hamartomas of melanocytic nevus cells. *Nevus cells* located in the dermis—*intradermal nevi*; at the dermoepidermal interface—*junctional nevi* or at both sites—*compound nevi.* Congenital. Or acquired—appearing in infancy, childhood and particularly adolescence or later.

Congenital Nevi

Small, medium or large pigmented macules. Degree of pigmentation variable—pale brown to dark brown or bluish black—and increases with age. Large, *giant*, nevi, generally on the trunk, lower back. Associated hairiness. Become thickened, large and nodular. Bilateral and symmetrical. Develop several small satellite pigmented nevi. Some associated with spina bifida or neurofibromas. Scalp nevi may develop a convoluted, cerebriform appearance—*cutis verticis gyrata*.

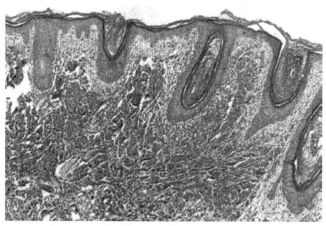

Histopathology of congenital melanocytic nevus: large collection of nevus cells and terminal hair.

Acquired Nevi

Common. Different variants. *Junctional nevus*: Pigmented macules—pigmentation variegated even within small lesion. May evolve into lightly or deeply pigmented (again variegated in color) dome-shaped, papulonodules—*compound nevus*; with or without a lightly pigmented halo. Smooth

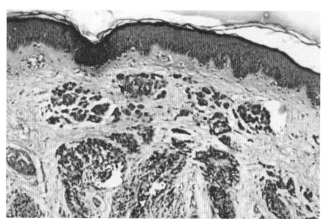

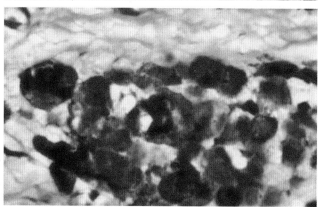

Histopathology of intradermal nevus: nevus cells containing melanin in superficial dermis; top (10x), bottom (40x).
Courtesy: Dr Meeta Singh, Assistant Professor, Department of Pathology, MAMC, Delhi.

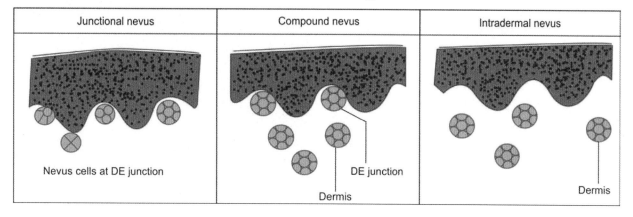

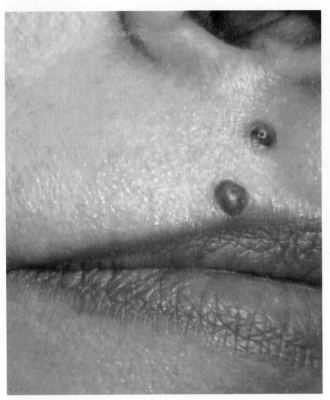

Acquired melanocytic nevi: dome shaped brown-black papules.

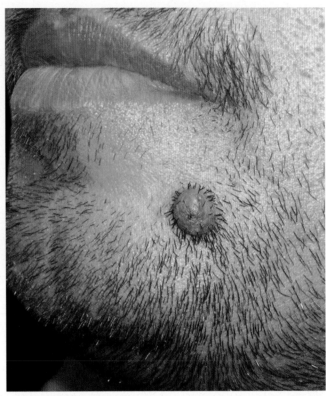

Dermal melanocytic nevus: skin colored pedunculated papule with normal hair growth (as rest of the beard).

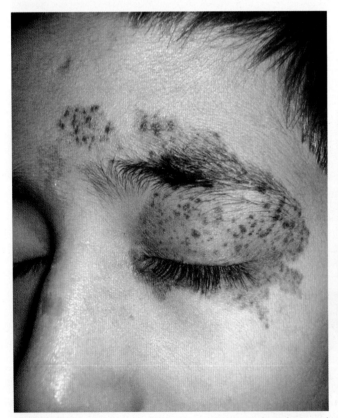

Nevus spilus: irregular edged light brown pigmented patch around left eye, studded with dark brown macules and few papules.

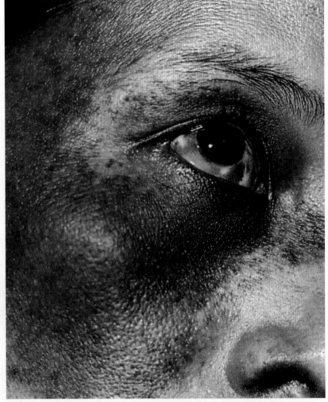

Nevus of Ota: slate-grey pigmentation of face and sclera.

or papillomatous surface with terminal hair on top. *Intradermal variant*—skin colored nodule.

Malignant potential of melanocytic nevi variable.

Nevus Spilus

Rare. Since infancy or early childhood. Initial lesion may be tan/light brown macule which increases in size and later many brown/black macules progressively develop over it. Conversely dark macules may appear earlier. Rarely, these darker macules may have hypertrichosis suggestive of compound melanocytic nevi.

Nevus of Ota
(Oculodermal Melanocytosis or Nevus Fuscocaerulius Ophthalmomaxillaris)

Uncommon. Young females more frequently affected. Brownish, slate-grey or bluish pigmentation of the skin; (often superimposed) conjunctiva (brown discoloration), sclera (slate grey discoloration), and palate. Speckled or diffuse. Generally unilateral and confined to trigeminal area.

Nevus Depigmentosus
(Nevus Achromicus)

Not uncommon. Well-defined, depigmented or hypopigmented macule of irregular configuration. On the trunk or elsewhere. Present at birth. Stable; no change in size.

OTHER LINEAR/NEVOID DISORDERS

Segmental Vitiligo

Variant of vitiligo in which one or more macules, more or less distributed according to a zosteriform

Difference between nevus spilus and Becker's nevus		
	Nevus spilus	*Becker's nevus*
Epidemiology Most common age group	Infancy/early childhood	2nd–3rd decade
Male:female	1:1	6:1
Prevalence	Approximately 0.2% (new born) to 2% (adult)	0.5% (adult)
Pathophysiology	Genetic field defect of melanocytic hyperplasia and neoplasia (most probable)	Sporadic > familial, androgen sensitivity
Clinical features		Anteroposterior chest, shoulder
Common sites	Trunk, extremities	Uniformly brown macule with irregular
Lesion	Tan to light brown background patch with scattered overlying darker macules and papules	block-like configuration, hypertrichosis and acneiform papules over the patch after puberty; center of the lesion may show thickening and perifollicular papules
Hypertrichosis	Very rare	Common; may not overlap with the area of hyperpigmentation
Associations	PHACES syndrome, phakomatosis pigmentokeratotica, phakomatosis pigmentovascularis	Developmental abnormalities such as hypoplasia of areola, nipple, and arm; lumbar spinal bifida; thoracic scoliosis; pectus carinatum; ipsilateral foot enlargement; accessory scrotum supernumerary nipples
Malignant melanoma	May develop.	Extremely rare (single case report)
Histopathology	Background patch: lentigine or café-au-lait macule Darker macules and papules; melanocytic nevus or lentigines	Increased basal pigmentation, elongation of rete ridges, hyperplasia of pilosebaceous unit, dermal melanophages; smooth muscle bundles in the dermis and hypertrophy of arrector pilorum
Treatment	Observation, pigmentation lasers (Q-switched neodymium-doped yttrium aluminum garnet, ruby, and alexandritic); Hair lasers (long-pulsed diode, alexandrite). Variable results. Excision of lesions with melanoma or small lesions for cosmetic reasons	Counseling. Pigmentation and hair lasers. Pigmentation more resistant to lasers because of prominent dermal component. Excision not indicated unless melanoma documented.

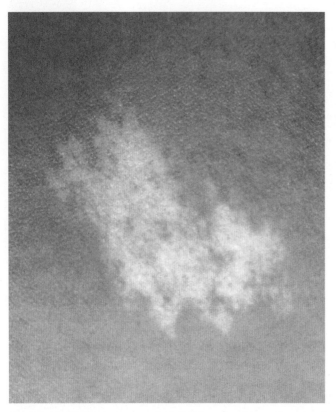

Nevus achromicus: characteristic depigmented irregular edged macule. Note feathered edge.

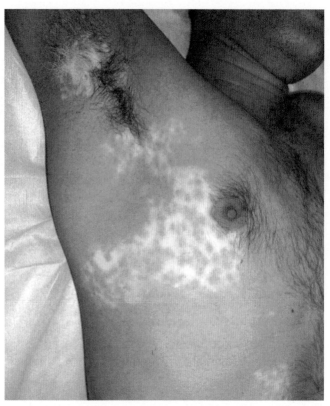

Segmental vitiligo: unilateral zosteriform distributed depigmented macules, islands of pigment within the lesion, leucotrichia also seen.

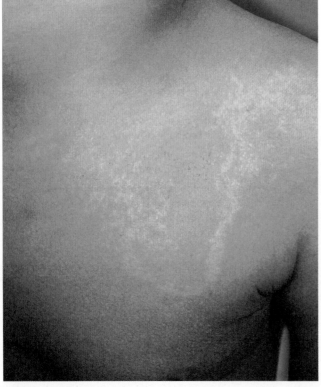

Lichen striatus: tiny hypopigmented papules grouped in a fine linear Blaschko's distribution over upper chest.

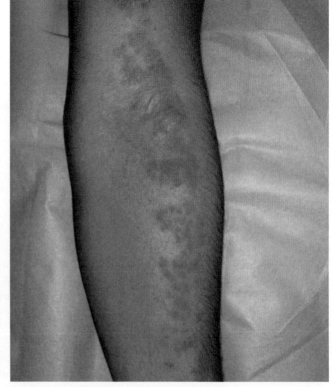

Linear spiradenoma: linearly arranged pinkish nodules over forearm.

distribution. Possible role of dysfunction of sympathetic nerves. Clinically, lesions are either unilateral zosteriform or blaschkoid or dermatomal or multifocal yet maintaining the distribution pattern. Variation in pigmentation more common than in non-segmental forms—islands of pigment inside the lesion, leucotrichia extending outside the margins. Common sites include head, trunk and limbs. Common associations: family history, atopic dermatitis, halo nevus.

Course

Static throughout after initial rapid spread. Spontaneous repigmentation known but partial or minimal. Rarely, evolves into generalized non-segmental variants.

Treatment

Good prognosis in early stages. Topical steroids, calcineurin inhibitors,PUVA/PUVA sol give relief to variable extent. Stable lesions best candidates for vitiligo surgeries like epidermal suspensions, suction blister grafting, etc.

Lichen Striatus

Idiopathic disorder of unknown etiology. Usually occurs during childhood, age of onset varying from infancy to 15 years. Possibly an eczematous disorder. Starts as erythematous or lichenoid, tiny papules arranged in a linear manner. Often occur along lines of Blaschko. Hypopigmented papules occur commonly in darker skin types. Usually asymptomatic, but may be itchy. Spontaneously subside in months to years. Subside with temporary hypopigmentation.

Histopathology

Variable. In active lesions, it may resemble lichen planus in form of band like dermal lymphoid infiltrate. Associated focal basal layer degeneration, acanthosis may be there. Infiltrate may go deeper to concentrate around appendages.

Treatment

Observation. Topical steroids for symptomatic relief.

Linear Spiradenoma

Extremely uncommon variant of a the uncommon tumor spiradenoma, which arises from sweat glands. Only few reports exist in literature, few in relation with malignant degeneration (spiradenocarcinoma). Lesions occur as skin colored or pinkish/greenish, dermal or subcutaneous nodules arranged linearly over a limb, more commonly on the lower limbs. As with the commoner non-linear variants, pain is associated. And histopathology is also similar. Complete excision curative. Ablation with radiofrequency or laser may benefit.

18

Cutaneous Tumors

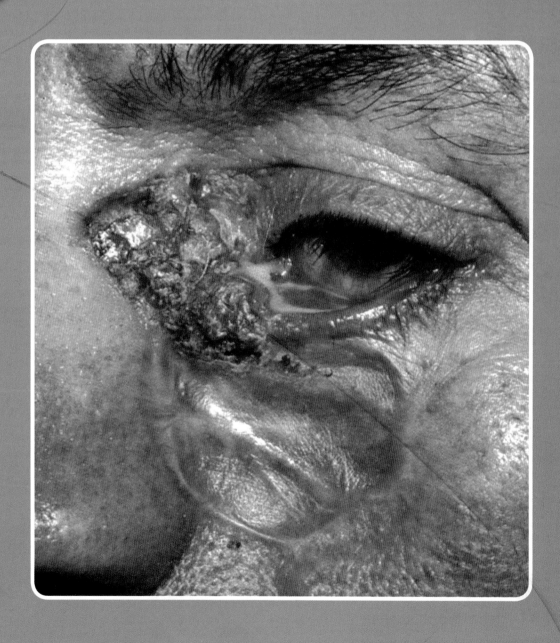

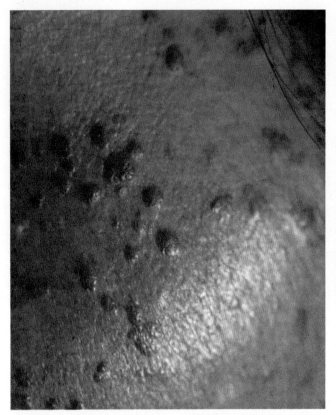

Seborrheic keratoses: dark brown, 'stuck on' papules.

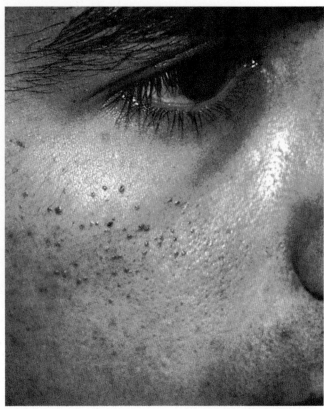

Dermatosis papulosa nigra: dark brown, dome-shaped papules.

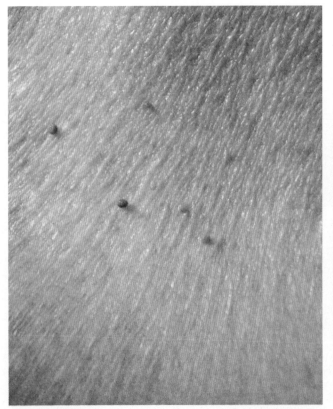

Acrochordon (Skin Tags): tiny pedunculated papules on side of neck.

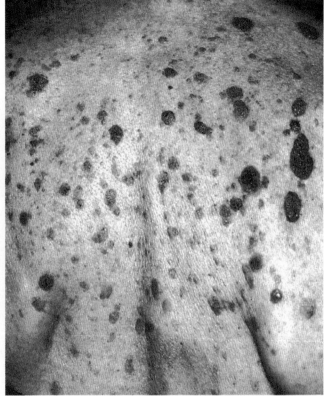

Seborrheic keratoses, eruptive: on the trunk—Leser-Trélat sign.

Tumors of the skin may arise in the epidermis, dermis or subcutis. *Epidermal tumors:* May be derived from keratinocytes, melanocytes or merkel cells. *Dermal tumors:* Adnexal (hair, sebaceous and sweat glands) fibrous, vascular, neural, muscular, or cellular (mast cells, lymphocytes, histiocytes) or others. *Subcutis tumors:* lipocytic. Tumors may be benign or malignant. Genetics and environment influence development of tumors.

Benign: well differentiated, expansile and slow growing. Non-metastatic. *Malignant:* poorly organized pattern. Individual cells show structural abnormalities in size, shape or nuclear pattern. Expansile and infiltrative growth. Metastatic spread. Division between benign and malignant not always clear cut. Tumors such as basal cell carcinomas, histologically malignant, biologically benign.

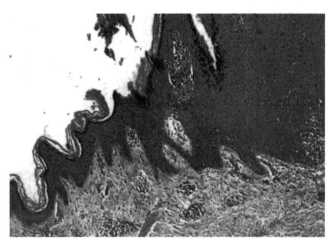

Histopathology of seborrhoeic keratosis: acanthotic epidermis containing basaloid cells.

EPIDERMAL TUMORS

Seborrheic Keratoses (SK)

Common, almost normal in elderly individuals. Both sexes affected. Well demarcated, light brown to brown black, flat or finely verrucous papules. Typically 'stuck on' appearance with keratotic plugs. Variable sized. Genetic predisposition present. Face, dorsa of the hands, trunk commonly involved. Eruptive appearance of seborrheic keratoses *Leser-Trelat sign* should raise suspicion of internal malignancy.

Acrochordon (Skin Tags)

Clinical and histological overlap with SK. Soft, usually 1 to 2 mm pedunculated papules in flexural sites—neck, axillae, inframammary. Predisposing conditions—familial, type 2 diabetes, obesity, etc.

Dermatosis Papulosa Nigra

A variant of seborrheic keratosis. More common in darker skin types. Younger adults. Bilateral, sessile, tiny 0.5 to 2 mm sized dark brown to brown black papules on the cheeks and temples.

Histopathology

Sharply defined basaloid epidermal tumor, may be exophytic or endophytic. Hyperkeratosis, follicular plugs and horn cysts are characteristic features. Variable, often pronounced, acanthosis.

Treatment

Shave off lesions—flush with the skin surface. Or radiofrequency ablation. Topical retinoids.

Keratoacanthoma

Exact nosological status uncertain yet. Some think it to be benign, some think it to be harbinger of SCC. Term abortive malignancy proposed.

Etiology

More common in whites, rare in pigmented population. UV, HPV, immunosuppression, genetic.

Clinical Presentation

Solitary or multiple; latter often familial. Usually solitary lesion with three phases—rapid growth over few weeks, stable for few weeks, spontaneous resolution over few months. Lesions is dome shaped/nodular with central firm keratin core. Usual sunexposed sites—face, forearms, hand dorsae, etc. Heal with hypopigmented scar.

Histopathology

Central keratotic core covered with an atrophic epidermis. Acanthotic epidermis, on either side. Well-differentiated cells with horn cysts. No atypia. Heavy lymphohistiocytic infiltrate in the upper dermis.

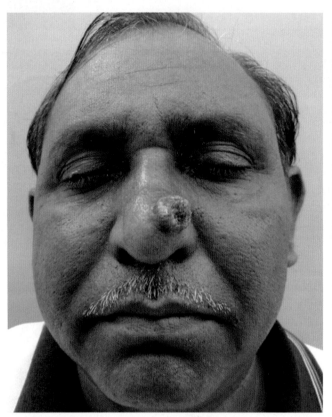

Keratoacanthoma: dome-shaped nodule with keratin filled crater, forehead.

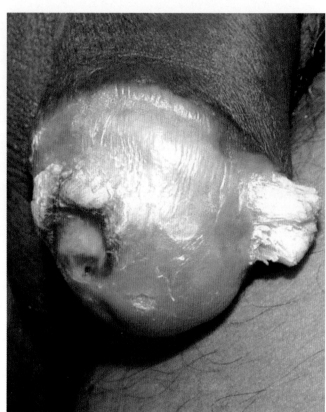

Cutaneous horn : on plaque of genital lichen sclerosus with associated squamous cell carcinoma.

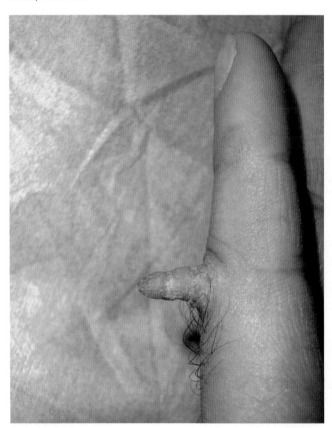

Cutaneous horn: over a verruca

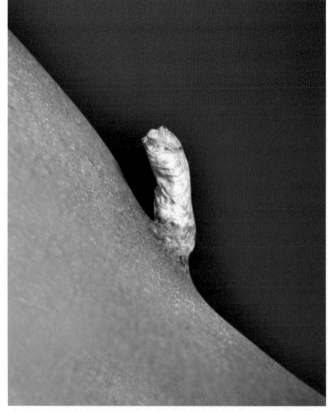

Cutaneous horn: over lichen planus.

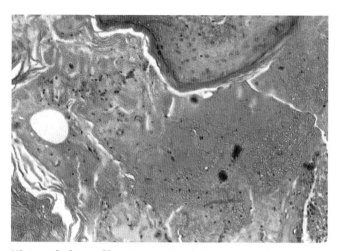

Histopathology of keratoacanthoma: keratin plug in the crater; acanthotic epidermis around; note horn cysts.

Treatment

Watchful waiting, complete surgical excision, electrosurgery, localized radiotherapy, intralesional chemotherapy.

Cutaneous Horn

Firm, hyperkeratotic, horn-shaped papule, height at least 2 times the diameter. Clinical entity, arising over a background pathology, rarely idiopathic. Common causes include actinic keratosis, seborrheic keratosis, verruca vulgaris and squamous cell carcinoma. Uncommonly over keratoacanthoma, basal cell carcinoma, epidermal nevus and angiokeratoma. Rarely on penis.

Histopathology

Keratinous material which may be lamellated or compact. Keratinization may be epidermal or tricholemmal (without granular layer). Base may reveal primary pathology. Epidermal hyperplasia may occur, usually without atypia.

Treatment

Rule out underlying malignancy. Radiosurgical ablation or surgical excision.

BENIGN APPENDAGEAL TUMORS

Syringomas

Uncommon. Young females more frequently affected. Asymptomatic. Multiple, skin colored or pale, flat angulated papules. Eyelids—upper, lower or both-affected, often symmetrically.

Infrequently present on the trunk. May also involve vulva, penis and flexors. Eruptive variant is generalized.

Histopathology

Variably shaped and sized eccrine ducts lined by two layers of cuboidal epithelium. May have comma like tails resembling tadpoles. Solid nests with basaloid appearance, embedded in sclerotic stroma.

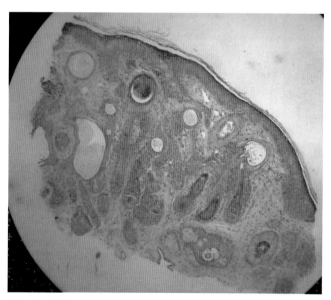

Histopathology of syringoma: basaloid aggregates with tubular differentiation, solid nests and horn cysts in a sclerotic stroma.

Treatment

Results not statisfying. Electrosurgery, dermabrasion, topical tretinoin, trichloroacetic acid.

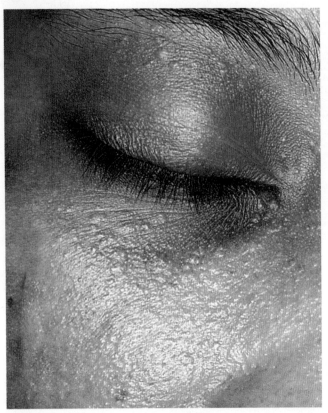

Syringomas: skin colored, flat, angulated papules on the lower eyelids.

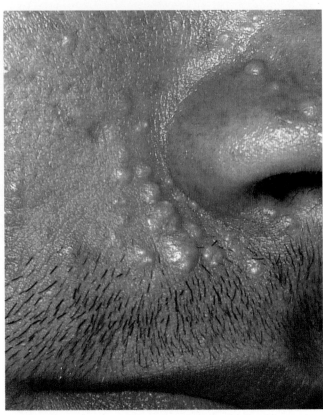

Trichoepithelioma: multiple skin colored to whitish, dome shaped papules over the nose tip and nasolabial fold.

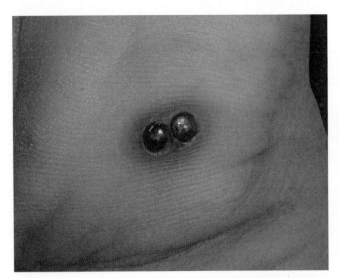

Eccrine poroma: shiny red nodule (bifurcated by a thin sleeve of epidermis) over the palm. Also note the peripheral collarette of thick skin, closely resembling pyogenic granuloma.

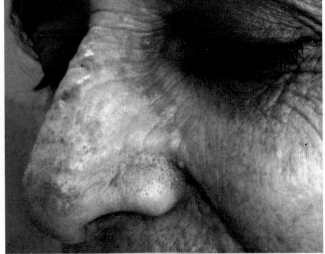

Eccrine hidrocystoma: multiple bluish papulo-vesicles over the dorsum of nose, side of nose, cheek and nasolabial fold.

Trichoepithelioma

Common hair follicle tumor with primitive follicular differentiation. Multiple tumors occur in inherited form. Solitary or few tumors occur sporadically. Pearly white to skin colored, dome shaped papules involving the centro-facial area—eyelids, nose, nasolabial folds, medial cheeks.

Histopathology

Basaloid islands in dermis which may show branching and peripheral palisading. Keratin cysts may be seen lined by basaloid aggregates.

Treatment

Ablation with radiofrequency, laser or trichloroacetic acid. Excision for larger lesions.

Eccrine Poroma

Uncommon tumors arising from the epidermal part of the eccrine duct (acrosyringium). Common sites include the palms and soles. Appear as red to pink nodules with glazed/moist surface. May mimic pyogenic granulomas.

Histopathology

Aggregates of cuboidal cells (paler, smaller than keratinocytes) projecting as columns or chords from the epidermis into the papillary dermis.

Treatment

Surgical excision.

Eccrine Hidrocystoma

Uncommon tumor arising from deformed eccrine sweat glands leading to dilatation of sweat ducts. Thought to be due to heat exposure due to the sites of predilection and since they show seasonal variation. Most common over cheeks and eyelids. More common in people exposed to heat (cooks, housewives, etc.). More in summers, may show tendency to resolve spontaneously in winters. Multiple 1–3 mm skin colored to bluish papules/papulo-vesicles. Fluid comes out on puncture. Common differential apocrine hidrocystomas but the latter are solitary, bigger (size in centimeters), more often bluish, deeper and on cheeks.

Histopathology

Thin twin cell-layer lined cysts—outer flat myoepeithelial cells and inner cuboidal cells.

Treatment

Topical applications usually do not help. Ablation using lasers, radiofrequency or excision.

Pilomatricoma

Uncommon tumor possibly arising from hair matrix. Common amongst hair follicle tumors. Usually over head and neck, and upper extremities. Solitary deep seated dermal/subcutaneous nodule with overlying skin being normal. More than 80% lesions undergo secondary calcification.

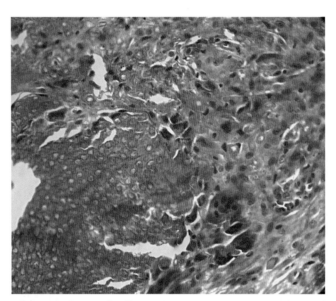

Histopathology of pilomatricoma: compact aggregate of eosinophilic cells with absent nuclei and smudged cell walls (ghost cells). Note foreign body type giant cells at the periphery.

Histopathology

Features depend on age of lesion. Well defined tumor islands with intervening soft tissue stroma. Two types of cells—compact basaloid aggregates at the periphery of lesion or in early lesions; compact eosinophilic aggregates with smudged cellular outlines and loss of nuclei (mummification or 'ghost cells'). Mummification and calcification starts from center of lesions. Foreign body giant cells in response to calcification.

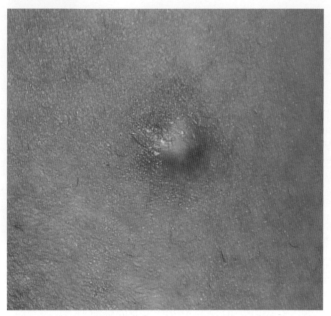

Pilomatricoma: solitary skin colored nodule over the upper arm. Note the whitish hue is due to dystrophic calcification within the tumor.

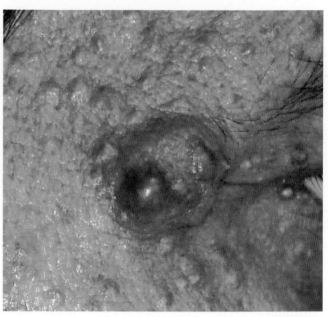

Eccrine spiradenoma: solitary dermal nodule with reddish blue hue. Few milia are studded over the nodule.

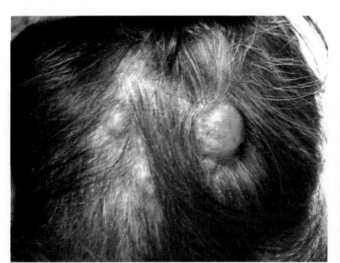

Cylindroma: multiple pinkish nodules and tumors over scalp causing overlying hair loss.

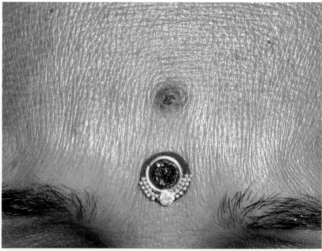

Hidradenoma: tiny red nodule over forehead.

Treatment

Complete surgical excision.

Eccrine Spiradenoma

Extremely uncommon tumor arising from sweat glands. Solitary, painful dermal nodules over trunk and upper limbs. Overlap may occur with cylindromas both clinically and histologically.

Histopathology

Well defined dermal nodules as islands and chords of basaloid cells. Two types of cells—dark cells (with hyperchromatic nuclei) present at periphery of islands and pale staining nuceli containing cells in the center. Many duct like structures seen in the nodules and sometimes with cystic spaces and vascular channels. Lymphocytic infiltration of tumor lobules may be seen.

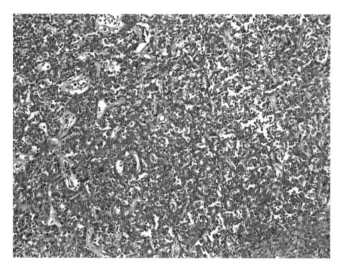

Histopathology of eccrine spiradenoma: tumor nodule of basaloid cells with numerous duct-like structures, dilated capillaries and some lymphocytic infiltration.

Treatment

Surgical excision.

Cylindroma

Uncommon tumor of uncertain origin. Frequently multiple, pink-red tumors or raised nodules over scalp causing hair loss, may cause discomfort due to large size. May be inherited in autosomal dominant manner (due to mutation in CYLD tumor suppressor gene) as part of Brooke Spiegler syndrome.

Histopathology

'Jigsaw puzzle' appearance on low power—multiple tumor lobules in dermis which appear to mould/fit into each other's shape. Prominent hyaline pink thickened basement membrane around tumor nodules which comprise of two types of cells (dark at the periphery and pale at the center), ductal differentiation may be seen.

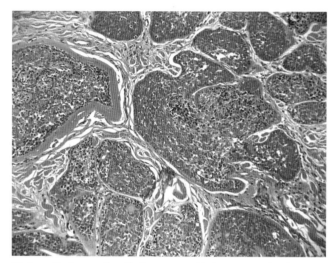

Histopathology of cylindroma: multiple tumor islands tending to fit into each other ('jigsaw puzzle appearance'), thick pink basement membrane lining these islands, duct like structures within the lobules.

Treatment

Excision or ablation using radiofrequency or lasers. Multiple or large tumors require excision and grafting. Topical salicylic acid tried anecdotally in multiple lesions.

Hidradenoma

Rare tumor of sweat gland origin. Now reclassified as either having apocrine or poroid differentiation. Solitary slow growing nodule occurring over scalp, face and trunk. More common in females.

Histopathology

Lobulated tumor masses in dermis composed of two types of cells—darker elongated cells at the periphery and light/clear cells towards the center. Stroma vascular with ectatic vessels surrounded by a sleeve of sclerotic collagen.

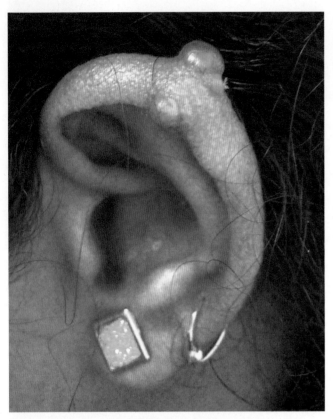

Keloid: after piercing of upper ear rim

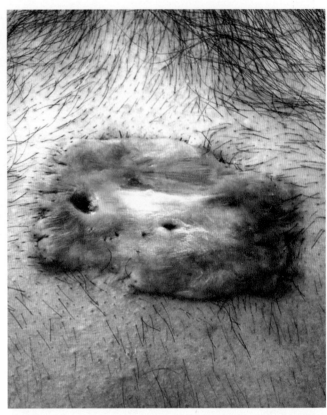

Keloid: red brown horizontal plaque on presternal area (classic location).

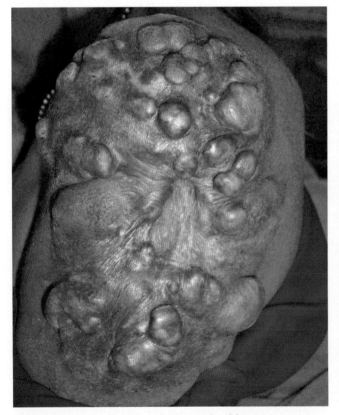

Keloid: Massive tumor-like keloid over shoulder.

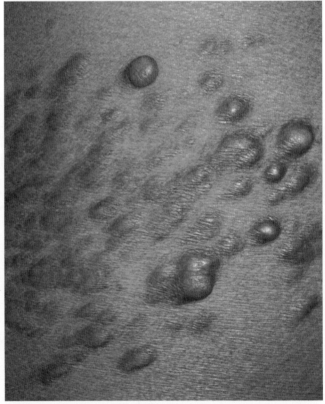

Multiple leiomyomas: grouped firm brown nodules and plaques in a segmental distribution over back.

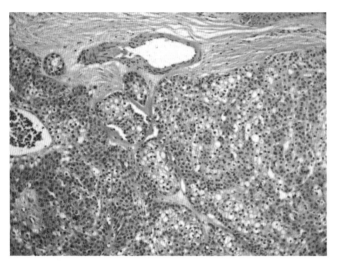

Histopathology of Hidradenoma: tumor mass comprised of darker cells at periphery and pale clear cells towards the center. Stroma showing numerous dilated capillaries.
(*Courtesy:* Dr Sudheer Arava, Assistant Professor of Pathology, AIIMS, New Delhi)

Treatment

Complete excision.

DERMAL TUMORS

Keloid

Common. Hyperplasia of fibrous tissue, history of trauma may or may not be there. Constitutional and racial susceptibility; blacks develop them frequently. Local factors such as an embedded foreign body may be responsible. Front of chest, shoulders, ear lobes, back, common sites. Itchy, hypersensitive flat, polygonal plaque. Smooth or 'striped' surface. Erythema extends beyond the scarred area.

Treatment

Prevention better than cure. Post operative intralesional (IL) steroid injections in patients with keloidal tendency. Combination therapy better than monotherapy. Intralesional steroids, 5 fluorouracil, bleomycin (tattooing), cryosurgery. Combination of surgical excison/laser ablation with intralesional steroids/localized radiotherapy. Maintenance with compression therapy. Other modalities with weaker evidence: topical imiquimod, silicone, onion products.

Leiomyoma

Uncommon tumor of smooth muscles. Based on origin, 3 types: piloleimyoma (from arrector pili), angioleiomyoma (from venous walls) and genital (from mammillary, dartos, vulvar muscles). Pilar most common, can be multiple and familial. Multiple leiomyomatosis has mutation in fumarate hydratase

Differences between keloids and hypertrophic scars		
Feature	*Hypertrophic scar*	*Keloid*
Incidence	Common	Less common
Race	All	Dark skin types
Genetic predisposition	Minimal	Strong
Trauma	Always (perpendicular to resting skin tension lines)	Sometimes
Lesions	Restricted to wound	Extend beyond wound ("pseudopodia-like" extension)
Sites	Any	Commonly pre-sternal, upper back, deltoid, ears
Histopathology	• Collagen fibers parallel to skin surface • Collagen fiber caliber and texture nearly normal • Vascularity increased • Capillaries perpendicular to skin surface • Minimal dermal mucin	• Collagen fibers arranged haphazardly • Thick hyaline eosinophilic collagen bundles • Decreased vascularity • Increased dermal mucin
Treatment required	Not usually	Always, usually resistant
Recurrence following excision	Usually none	Invariably
Spontaneous resolution	Usual	Rare

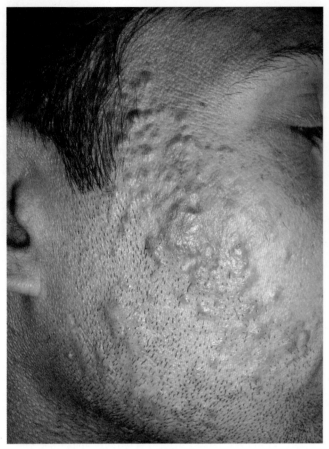

Multiple leiomyomas: grouped firm brown nodules and plaques in a segmental distribution over face.

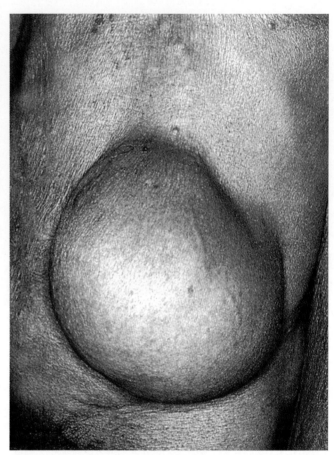

Lipomatosis: large, soft, lobulated subcutaneous nodule—trunk.

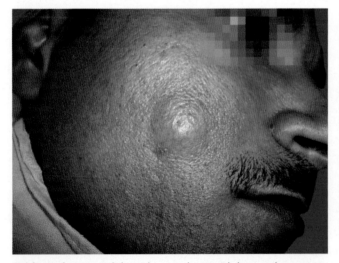

Epidermal cyst: nodule with central greenish hue and punctum.

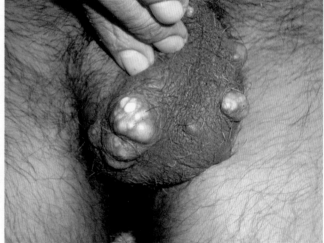

Epidermal cyst: multiple whitesh nodules on scrotum.

on 1q. Syndromes include MCUL (multiple cutaneous and uterine leiomyomatosis, aka, Reed syndrome); hereditary leiomyomatosis and renal cell cancer. Both genital and angioleiomyoma usually solitary. Firm, erythematous to brown colored nodules. Angioleiomyoma deeper or subcutaneous nodules. Painful and tender to touch and on exposure to cold.

Histopathology

Piloleimyomas are poorly circumscribed dermal tumors with haphazard arrangement of smooth muscle bundles. Angioleiomyomas well-defined tumors rich in vessels. Genital tumors similar to pilar tumors.

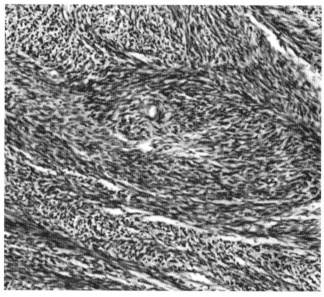

Histopathology of piloleimyoma: hapahazardly arranged smooth muscle bundles in dermis.
(*Courtesy:* Dr Meeta Singh, Assistant Professor of Pathology, MAMC, Delhi).

Treatment

Surgical excision. Or laser ablation. Palliative pain relieving therapies include calcium channel blockers (nifedipine, amlodipine, etc), gabapentin, nitroglycerin, phenoxybenzamine, intralesional botulinum toxin, etc.

Lipoma

Common. Single or multiple. Freely movable (slipping) subcutaneous masses of varying size. Distributed over the neck, arms, shoulders, back.

Multiple lipomatosis may be familial—autosomal dominant hereditary lipomatosis. May be associated with metabolic abnormalities of lipids. Angiolipoma contains blood vessels; painful and tender.

Treatment

None required. Remove if painful or cosmetically objectionable.

CYSTS OF EPIDERMAL ORIGIN

Epidermal Cyst (Epidermoid Cyst/Epidermal Inclusion Cyst)

Common. Single or multiple. Males more frequently affected. Origin from follicular infundibulum. Face, trunk, scrotum, earlobes involved. Firm, pale yellow, spherical dermal cysts attached to the epidermis. May have a central blue-black punctum. Asymptomatic unless inflamed. May get calcified.

Course

Fibrosis of wall, calcification, rupture, secondary infection.

Histopathology

Cyst wall made of stratified squamous epithelium with epidermal keratinization (keratin formation through presence of granular layer). Cyst contains laminated keratin. Older cyst may show fibrosis of wall, calcification/cholesterol crystals in cavity.

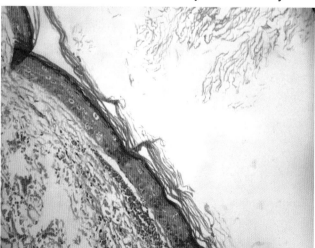

Histopathology of epidermoid cyst: wall showing stratified squamous epithelium with granular layer and lumen containing laminated keratin.

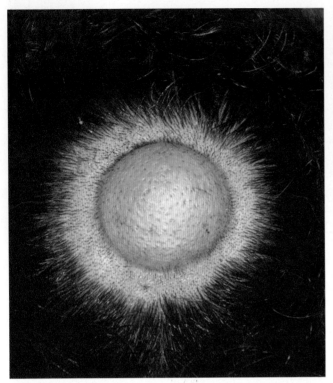

Trichilemmal cyst: solitary well-defined nodule over scalp (with overlying hair shaved)

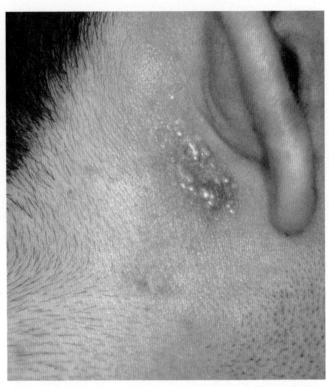

Milia en plaque: grouped milia over an inflamed plaque behind the ear

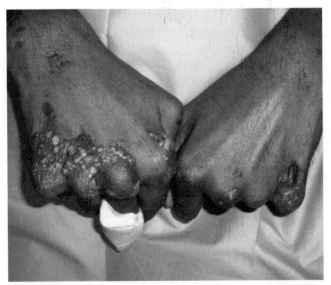

Secondary milia: in a case of epidermolysis bullosa acquisita

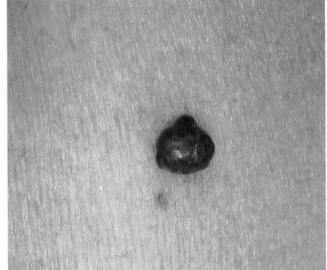

Cherry angioma: over chest

Treatment

Mostly left alone. If symptomatic or disfiguring, complete elliptical excision including overlying skin with punctum. Recurrence common if wall portion left. Some authors tried aspiration followed by intralesional sclerosant injection with success.

Trichilemmal Cyst (Pilar Cyst)

Probable origin from isthmic region of follicle. Firm, well circumscribed nodules predominantly present on scalp. Majority have multiple lesions. Usually asympatomatic, occasionally secondary infection or rupture occurs. Proliferating trichilemmal cyst may mimic malignancy.

Histopathology

Lining composed of startified squamous epithelium without granular layer. Plump, pale columnar keratinocytes at inner lining have interdigitating edge with the compact eosinophilic keratin filling the lumen.

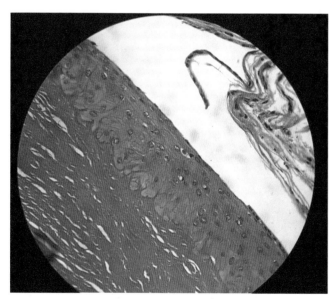

Histopathology of trichilemmal cyst: startified squamous epithelial lining without granular layer, plump inner keratinocytes interdigitating with compact pink keratin in lumen.

Treatment

Complete surgical excision.

Milia

Tiny epidermal cysts, 1 to 2 mm dome-shaped white papules. May be congenital/inherited or acquired. Scattered or grouped. Primary or secondary (following healing of dermatoses or trauma). Secondary causes include epidermolysis bullosa, porphyrias, linear IgA disease, etc. Common sites of primary lesions cheeks, eyelids. Variants include eruptive milia, milia en plaque (common behind ears), etc.

Histopathology

Identical to epidermal cysts.

Treatment

Congenital subside on their own, acquired removed by needle/blade/electrodessication.

BENIGN VASCULAR TUMORS

Cherry Angiomas (Campbell de Morgan Spots)

Common. Benign. Innocuous. Elderly or middle aged adults. Pinhead to slightly larger nodules. Verrucous surface. Purple color. May persist or resolve.

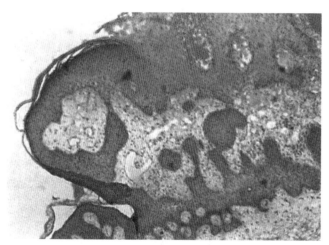

Histopathology of Cherry angioma: multiple dialated capillaries in the dermis.

Treatment

Best left alone.

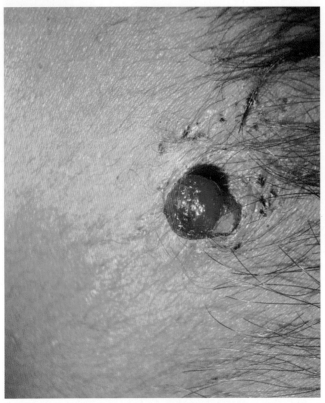

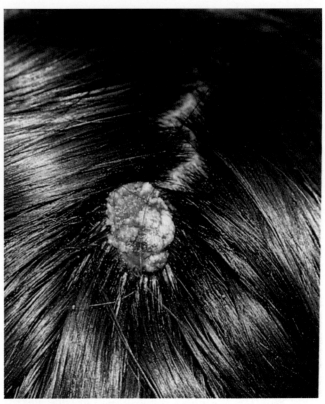

Pyogenic granuloma: solitary bright red moist pedunculated papule (side of neck) with acanthotic skin collar at base

Pyogenic granuloma: a pedunculated vascular lesion on scalp. Has a collarette at base.

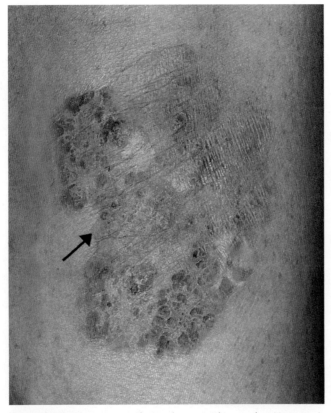

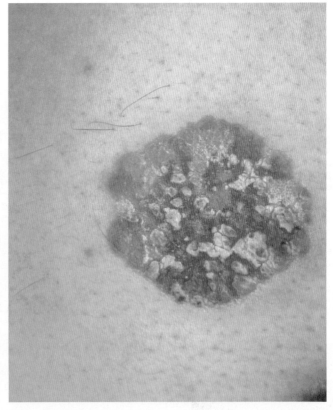

Bowen's disease: psoriasiform plaque with atrophy. Note reniform notch.

Bowen's disease: crusted inflamed plaque with renifrom borders.

Granuloma Pyogenicum (Lobular Capillary Hemangioma)

Uncommon angiomatous lesion. Any age, both sexes affected. Generally follows an injury. Bright or brownish red pedunculated lesion that bleeds easily. Collarette of acanthotic skin at base. Gradual enlargement. Spontaneous resolution uncommon. Common sites fingers, feet, lips, head and neck, oral and anal/perianal mucosae.

Histopathology

Lobular aggregate of proliferating capillaries, more compact in deeper dermis and loose in upper dermis. Thin slit like spaces in place of lumina when compact. Thinned out epidermis and margins of lesion show collarette of epidermis in the form of elongated rete ridges or sweat ducts.

Treatment

Electrocauterization or surgical excision. Recurrence likely if deeper portion left.

PREMALIGNANT SKIN CONDITIONS

Diverse dermatological conditions that have the potential to transform into invasive tumors. Classification in table.

Classification of some premalignant conditions in dermatology	
Cutaneous	**Mucosal**
• Bowen's disease	• Erythroplasia of Queyrat
• Actinic keratosis	• Leukoplakia
• Arsenical keratosis	• Erythroplakia
• Thermal keratosis	• Oral lichen planus
• Hydrocarbon keratosis	• Chronic hyperplastic candidiasis
• Chronic radiation keratosis	
• Chronic scar keratosis	
• Reactional keratosis	
• PUVA keratosis	
• Bowenoid papulosis	
• Epidermodysplasia verruciformis	
• Lentigo maligna	
• Congenital giant melanocytic nevus	

Bowen's Disease

Rare. Intraepidermal squamous cell carcinoma. Elderly individuals. Sunlight causally important in lesions on light exposed parts. Arsenic toxicity suspected when unexposed parts of body involved; toxicity often associated with systemic malignancies. Solitary or multiple. Superficial, irregularly circinate, scaly, at places atrophic, psoriasiform plaques. Trunk, face commonly affected.

Histopathology

Hyperkeratosis, parakeratosis, acanthosis with broad rete ridges. Full thickness dysplasia (disorganization of epidermal cells). Characteristic *dyskeratotic* and vacuolated cells. Basement membrane intact. Dermis shows heavy inflammatory infiltrate.

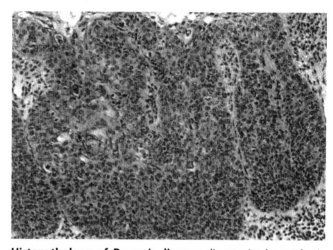

Histopathology of Bowen's disease: disorganized acanthotic epidermis with dyskeratotic cells (Bowenoid cells).

Treatment

Topical imiquimod 5% cream or 5 fluorouracil 5% cream or photodynamic therapy. Cryosurgery or Moh's micrographic surgery or complete excision.

Leukoplakia

Common. An adherant white plaque in the mouth. Elderly males more frequently affected. Betel or tobacco chewing, smoking, sharp, jagged teeth or poorly fitting dentures responsible. Rarely late syphilis. Variable clinical presentation: small or large plaques, with sharp or poor demarcation.

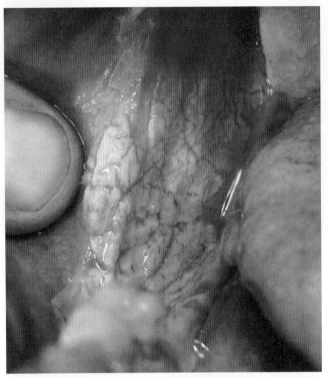

Oral leukoplakia: whitish elevated plaque over right buccal mucosa in a tobacco chewer (prominent mucosal markings).

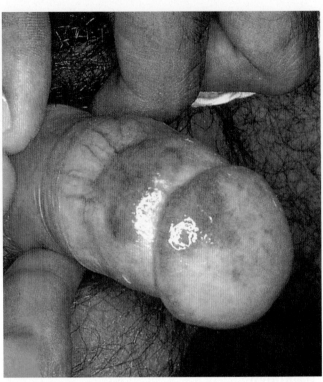

Erythroplasia of Queyrat: shiny well-marginated erythematous plaques; glans penis and prepuce.

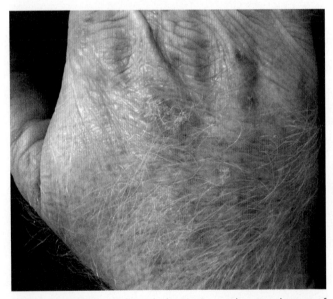

Actinic keratosis: rough, scaly, keratotic papules over dorsum of hand in an albino man.

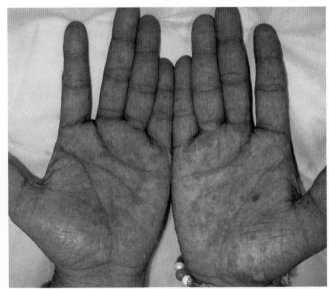

Arsenical keratosis: punctate keratosis of palms.

Smooth or rough surface. Greyish white color. Induration, inflammation or ulceration indicate evolution to squamous cell carcinoma.

Histopathology

Always biopsy acanthotic epidermis with or without atypia. Dysplastic lesions more likely to progress to squamous cell carcinoma. Non-specific inflammatory infiltrate in the submucosa.

Treatment

Several lesions resolve simply by removing the causal agent. Treat syphilis if evidence present. Indurated lesions ought to be excised.

Erythroplasia of Queyrat

Uncommon. Elderly, uncircumcized males affected. Sharply demarcated, brightly erythematous, velvety smooth, oval, round or patterned plaques on the glans penis and/or the foreskin. Little induration. Occasionally evolves into squamous cell carcinoma.

Histopathology

Bowenoid picture.

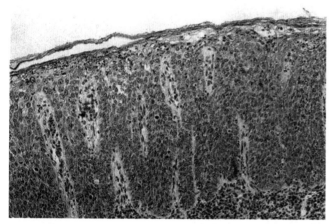

Histopathology of erythroplasia of Queyrat: bowenoid picture.

Actinic Keratoses

Sun induced. Common in whites, particularly blue eyed, red haired elderly individuals. Also in patients with xeroderma pigmentosum or albinism. Irregular, keratotic papules with surrounding erythema on the face, dorsa of hands or other light exposed parts.

Histopathology

Hyperkeratosis with irregularly atrophic and acanthotic epidermis. Epidermal cellular atypia. May have bowenoid picture with dyskeratotic cells but mainly limited to lower layers of epidermis. Variable inflammatory infiltrate in the dermis.

Treatment

Photo-protection. Medical therapies: imiquimod, 5 fluorouracil, tretinoin, diclofenac, cidofovir, systemic retinoids. Surgical therapies: chemical peeling, electrosurgery, cryosurgery, curettage, laser, dermabrasion, excision.

Arsenical Keratosis

Due to chronic exposure to arsenic in the form of indigenous medications for rheumatological or dermatological illnesses or through arsenical impurities in drinking water or occupational exposure. Manifestation of chronic arsenic toxicity, hence arsenic not detectable in blood. Sites: palms and soles, trunk, extremities, genitalia, eyelids. Punctate keratosis of palms and soles. Invasive tumors may develop like basal cell and squamous cell carcinomas. Other findings of chronic arsenism: rain drop pigmentation, diffuse alopecia, blackfoot disease, hepatic cirrhosis, internal malignancies, etc.

Treatment

Stopping further exposure. Systemic retinoids for prevention of malignancies. Specific lesions treated with topical 5 FU or ablative or surgical therapies.

PUVA Keratosis

Chronic exposure to PUVA. Uncertain etiology but possibly to UVA induced mutation in p53 or H-ras. Keratotic papules and plaques at sites of UVA exposure. Malignant transformation into SCC may occur. Virtually unknown in Indian skin.

Lentigo Maligna (Melanotic Freckle of Hutchinson)

Uncommon. Elderly individuals affected. Light exposed areas, most frequently the face. Solitary large, pigmented macule with irregular margins.

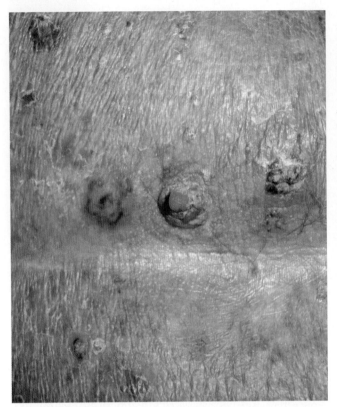

Arsenical keratosis and cutaneous: horns over the natal cleft in chronic arsenic poisoning.

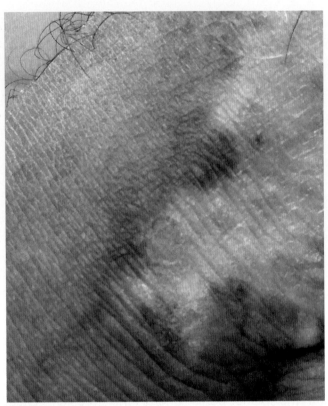

PUVA keratosis: yellowish keratotic papule over vitiligo lesion chronically exposed to PUVA.

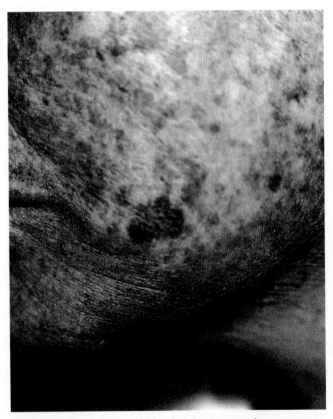

Lentigo maligna: flat, irregular dark brown macule.

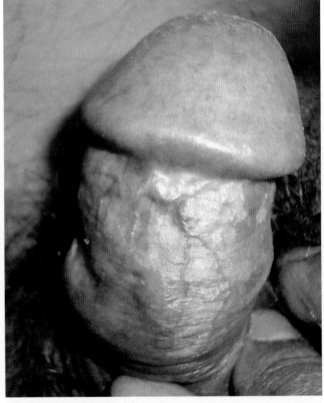

Bowenoid papulosis: pink barely elevated papules over glans penis and coronal sulcus.

Varying shades of brown or black color. Melanoma *in situ*. Gradual progression. Nodulation or verrucosity of surface, mottled pigmentation, ulceration or bleeding arouse suspicion of a malignant change.

Histopathology

Nests of atypical melanocytes at the dermo-epidermal interface. Inflammatory infiltrate in the dermis.

Treatment

Surgical excision if feasible. Electrodessication or other destructive measures in carefully selected patients. Imiquimod 5% cream also effective. Alternatively careful follow-up for development of any suspicious change.

Bowenoid Papulosis

Pigmented or pinkish plane topped or verrucous papules involving the genitalia and showing changes of carcinoma in situ (Bowen's) on histopathology. Commonly caused by high risk human papilloma viruses types 16 and 18.

Treatment

Topical imiquimod, 5 fluorouracil, cidofovir. Ablation using radiofrequency, cryosurgery, laser or complete excision.

Paget's Disease of the Nipple

Uncommon. Breast, rarely other sites (extra-mammary). Males also affected, females far more frequently. *Primary:* an intraductal carcinoma. Involvement of nipple and areola, secondary— by contiguity. Unilateral itchy, sharply delineated, eczematous or indurated plaque. Margin irregular and often slightly elevated. Psoriasiform or shiny glazed surface. Nipple retracted or obliterated. Associated lump in the breast, with or often without regional lymphadenopathy.

Histopathology

Presence of Paget's cells in an acanthotic epidermis. *Paget's cells:* large rounded cells with large regular nuclei, prominent nucleoli and

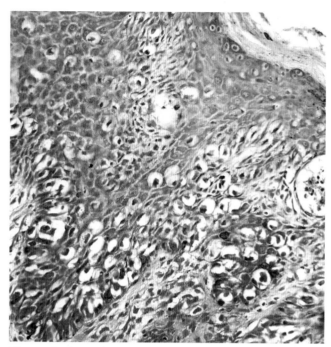

Histopathology of Paget's disease: typical Paget's cells (large round cells with large nucleus and vacuolated cytoplasm), arranged lalong the basal epidermal layer and focally scattered [CK 20 stain].
Courtesy: Dr Sarita Singh, Gynecologist, Safdarjung Hospital, Delhi and Dr Meeta Singh, Assistant Professor of Pathology, MAMC, Delhi.

vacuolated cytoplasm. Atypia present. Dermis shows chronic inflammatory infiltrate.

Treatment

Conservative surgery as far as possible, depending on underlying breast lump and lymph node status.

Summary of treatment modalities used in treatment of premalignant conditions of skin	
Medical treatment	*Surgical treatment*
• 5-Fluorouracil	• Chemical peeling/cautery
• Imiquimod	• Dermabrasion
• Photodynamic therapy	• Curettage
• Tretinoin	• Electrosurgery
• Diclofenac	• Cryosurgery
• Cidofovir	• Laser
• Systemic retinoids	• Shave excision
	• Complete excision
	• Moh's micrographic surgery

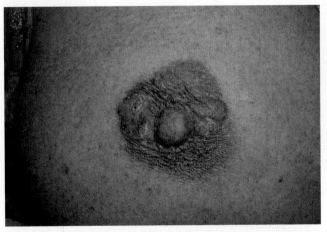

Paget's disease, early: scaly plaques involving the areola.

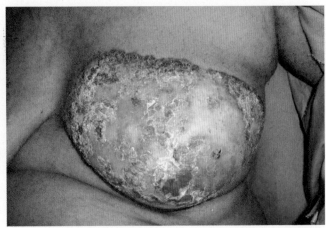

Paget's disease, advanced: thin scaly plaque over the left breast with destruction of the nipple-areola complex (moist erosion in center).

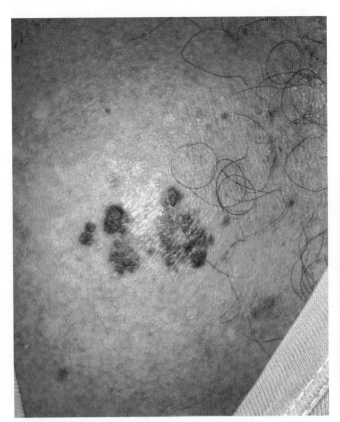

Superficial basal cell carcinoma: irregulalry arcuate plaque with thin edge and scaly papule at the margins.

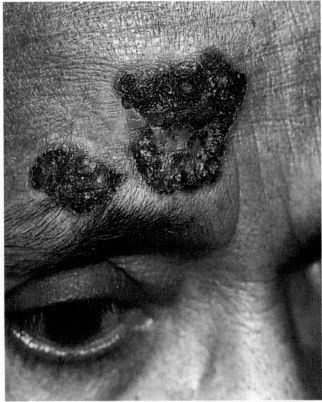

Pigmented basal cell carcinoma: pigmented scaly plaques over forehead with atrophic center.

MALIGNANT TUMORS OF EPIDERMAL ORIGIN

Basal Cell Carcinoma (Basal Cell Epithelioma)

The most common form of skin cancer across all races and skin types. Elderly individuals. Sunlight, an important causal factor. Face, temples, eyelids, cheeks, nose commonly affected. Variable clinical types: *superficial, pigmented, nodulo-ulcerative, sclerosing (morphea-form) and fibroepithelioma of Pinkus*. Small translucent nodule, extends peripherally. with atrophy and scarring in the middle. Pearly border almost diagnostic. The nodulo-ulcerated form (*rodent ulcer*) locally destructive. May invade the bones and cartilage. Does not metastasize generally. Not even to local lymph nodes.

Histopathology

Characteristic multilobular mass of basaloid cells (cuboidal cells with deeply basophilic nuclei) lying in the dermis. May maintain continuity with the epidermis. Peripheral cells palisade with clear space between the tumor mass and the surrounding fibrotic stroma (artefactual clefting). Much present in the stroma. Some differentiation towards adnexal structures. Tumor cells may contain melanin or dendritic melanocytes.

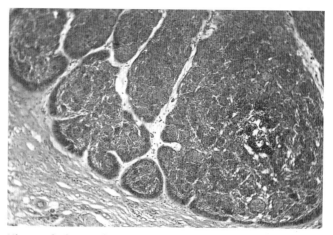

Histopathology of nodular basal cell carcinoma: grouped nodular aggregates of basaloid cells with prominent peripheral palisading.

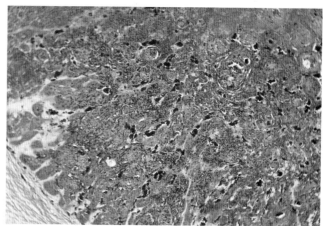

Histopathology of pigmented basal cell carcinoma: melanin and dendritic melanocytes (note fine dndritic processes) within a basaloid cell tumor aggregate.

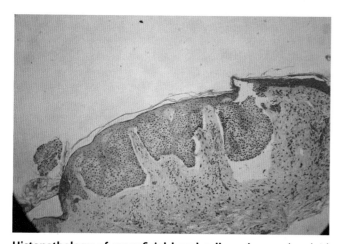

Histopathology of superficial basal cell carcinoma: basaloid cell nests extending in form of bulbous protrusion from the epidermis into the papillary dermis with artefactual clefting.

Treatment

Several modalities available. Choice depends on clinical type, size of tumor and site involved. Moh's micrographic surgery ideal. Standard treatment is excision with 2–4 mm free margin. About 1 cm margin required for tumors >2 cm in size. Other modalities include curettage and electrodessication, cryosurgery, radiotherapy, topical 5 fluorouracil, topical photodynamic therapy. Imiquimod, 5% cream in superficial type gives cure with excellent esthetic results. Recently vismodegib, a hedgehog pathway inhibitor, FDA approved for metastatic basal cell carcinoma.

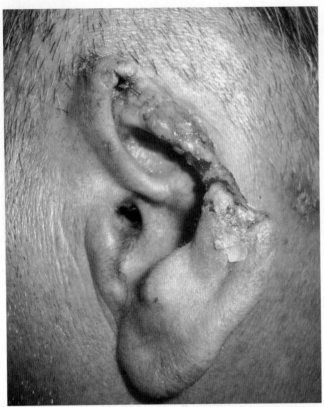

Nodulo-ulcerative basal cell carcinoma (rodent ulcer): plaque destryoing the ear helix.

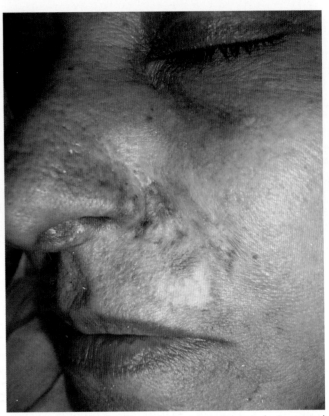

Morpheaform basal cell carcinoma: small crusted pigmented papule in the nasolabial fold with a large area of scarring and depigmentation around it.

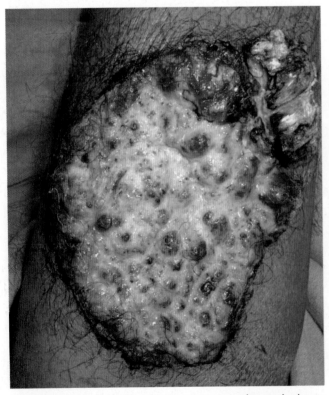

Squamous cell carcinoma: large verrucous ulcerated plaque over thigh.

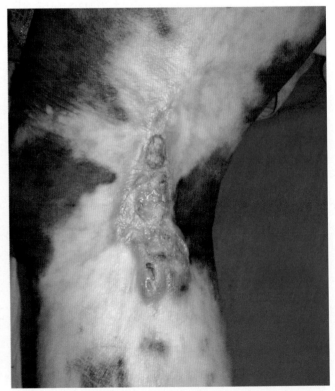

Marjolin ulcer (squamous cell carcinoma in scar): indurated non-healing ulcer on a chronic burn scar.

Squamous Cell Carcinoma

Fairly frequently. Seen in Whites subjected to chronic sunlight exposures. Uncommon in pigmented people. Develops *de novo* or on solar keratoses, Bowen's disease, bowenoid papulosis, leukoplakia, erythroplakia, arsenical keratoses or radiodermatitis. Also secondary to: burns or chronic heat injury (Kangri cancer). Or chronic ulcers as in leprosy. Or granulomas such as lupus vulgaris. Or other dermatoses—discoid lupus erythematosus, lichen planus hypertrophicus lichen sclerosus, oral lichen planus, hyperplastic oral candidiasis. Also in individuals with uncircumcized prepuce. Viral etiology in some: onchogenic human papilloma virus infection especially in immunosuppressed individuals (HIV or iatrogenic). Or patients with epidermodysplasia verruciformis.

Asymptomatic ulceration with rolled-out edges. Or verrucous growth. Variable presentations-nodule, abcess (especially in periungual location), cutaneous horn, etc. Always indurated—indicating dermal (or deeper involvement). Variable course. Metastatic spread through lymphatics. High risk or poor prognostic factors include carcinomas arising on ears/lips, scars, size > 2 cm or depth > 4 mm, Broders grade 3 or 4, immunocompromised state, involvement of nerve/bone/muscle. Perineural invasion is uncommon and vascular invasion is rare. Spread through lymphatics more common in SCCs of head and neck and genital region.

Histopathology

Hyperkeratosis and acanthosis, dermal invasion by well differentiated keratinizing or anaplastic cells. Nests of keratinocytes in dermis; well differentiated ones form keratin horn cysts ('keratin pearls'). Difficult to diagnose if poorly differentiated or of spindle cell type. Immunohistochemistry helps in these:using cytokeratin 5/6, epithelial membrane antigen; p63 is very specific marker. Broders' grading system on basis of percentage of undifferentiated cells in tumor nests. Inflammatory infiltrate pronounced in the dermis.

Treatment

Eradicate the tumor. Any modality employed should ensure good cosmetic results. Topical

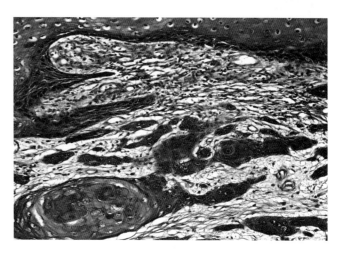

Histopathology of squamous cell carcinoma: infiltrating islands of squamous cells in upper dermis, few tending to form keratin pearls (suggestive of well diffrentiated squamous cell carcinoma). (*Courtesy*: Dr Meeta Singh, Assistant Professor of Pathology, MAMC, Delhi)

imiquimod or 5 fluorouracil only for SCC *in situ*. Moh's micrographic surgery is ideal. Conventional excision standard in most cases. Tumor free margin of 4 mm for tumors with depth <2 mm or low risk lesions and 6 mm for lesions larger >2 cm in size. For high risk lesions, Moh's recommended. Early lesions treated with curettage and electrodessication, cryosurgery. Radiotherapy in moderate risk lesions or patients unable to undergo surgery. Metastatic SCC treated with chemotherapy—platins, 5 fluorouracil, taxanes, cituximab (epidermal growth factor receptor inhibitor).

Malignant Melanoma

Tumor arising from melanocytes. Widely varying incidence. Common in Whites, particularly blue-eyed, red haired or blondes of Celtic descent. Also in patients with xeroderma pigmentosum and albinism. Sunlight, an important causal factor. Genetics also plays a role. May arise *de novo* or develop in a pre-existing lesion—melanocytic nevus or lentigo maligna.

Initially confined to the epidermis, epidermo-dermal junction or papillary dermis. Later invades deep dermis, subcutis and spreads to lymph nodes and viscera.

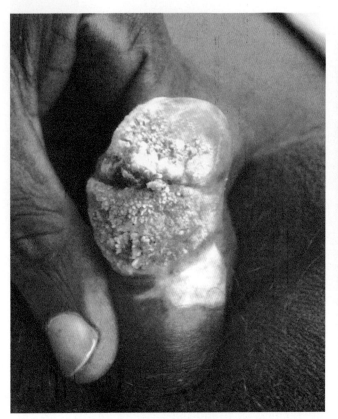

Genital squamous cell carcinoma: verrucous plaque over genital lichen sclerosus.

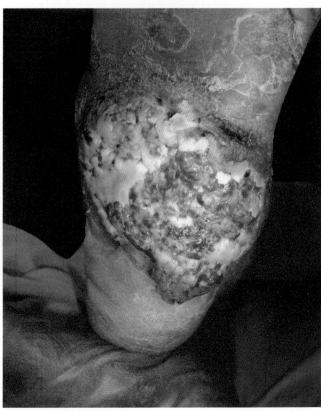

Epithelioma cuniculatum (verrucous carcinoma sole): verrucous plaque over the sole.

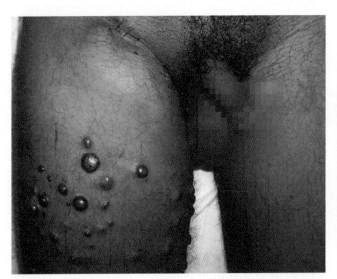

Malignant melanoma: in transit metastasis from a foot lesion with lymph node mass in right inguinal region.

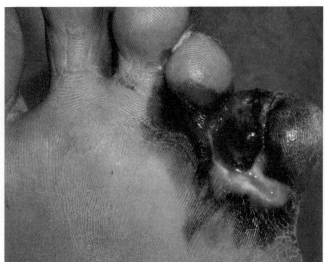

Malignant melanoma, acral lentiginous type: ulcerated nodule in web space.

Four types: *nodulo-ulcerative; superficial spreading, acral lentiginous melanoma and lentigo maligna melanoma. Nodulo-ulcerative type*, the most malignant form. Males more frequently affected. Rapid growth. Pigmented nodule. May ulcerate or bleed. Satellite lesions present. *Superficial spreading melanoma* commonest; less malignant than nodular form. Females more frequently affected. Back and lower limbs. Slightly elevated plaque with varying shades of pigmentation. Irregular border. Slow, asymmetric progression. May develop nodule after several years. *Lentigo maligna melanoma:* papulation or nodulation in a pre-existing melanotic freckle of Hutchinson. Face, the site of predilection. Elderly individuals. Slowly progressive. Least malignant of all melanomas; women fare better.

Acral Lentiginous Melanoma

The most common type in darker individuals including Indians. More in elderly, commonest site sole. Delay in diagnosis due to confusion with benign conditions.

Course

Progressive at variable pace. Lymphatic, later hematogenous, spread. Course depends on the type and depth of the tumor.

Histopathology

Atypical melanocytic aggregates. Location and extent differs amongst the variants. Nodular melanoma has dermal nodule invading the basal epidermal layer. Lentigo maligna melanoma has atypical melanocytes singly or nesting in basal layers of epidermis. Superficial spreading has pagetoid scatter of melanocytic nests ('buckshot scatter') at all levels of epidermis causing consumption of epidermis. Acral lentiginous melanoma has lentiginous melanocytic nesting with vertical growth phase, epidermal changes appear benign with minimal pagetoid scatter. Among immunohistochemistry markers, Melan-A is more sensitive than HMB-45 and more specific than S-100 for melanoma. A variant of melanoma, desmoplastic melanoma is negative with HMB-45 but positive with S-100 and vimentin. Amount of melanin variable, may be absent. Inflammatory infiltrate inversely proportional to the invasiveness of the tumor.

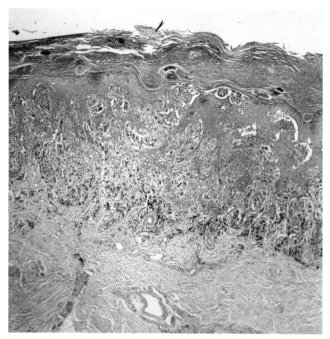

Histopathology of malignant melanoma, superficial spreading type: papillary dermal melanocytic aggregates, pagetoid scatter of pigmented melanocytic nests in epidermis, melanocytes and melanin also in the startum corneum.

Treatment

Wide surgical excision: 0.5 cm margin for *in situ*, 1 cm margin for depth <1 mm, 1–2 cm margin for depth of 1–2 mm and 2 cm margin for depth >2 mm. Sentinal lymph node dissection done in all cases with depth >1 mm and cases with depth <1 mm having-ulcerated lesions in young patients showing evidence of angiolymphatic invasion. Positive sentinal lymph node warrants complete node dissection. Regional metastasis treated by interferon alpha 2b or isolated limb perfusion with melphalan. Distant metastasis or dissemination treated with dacarbazine/interleukin-2 alone or in combination with cisplatin and vinblastine.

CUTANEOUS T CELL LYMPHOMA (CTCL)

Mycosis Fungoides (MF)

Three fourth of cutaneous lymphomas are of T cell type (CTCL). Out of these, more than 50% are MF (commonest CTCL subtype). An uncommon dermatosis characterized by infiltration of skin with T lymphocytes. Middle aged or elderly individuals, often males. Several distinct or overlapping stages:

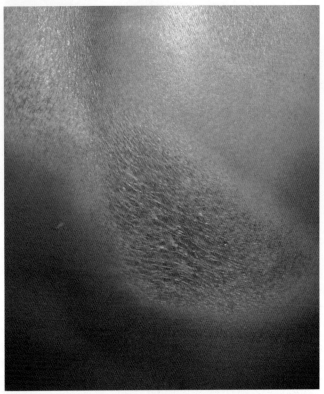

Mycosis fungoides, patch stage: atrophic (shiny, wrinkled) hyperpigmented patches over back.

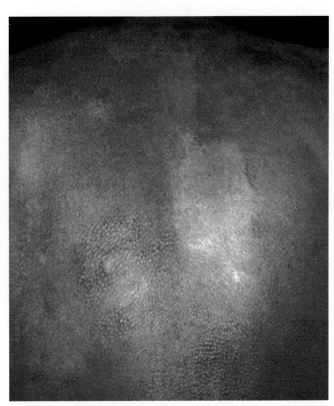

Mycosis fungoides: hypopigmented patches along with follicular papules over the back.

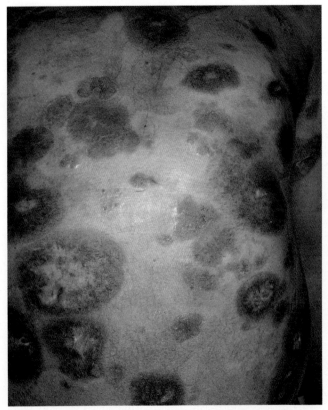

Mycosis fungoides, patch/plaque stage: few moist eczematous plaques over background of patches and post inflammatory hyperpigmentation.

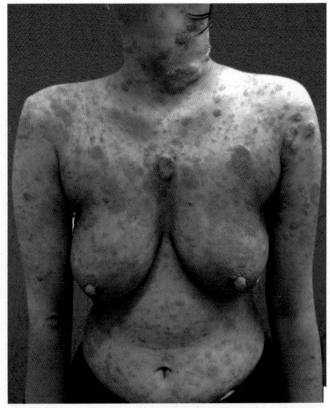

Mycosis fungoides, tumor d' emblee: multiple nodules and tumors developing on trunk and neck, *de novo*.

patch stage, plaque stage and *tumor stage. Patch stage:* itchy circular or oval, rather large, finely wrinkled, atrophic lesions with little infiltration. May partially or completely resolve spontaneously leaving atrophic hypo/hyperpigmented areas. Patch stage MF most difficult to diagnose and differentiate, both clinically and histologically, from other papulosquamous conditions. *Plaque stage:* may get elevated and acquire an infiltrated appearance. Covered parts—trunk. *Tumor stage:* may start *de-novo-tumor d'emblee*. Or more often, evolve from plaque stage. Face and flexures preferentially affected. May become confluent and ulcerate.

Several clinical variants recognized: pagetoid reticulosis, granulomatous slack skin, poikilodermatous, ichthyosiform, hypopigmented and folliculotropic and histological variants— granulomatous, syringotropic, large cell transformation.

Evaluate for extent of involvement: lymph nodes, hepatosplenomegaly and bone marrow.

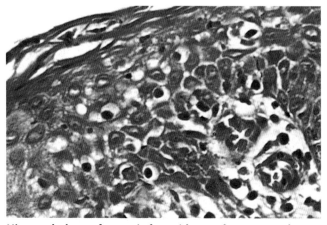

Histopathology of mycosis fungoides, early: tagging of atypical lymphocytes along basal epidermal layer. Few lymphocytes also in spinous layer.
Courtesy: Dr Sudheer Arava, Assistant Professor of Pathology, AIIMS, New Delhi.

Histopathology

Early MF shows non-specific features but important to note: lymphocytic tagging of basal layer, epidermotropism, epidermal lymphocytes

TNM staging of mycosis fungoides						
Cutaneous involvement (T)		*Stage*	*T*	*N*	*M*	*B*
T0	Lesions clinically and/or histologically suspicious but not diagnostic	IA	T1	N0	M0	B0–1
T1	Patches, papules or plaques					
T2	T1a - Patches only					
T3	T1b - Plaques with or without patches involving less than 10% of skin					
T4	Patches, papules or plaques					
	T2a - Patches only					
	T2b - Plaques with or without patches involving more than 10% of skin					
	≥ 1 tumor of ≥ 1 cm					
	Erythroderma (BSA > 80%)					
Lymph nodes (N)		IB	T2	N0	M0	B0–1
N0	Clinically and pathologically normal	IIA	TI–T2	N1–2	M0	B0–1
N1	Palpable; pathologically not involved					
N2	Palpable histological evidence of lymphoma, node architecture maintained					
N3	Palpable histological evidence of lymphoma, node architectural effacement					
Viscera (M)		IIB	T3	N0–2	M0	B0–1
M0	No visceral spread	IIIAB	T4	N0–1	M0	B0
M1	Visceral spread present					B1
Peripheral blood (B)		IVA12	T1–4	N3	M0	B2
						B0–2
B0	Peripheral blood atypical lymphocytes <5%	IVB2	T1–4	N0–3	M1	B0–2
B1	Peripheral blood atypical lymphocytes >5% but <20%					
B2	Peripheral blood atypical lymphocytes (sezary cells) >20%/> 1000 cells/microliter with positive TCR clone or one of the following: CD4/CD8 >10:1 or CD4+ CD7- ≥ 40% or CD4+ CD26- ≥30%					

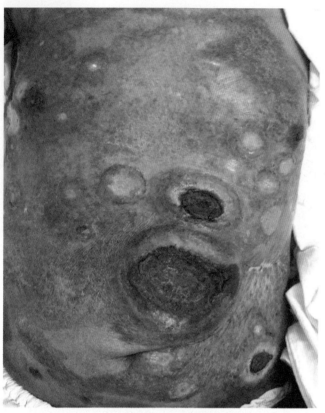

Mycosis fungoides, tumor stage: multiple ulcerated plaques and nodules over background of hyperpigmented patches.

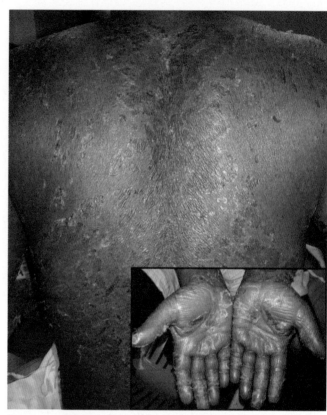

Sezary syndrome: generalized erythroderma with palmar scaling and thickening.

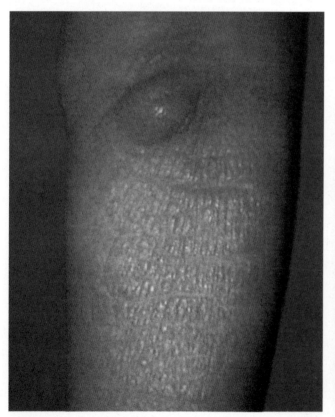

Sezary syndrome: infiltrated skin, forearm, nodule in the elbow.

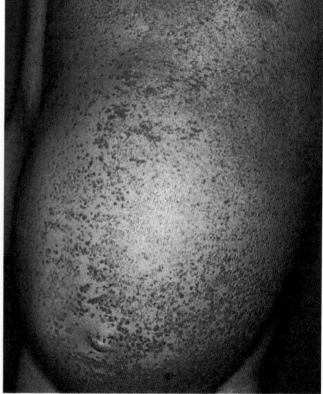

Langerhans' cell histiocytosis: papules, many purpuric, distributed in seborrhiec distribution. Abdominal distension due to hepatosplenomegaly.

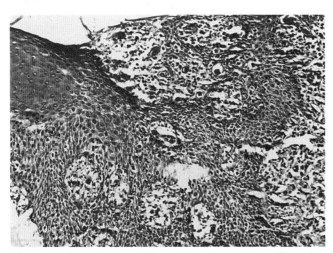

Histopathology of mycosis fungoides: intra-epidermal lympho-
cytic aggregates (Pautrier's microabscesses, 10x).
Courtesy: Dr Sudheer Arava, Assistant Professor of Pathology,
AIIMS, New Delhi.

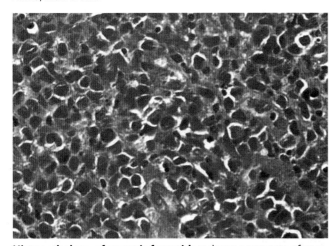

Histopathology of mycosis fungoides: dense aggregate of atyp-
ical lymphocytes. Many cells show mitoses and karyorrhexis (40x).
Courtesy: Dr Sudheer Arava, Assistant Professor of Pathology,
AIIMS, New Delhi.

with hyperconvoluted and larger nuceli, reticular
fibroplasia of papillary dermis. Lymphocytic infiltrate
in the upper dermis with pronounced invasion of
the epidermis—*epidermotropism*. Collection of
lymphocytes in epidermis to form abscesses–*Pautrier
microabscesses*. Epidermotropism less pronounced
and atypia more marked, as disease progresses.
Epidermotropism and Pautrier microabcesses
difficult to find in tumor and erythrodermic stages.

Sezary Syndrome

Erythrodermic form of CTCL. Triad of erythroderma
(> 80% body surface area of involvement), sezary
cells (T cells with cerebriform or convulted nuclei)
in peripheral blood >20% or absolute sezary cell
count >1000 cell/microliters and severe pruritus
with or without lymphadenopathy. May evolve from
MF or *de novo* (more commonly arises *de novo*).
Develop infiltration and nodulation. Evaluate
for extent of involvement. *Course:* Progressive.
Prognosis generally poor.

Treatment of CTCL

Treatment of mycosis fungoides and sezary syndrome according to staging	
Stage and therapy type	*Agent*
• Early stage MF (stage IA-IIA)	
– Topical/skin-directed therapy	Steroids
– Refractory early stage MF (stage IA-LA) Combination therapy	PUVA or NBUVB and I-Nα (low-dose) PUVA or NBUVB and bexaro- tene (Low-dose)
• Advanced MF/SS (stage IIB-IVB)	
– Skin-directed therapy Immunomodulators	TSEB Interferons (IFNα and IFNγ) Retinoid/rexinoid (bexarotene) ECP
– Biologic/targeted therapies	Alemtuzumab HDACis (e.g. romidepsin and vorinostat) Antifolates (e.g. methotrexate and pralatrexate)
– Combined therapy	IFNα and phototherapy IFNα and retinoids/rexinoids Retinold and phototherapy ECP and IFNα ECP and retinoids/rexinoids
– Systemic chemotherapy Single-agent	Pegylated doxorubicin Purine/pyrimidine analogs (e.g. gemcitabine)
– Multiagent	CHOP and CHOP-like
– Stem cell transplant	Autologous Allogeneic Non-myeloablative allogeneic

Key to Abbreviations:
PUVA: Psoralen with ultraviolet A; NBUVB: Narrowband ultraviolet B;
TSEB: Total skin electron beam therapy; ECP: Extracorporeal
photopheresis; HDACis: Histone deacetylase inhibitors;
CHOP: Cyclophosphamide doxorubicin vincristine and prednisolone

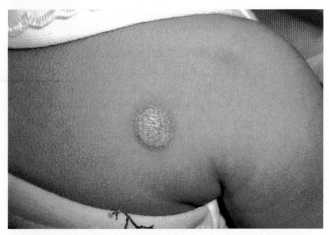

Juvenile xanthogranuloma: solitary yellowish plaque over upper back.

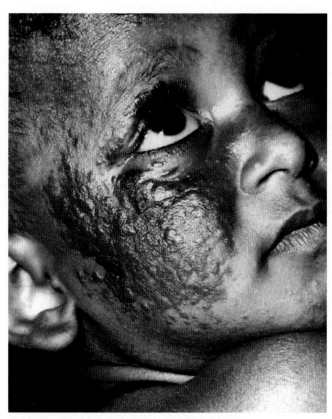

Juvenile xanthogranuloma: erythematous plaque on cheek.

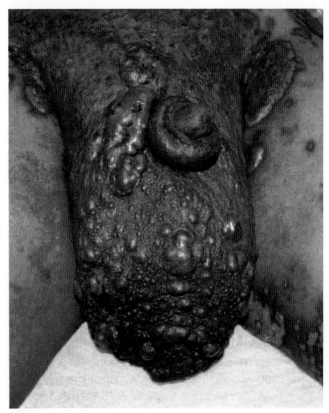

Rosai Dorfman syndrome: yellow to erythematous papules, nodules and plaques in genital area.

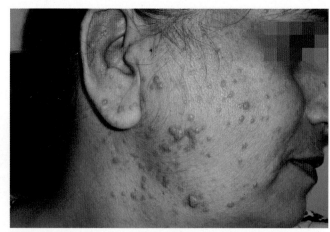

Generalized eruptive histiocytosis: tiny erythematous papules scattered over face.

REACTIVE TUMOROUS CONDITIONS

Histiocytoses

Diverse group. Classification in table. Mostly reactive conditions characterized by activated histiocytes. Cutaneous manifestations mainly limited to class I (Langerhans' cell histiocytosis) and class II (non-Langerhans' cell histiocytosis).

Langerhans' Cell Histiocytosis

Uncommon. Uncertain etiology. Current classification disregards classic eponyms. Stratification into single system disease (single site-isolated skin, lymph node, monostotic bone; or multiple site-multiple lymph nodes, multifocal bone, polyostotic bone) and multisystem disease (low risk group—skin, lymph node, pituitary, bone; or high risk group—hematopoietic system, lung, liver, spleen).

Skin lesions: seborrheic dermatitis-like lesions on the scalp: greasy, yellow-brown scaly papules on the trunk. May be purpuric healing with hypopigmented atrophic scars. May present as vesicules and pustules or nodules and ulcers. Flexures frequently affected. Noduloulcerative lesions over gingiva, perianal area. Nails show purpuric striae on nail bed, onycholysis, nail fold destruction. *Bones* show osteolytic areas. Most commonly involved bones—skull, femur, mandible, pelvis, spine. Stunted growth. *Diabetes insipidus* often present due to involvement of skull bone.

Hepatosplenomegaly, bone marrow involvement occurs late, indicates poor prognosis. Course and prognosis dependent upon age of patient and extent of the disease. Since internal involvement is mostly asymptomatic, exhaustive systemic screening investigations required.

Histopathology

Histiocytic cells with abundant eosinophilic cytoplasm, indented or reniform nucleus, present in papillary dermis and invading the epidermis focally. Extravasation of red blood cells in upper dermis, indicative of purpura. Intra-epidermal small aggregates of histiocytes may be there CD1a +, S100 +, CD 207 (langerin) +.

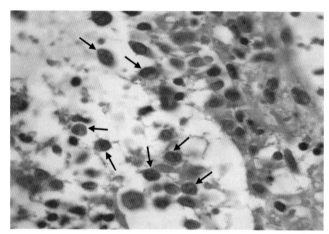

Histopathology of Langerhans' cell histiocytosis: plump histiocytes with large indented/reniform nuclei (black arrows) [40X].

S.No	Class	Group	Disorders
		Modified classification of histiocytosis	
1	I	Langerhans' cell histiocytosis (LCH)	Letterer-Siwe disease, Hand-Schuller-Christian disease, eosinophilic granuloma, Hashimoto Pritzker disease
2	II A	Histiocytosis involving dermal dendrocytes	Juvenile xanthogranuloma, generalized eruptive histiocytosis, benign cephalic histiocytosis, progressive nodular histiocytosis, xanthoma disseminatum, Erdheim Chester disease
	II B	Histiocytosis involving cells other than Langerhans' cells and dermal dendrocytes	Reticulohistiocytoma, multicentric reticulohistiocytosis, necrobiotic xanthogranuloma, Rosai Dorfman disease, familial hemophagocytic lymphohistiocytosis, malakoplakia, progressive mucinous histiocytosis, virus induced hemophagocytic syndrome
3	III	Malignant histiocytosis	Monocytic leukemias, histiocytic sarcomas, histiocytic lymphoma

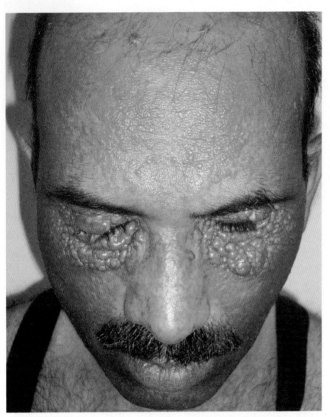

Xanthoma disseminatum: diffuse infiltration of face with erythematous papules, infiltrated papules and nodules over the eyelids.

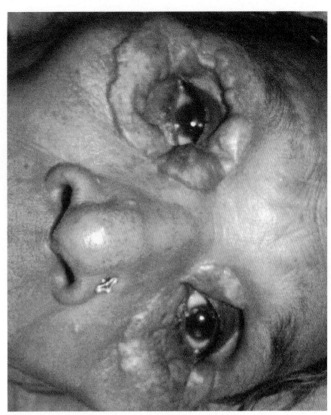

Adult xanthogranuloma: yellowish papules and nodules arranged symmetrically in periocular area; patient had vision loss. Note dilated pupils.

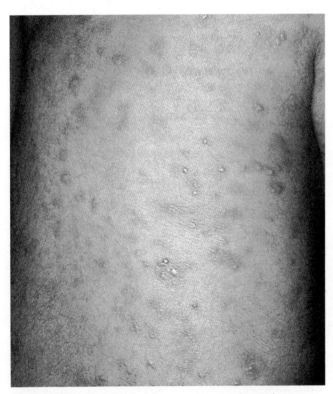

Mastocytosis: irregular dark brown pigmented macules.

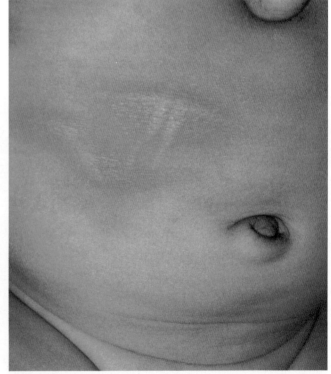

Darier sign: erythema and urtication in a patient of urticaria pigmentosa.

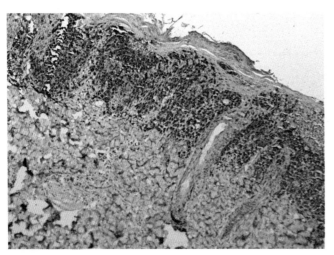

Histopathology of Langerhans' cell hsitiocytosis: sheets of Langerhans' cells (stained brown) invading the epidermis, showing strong positivity for langerin (CD 207) [10X, H&E].
Courtesy: Dr Ashok Singh, Pathology, AIIMS, New Delhi.

Treatment of LCH

Skin Disease Alone

- **Children:** observation, topical steroids/ tacrolimus/imiquimod.
- **Adults:** topical nitrogen mustard, psoralen with ultraviolet A, narrow band ultraviolet B, CO_2 laser, systemic prednisolone, thalidomide and isotretinoin.

In case of extensive, life-threatening skin disease with low risk multisystem involvement, LCH protocol III in form of prednisolone, vinblastine for initial 6 weeks, those who respond favorably get same drugs in pulse form along with 6 mercaptopurine for total 12 months. Those who do not respond well to 12 week prednisolone plus vinblastine or have high risk organ involvement, treated with cladribin and cytarabine.

Class II Histiocytosis or Non-Langerhans' Cell Histiocytosis

Juvenile Xanthogranuloma

Commonest non-Langerhans' cell histiocytosis. Infants and children (rarely adults). Solitary or multiple, asymptomatic, self-healing, red to yellow papules and nodules. Head and neck; sometimes trunk and extremities. Eyes (periorbital area and iris), lungs, liver and other visceral organs less frequently involved.

Histopathology

Dense dermal monomorphous histiocytic infiltrate with foam cells; Touton giant cells and foreign body giant cells typical.

Treatment

Reassurance and regular ophthalmological examination. Ocular and visceral involvement: treat with oral steroids.

Rosai Dorfman Disease (Sinus Histiocytosis with Massive Lymphadenopathy)

Etiology unknown (? reactive phenomenon). Young adults. Painless lymphadenopathy (mostly cervical) with constitutional symptoms. Skin, most common 'extranodal' site: yellow papules, plaques or nodules. Lung, liver, heart and other visceral organs also involved.

Histopathology

Pathognomonic—large pale histiocytes with *emperipolesis* (phagocytosis of lymphocytes).

Treatment

Spontaneous regression common. Cytotoxic agents help.

Generalized Eruptive Histiocytosis

Asymptomatic eruption of multiple papules scattered all over body. Involvement of mucosae more common in adults.

Xanthoma Disseminatum

Asymptomatic papules over eyelids, face, trunk. Initially red-brown then turn yellowish. Tendency to coalesce. Commonly associated with diabetes insipidus. Erdheim Chester disease is variant with chronic bone pain and visceral involvement.

Necrotic Xanthogranuloma

Nodules and plaques with central atrophy and ulceration. Involvement of face, trunk and extremities. Periorbital involvement characteristic. Underlying paraproteinemia/myeloma.

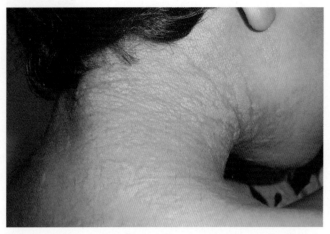

Diffuse cutaneous mastocytosis: pale infiltrated skin with peau-d-orange appearance over the neck and suprascapular area.

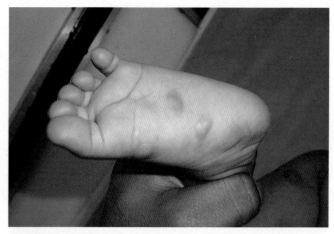

Mastocytoma: tan colored nodules over sole of an infant.

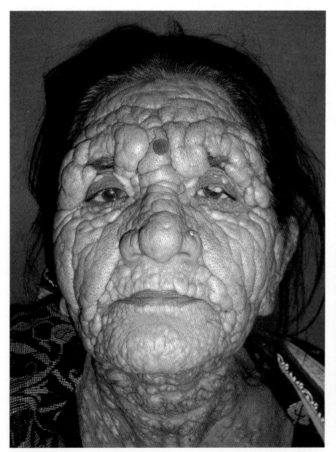

Diffuse cutaneous mastocytosis, pseudoxanthomatous type: diffuse facial infiltration along with waxy yellow plaques and nodules.

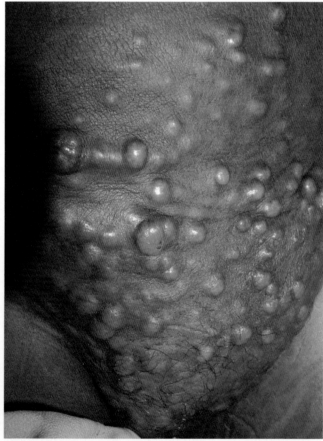

Metastatic tumor: stony hard nodules on lower abdomen; primary tumor in the breast.

Treatment

Juvenile xanthogranulomas and Rosai Dorfman self limiting. For others, treatment usually unsuccessful. Systemic steroids and immunosupressants (methotrexate, azathioprine, chlorambucil, cyclophosphamide, melphalan) used with variable response. Destructive therapies for cosmetic relief.

Mastocytosis

Uncommon proliferative disorder of mast cells. Generally benign. Onset, infancy or early childhood. Generalized cutaneous (urticaria pigmentosa), diffuse cutaneous or systemic forms. Occasionally solitary tumor mastocytoma. Rarely malignant.

Urticaria Pigmentosa

Commonest form. Onset: infancy or childhood. Yellowish brown or brown-black illdefined macules or plaques that urticate easily Darier's sign. Bullous lesions in some. Self limiting. Pigment fades around puberty. Diffuse cutaneous form: diffuse infiltration of the skin. Yellowish discoloration, doughy feel. May have associated systemic involvement: hepatosplenomegaly, osseous lesions, hematological abnormalities.

Histopathology

Biopsied with care to avoid degranulation. Sheets of mast cells in dermis which stain metachromatically with toluidine blue or Giemsa stain.

Treatment

Excise solitary tumors. For generalized or diffuse cutaneous forms, use antihistamines combined with H2 antagonists. PUVA helpful in some patients. Systemic steroids, if bullous lesions.

Diffuse Cutaneous Mastocytosis

Exclusively seen in infants. Thick skin with peau-d-orange appearance, yellowish brown discoloration. Hemorrhagic bullae develop in early phase, diffuse skin thickening persists.

Mastocytomas

Usually in infants, over extremities. More commonly solitary.

Histopathology

Demonstration of mast cells—'Fried egg' appearance round central nucleus and surrounding amphophilic granular cytoplasm. Number of cells dependent on subtype. Upper dermal infiltrate in urticaria pigmentosa and sheets of mast cells in mastocytoma and diffuse cutaneous variants. More compact and deeper aggregates in mastocytoma as compared to diffuse cutaneous variant. Toludine blue stain and CD117 immunostains for mast cells.

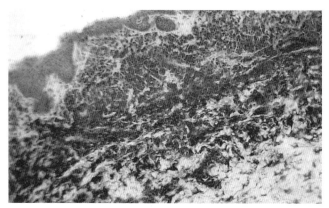

Histopathology of mastocytosis: sheets of mast cells in diffuse cutaneous variant, staining strongly with toludine blue.

Treatment

Frequently no treatment required. Oral antihistaminics for symptomatic relief. For persistent lesions: topical/intralesional steroids, calcineurin inhibitors, excision of mastocytomas, oral psoralen plus ultraviolet therapy, orals steroids and mast cell stabilizers. Avoidance of vigorous exertion/emotions, food items like raw fish/peanut/cheese/alcohol/hot beverages, etc.

METASTATIC MALIGNANT TUMORS

Uncommon. Single or multiple. Rather late lymphogenous or hematogenous spread. Primary site variable: breast, prostate, lungs, kidney, stomach, intestine, liver, bone. Or cutaneous malignant melanoma. Commonly localized to scalp, trunk. Asymptomatic. Skin colored or erythematous, firm nodules or plaques.

Course

Generally unfavorable. Occasional cure on removal of primary and metastasis.

19

Sexually Transmitted Diseases

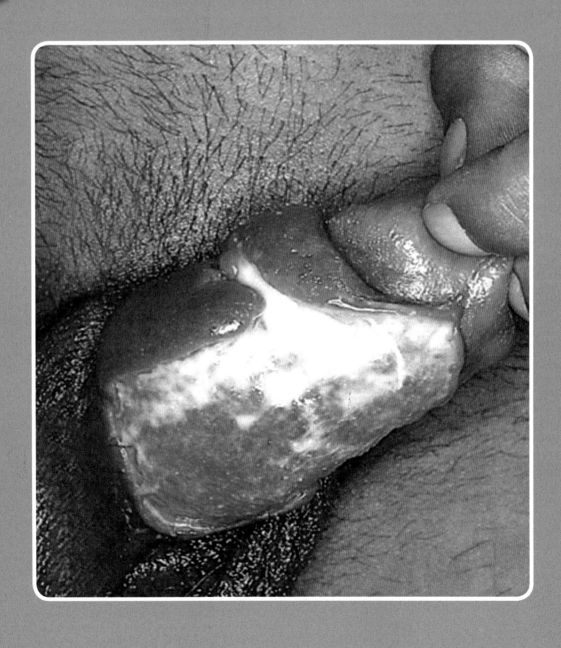

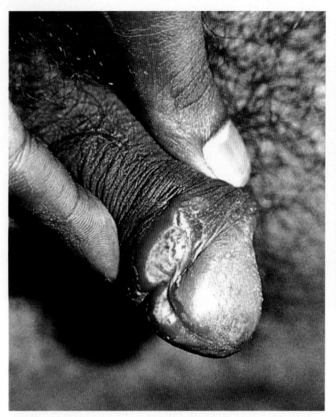

Primary syphilis: solitary indurated ulcer.

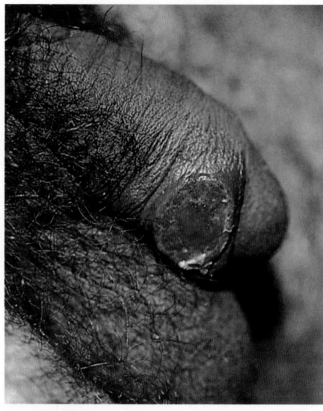

Primary syphilis: indurated, ulcerated, clean ulcer.

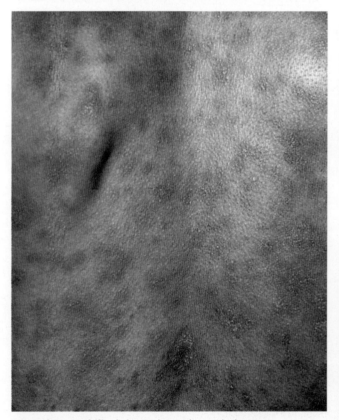

Secondary syphilis: lichenoid papules and plaques.

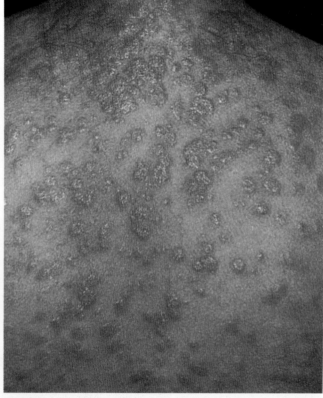

Secondary syphilis: nodular lesion. Rare symmetrical pattern.

Infective disorders, in which *sexual transmission is epidemiologically important*. The old term venereal diseases (VD) included syphilis, gonorrhea, chancroid, donovanosis and lymphogranuloma venereum (LGV)—*the infamous five*! The scope enlarged to include others such as herpes genitalis, genital molluscum contagiosum, anogenital warts, genital candidiasis, hepatitis B, pediculosis pubis, scabies and the latest and most dreaded of them all—acquired immunodeficiency syndrome (AIDS).

Laxity in sexual standards, permissiveness of the society in general, easy access to sex, economic independence and breakdown of family structure have all helped promote the spread of sexually transmitted diseases (STDs). Males report more frequently and earlier. Females, may be asymptomatic or have lesions on concealed genital parts. Heterosexual or homosexual contact—genital, anogenital or orogenital—causal.

SYPHILIS

The classical sexually transmitted disease. Ancient, fascinating, capricious. Causative organism—*Treponema pallidum*—subsp. pallidum a spirochete, 5–15 μ × 0.1–0.2 μ. Characteristic undulating *to-and-fro* and bending movements with little translational motion. Unable to grow on artificial media. Grown in rabbit testicles.

Incubation period—long and variable: 9–90 days, generally 3–5 weeks. Estimated rate of transmission from infected partner for a single sexual exposure about 30%.

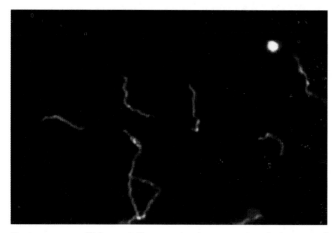

Treponema pallidum: delicate spirochetes under dark ground microscopy.

Divided into *early* and *late syphilis*. Or *primary, secondary, latent* and *tertiary* stages. Early syphilis comprises primary, secondary and early (<1 year) latent stages. Late syphilis, late latent (>1 year) and tertiary stages. Various stages, overlapping and arbitrary.

Primary Syphilis

The first manifestation, the *chancre:* the lesion at the point of entry of organisms. Solitary, *asymptomatic*, non-tender, *indurated*, erosive papulo-nodule or a shallow ulcer—moist, smooth, non-bleeding with sharply defined border. Genital, extragenital or perianal location. Glans or shaft of penis, prepuce, coronal sulcus, cervix, clitoris, vagina and vulva—frequently affected. Extragenital sites, lip, areola of breast, finger. Self healing—with a hyperpigmented macule or a superficial scar within 3–6 weeks. Unilateral or bilateral regional lymphadenopathy: small, rubbery, discrete, firm.

Secondary Syphilis

Systemic disease. Spirochetemia present. Develops 6 weeks to 6 months after onset of primary syphilis—may overlap with healing primary sore. Generalized, bilateral, symmetrical rash—macular, papular, papulosquamous or psoriasiform. And nodular (often asymmetrical). *Never vesicular*. Asymptomatic. Mucocutaneous lesions, *moist papules*. Intertriginious, perianal and genital lesions often florid and vegetative—*condylomata lata*. Mucosal and mucocutaneous lesions, particularly infectious—buccal, labial, faucial, tonsillar. Generalized lymphadenopathy—painless, discrete, non-tender. 'Moth-eaten' alopecia over scalp with or without telogen effluvium. *Systemic symptoms*—malaise, fever, bone pains, headaches. Treponemal and non-treponemal serological tests for syphilis invariably positive. Secondary stage lasts 1–3 months. Relapses infrequent—generally within 6 months; not beyond 2 years. Transplacental transmission to fetus significant.

Latent Syphilis

No clinical or laboratory (radiological and CSF examination included) evidence of syphilis, except a positive blood serology.

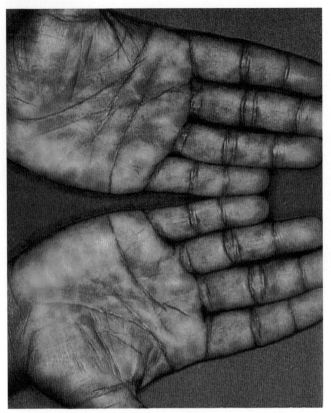

Secondary syphilis: pigmented palmar scaly macules.

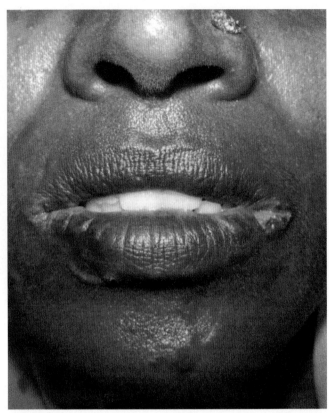

Secondary syphilis: characteristic 'split papules'.

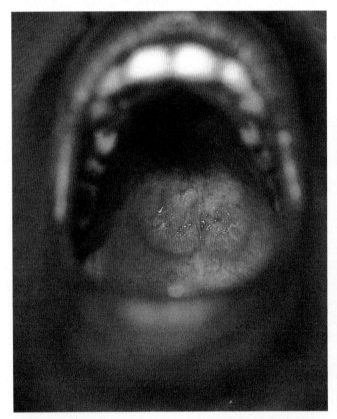

Secondary syphilis: erosive mucosal lesions.

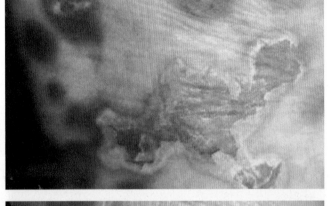

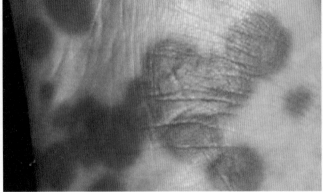

JH reaction to penicillin in secondary syphilis: bright red plaques over sole at baseline (top) and after (bottom) oral steroid therapy.

Arbitrarily divided into potentially infectious: *early* (less than 1 year) or *late* (more than 1 year) post infection stages.

Tertiary Syphilis

Classified as *benign:* involves the skin, subcutaneous tissue, bones or joints. Or *neurosyphilis*. Or *cardiovascular* syphilis (indicating respectively involvement of the nervous or cardiovascular systems). Develop 5, 10 or 20 years after infection, respectively.

Characteristic lesion, *gumma*—a granulomatous lesion rich in lymphocytes and plasma cells and associated with endarteritis. Treponemes not demonstrable. Serological tests for syphilis almost always positive in blood.

Mucocutaneous gummata: asymptomatic nodules or plaques. Asymmetrical. Arranged in polycyclic and arcuate configuration; variable in size and number. Break down into indolent ulcers— heal with atrophic scars. Mucosal involvement common—gumma of palatal bone and overlying mucosa-perforation of the hard palate; 'eating' away of uvula or depression of bridge of the nose.

Diagnosis

Primary and secondary stages, diagnosed most specifically by demonstration of *Treponema pallidum* on dark ground microscopy from ulcer transudate or lymph node aspirate. If negative, syphilitic serology along with clinical features of presumptive value. Latent syphilis shows serological positivity in blood alone (no other evidence of syphilis).

Late syphilis, by quasi-specific histology of syphilis together with positive serology in blood (and CSF in neurosyphilis).

Treatment

Penicillin, always the drug of choice. 0.1 µg/mL effective treponemicidal serum levels. Parenteral route preferred because of compliance and consistent absorption. To be administered after intradermal sensitivity testing before each dose.

Early syphilis: benzathine penicillin, total of 2.4 million IU—1.2 in each buttock. Or procaine benzyl penicillin, 1.2 million IU, once daily for 10 days.

Late syphilis: 2.4 million IU of benzathine penicillin weekly for 3 successive weeks. For neurosyphilis, aqueous benzyl penicillin, 3–4 million IU, intravenously (IV), every 4 hours for 14 days.

Congenital syphilis: treat syphilitic mother at earliest to prevent congenital syphilis. Procaine penicillin 50,000 IU/kg daily for 10 days or aqueous benzyl penicillin 1 lakh IU/kg in two divided doses, daily for 10 days. The infant may be treated with a single dose of benzathine penicillin G 50,000 IU/kg single dose IM of the baby is normal clinically, with a non-treponemal titer <4 fold of mother's titer and the mother has been treated adequately with penicillin regimen for syphilis during pregnancy.

In penicillin sensitive individuals: tetracycline or erythromycin, a total dose of 30 g (2 g a day for 15 days) or doxycycline 100 mg twice a day for 15 days for early and late benign syphilis. For neurosyphilis 60 g (2 g per day for 30 days). Tetracyclines should not be used in pregnant women or in children under 8 years.

Jarisch-Herxheimer reaction: develops within a few hours of administration of penicillin or other treponemicidal drugs. More common in early syphilis, more serious in late. Fever, malaise, body aches. Also exacerbation of syphilitic lesions. Useful as presumptive evidence of syphilis.

GONORRHEA

Extremely common. Almost always sexual transmission, rarely accidental. Caused by *Neisseria gonorrhoea*—an intracellular Gram negative diplococcus. Incubation period 2–7 days, occasionally less or more. Males present with acute urethritis, females asymptomatic. Or with cervicitis.

Acute urethritis: copious, purulent or mucopurulent discharge with dysuria and burning micturition in males. Some males and most females asymptomatic.

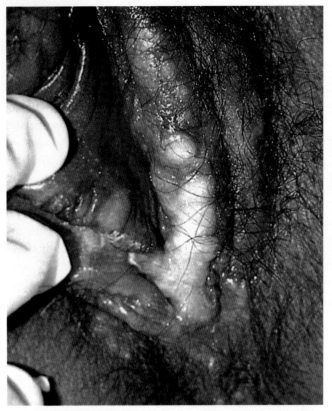

Condylomata lata: flat papules and plaques, vulva.

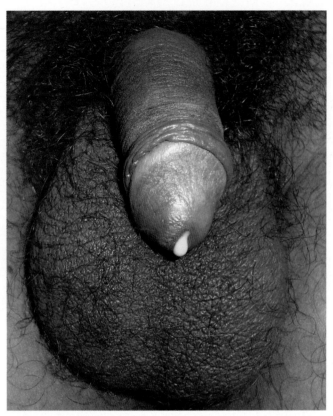

Frankly purulent urethral discharge in gonococcal urethritis.

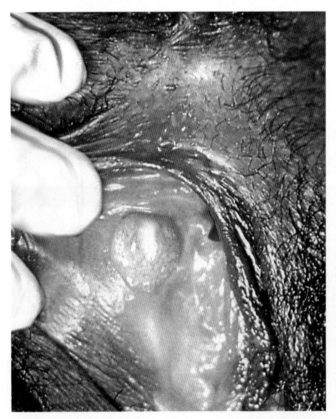

Gonorrhea: urethritis, purulent discharge.

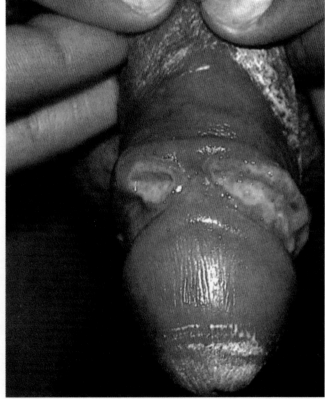

Chancroid: 'dirty' deep necrotic ulcers.

Cervicitis: purulent cervical discharge. Salpingitis and pelvic inflammatory disease (PID) may complicate.

Vulvo-vaginitis: in female children—suspect sexual assault. Acute painful swelling of the vulva with purulent vaginal discharge.

Pharyngeal gonorrhea: orogenital contact. Asymptomatic or mildly painful throat with muco-purulent discharge; hoarseness due to laryngitis.

Diagnosis: clinically suspected, in males, by the presence of purulent discharge. Demonstration of pus cells and intracellular Gram negative diplococci in urethral discharge generally adequate evidence. Culture and biochemical tests essential for confirmation in females and preferably in males.

Treatment

Choice of antimicrobial therapy depends on antibiotic sensitivity and resistance pattern in the geographic area.

Uncomplicatd gonorrhea: cefixime 400 mg or azithromycin 2 g, single dose orally. Or ceftriaxone 250 mg, single IM injection.

Complicated and disseminated gonorrhea: ceftriaxone 1 g, once daily IM or IV for 7 days. Or cefixime 400 mg, twice daily, orally for 7 days.

NON-GONOCOCCAL URETHRITIS

Extremely common; commoner in the West, particularly in Whites. Basically, urethritis (in males) that is not *gonococcal. Causative organisms: Chlamydia trachomatis, Mycoplasma genitalium*; less important *Ureaplasma urealyticum*, and *Trichomonas vaginalis*. Incubation period: 2–3 weeks. Mild dysuria and mucopurulent discharge. Females: symptomatic sterile pyuria (*urethral syndrome*). Reiter's syndrome, a serious but rare complication.

Diagnosis: essential prerequisite demonstration of polymorphonuclear leukocytes and absence of *N. gonorrhoeae* in the urethral smear. Culture and immunoconfirmation of antigen.

Treatment

Doxycycline,100 mg orally, twice daily for 7 days or azithromycin 1 g orally, single dose. Erythromycin base/stearate, 500 mg orally, 4 times a day for 7 days in pregnant females. Treat sexual partner(s). Condom, a good prophylactic measure against gonococcal and non-gonococcal urethritis.

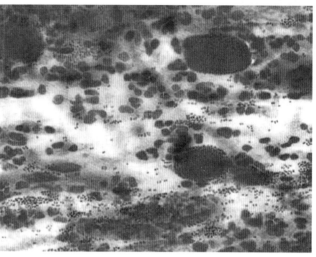

Histopathology of *Neisseria gonorrhoea*: Gram negative intra-cellular and extracellular diplococci in urethral discharge.

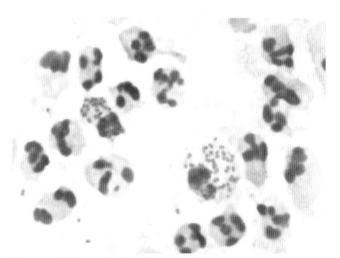

Histopathology of *Neisseria gonorrhoea*: Gram negative pre-dominantly intracellular ocucci in purulent urethral discharge.

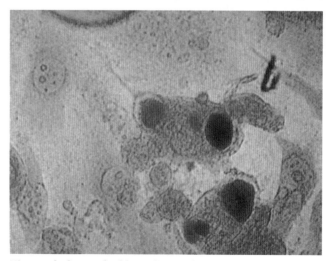

Histopathology of *Chlamydia trachomatis*: inclusion bodies stained with iodine.

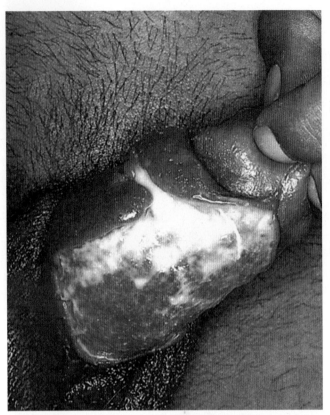

Chancroid, phagedenic ulcer: most of the shaft of penis destroyed.

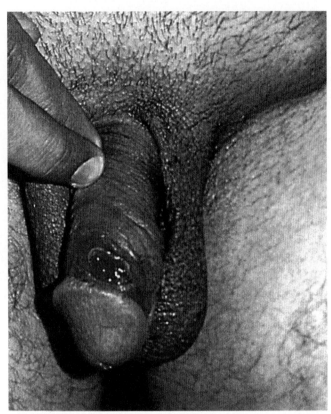

Chancroid: with bubo. Inflammatory inguinal lymphadenopathy.

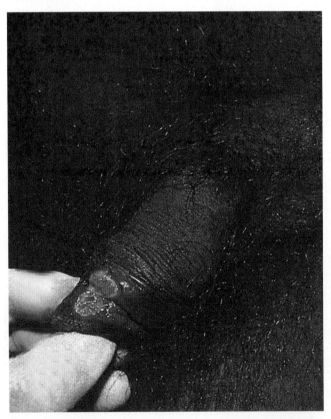

Donovanosis: clean shiny beefy red lesions with a pearly border.

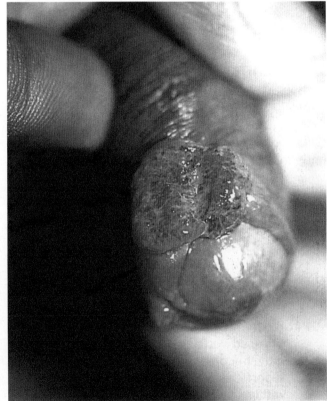

Donovanosis: multiple, clean fleshy lesions.

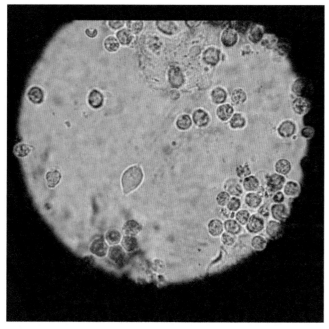

Wet mount from vaginal discharge: a central pear shaped structure with tapering ends suggestive of Trichomonas. The more tapered ends suggest location of axostyle and the rounded end shows filamentous projection suggestive of the flagellae (400x).

CHANCROID

Common in tropics and subtropics. Bacterial infection; autoinoculable. Causative organism: *Haemophilus ducreyi*, Gram-negative bacillus. Characteristic chain formation. Uncircumcised males with poor personal hygiene more frequently affected. Incubation period: 2–6 days. Multiple, superficial, dirty sloughed ulcers with ragged margins; bleed easily. Coronal sulcus, prepuce, shaft and glans penis affected. Secondary infection with fusospirochetal organisms results in rapidly destructive *phagedenic* ulcer. Inguinal lymphadenitis, 1–2 weeks later; unilateral, painful, fluctuant; may rupture.

Diagnosis: difficult to confirm. Demonstration of *H. ducreyi* in a Gram stained smear—bacilli arranged in '*a school of fish*' configuration, not specific or sensitive. Culture of fastidious bacillus difficult.

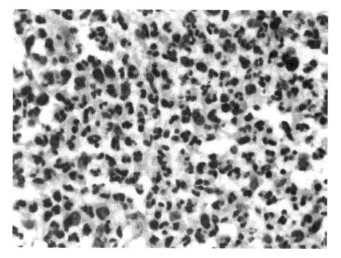
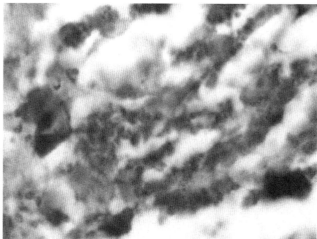

Histopathology of donovanosis: Giemsa stained crushed tissue preparation showing intracytoplasmic and extracellular bipolar (safety pin appearance) staining *Calymmatobacterium granulomatis* (Donovan bodies); top (10x), bottom (40x)

Treatment

Azithromycin, 1 g orally, single dose. Or ceftriaxone 250 mg, IM single dose. Or ciprofloxacin 500 mg, twice a day for 3 days. Sexual partners should also be treated to avoid relapses. Fluctuant lymph nodes should be aspirated, through non-dependent normal skin.

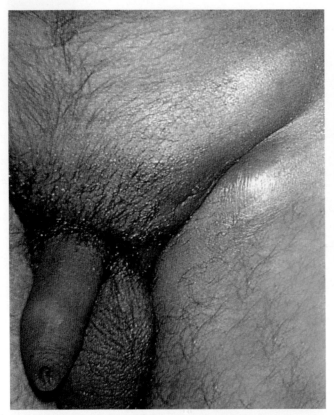

Lymphogranuloma venereum: typical groove sign due to enlargement of femoral and inguinal lymph nodes.

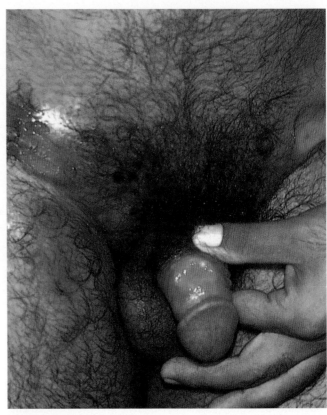

Mixed infection: lymphogranuloma venereum and syphilis.

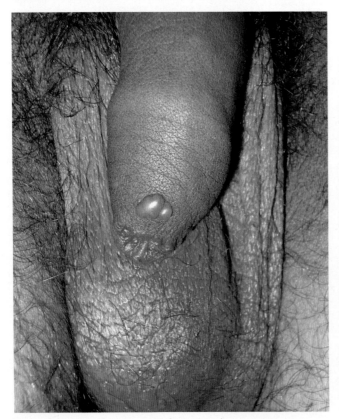

Vesicular primary herpes genitalis in a male.

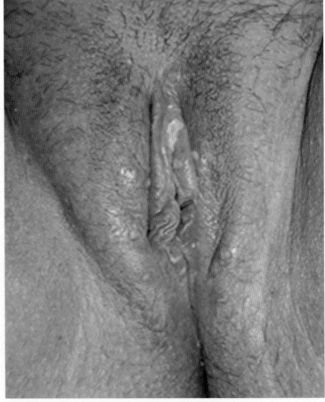

Primary ulcerative herpes genitalis in a female.

DONOVANOSIS (GRANULOMA INGUINALE)

Endemic in tropical countries—parts of Africa, South East Asia and South India. Causative agent: a bacterium, *Klebsiella granulomatis (previously known as Calymmatobacterium granulomatis)* small, Gram negative and pleomorphic. Incubation period: 2–8 weeks. Asymptomatic papule that breaks down to form an ulcer with characteristic *rolled edges* and a red beefy floor made of granulation tissue. *Sites of involvement:* coronal sulcus, shaft of penis, vulva. No lymphadenopathy. Subcutaneous granulomas in the inguinal region may resemble a bubo—'*pseudobubo*'. Squamous cell carcinoma, an occasional complication.

Treatment

Doxycycline, 100 mg twice a day for 14 days. Or tetracycline 500 mg, 4 times a day for 14 days. Or erythromycin stearate/base 500 mg 4 times a day for 14 days. Or azithromycin 500 mg twice a day for 2 weeks. All drugs given orally.

LYMPHOGRANULOMA VENEREUM

Lymphogranuloma venereum (LGV), an uncommon *Chlamydia trachomatis* infection (caused by either of the serovars L1, L2 or L3). Trophism for lymphoid tissue characteristic. Incubation period; 3–30 days.

Primary lesion: a transient, herpetiform (vesicular) lesion. Asymptomatic—often not noticed. Glans penis, vagina, vulva common sites. Heals without residue. *Lymphadenopathy:* a conspicuous feature. Painful, multiple, bilateral, matted inguinal and femoral lymph nodes—may form a furrow—'*the groove sign*', considered pathognomonic. Lymph nodes burst, unilaterally or bilaterally to form sinuses discharging seropurulent material. Constitutional symptoms—fever, malaise, headache and anorexia accompany lymphadenopathy.

Females: internal iliac nodes, apart from the inguinal, also commonly involved. Late sequelae: lymphedema of the vulva with elephantiasis and ulcerations—*esthiomene*. Anorectal syndrome, more frequent in females; results in anal strictures.

Treatment

Doxycycline, 100 mg twice a day for 3 weeks. Or tetracycline, 500 mg 4 times a day for 3 weeks. Or erythromycin stearate/base 500 mg orally 4 times a day for 3 weeks. *Bubo should be aspirated, not incised.*

GENITAL HERPES

Common, particularly in the uncircumcised males. Caused more frequently by herpes simplex virus 2 (HSV 2) and sometimes HSV 1. Primary (first exposure) or recurrent disease. Incubation period: 3–7 days, sometime longer. *Primary disease:* extensive grouped vesicles on an erythematous base. Vulva, vagina, glans, prepuce, shaft of penis, pubic area or perianal area affected. Preceding local discomfort or burning sensation. *Systemic symptoms:* headache, fever, malaise present. Associated lymphadenopathy. Heal in 2–3 weeks. Prior HSV 1 infection reduces severity of systemic symptoms. HSV 1 genital infection less symptomatic.

Recurrent herpes genitalis: less severe. Prodromal paresthesia or burning sensation. Grouped vesicles on an erythematous base; may become pustular or erode to form superficial ulcerations. Heal spontaneously within a few days to a couple of weeks. Recurs with varying, but decreasing, frequency. HSV 2 infection more likely to be recurrent.

Neonatal herpes simplex: acquired during passage through infected birth canal.

Treatment

First clinical episode: acyclovir 200 mg five times a day or 400 mg three times a day for 7 days.

Recurrent episode: acyclovir either 200 mg five times a day or 400 mg three times a day for 5 days. Or famciclovir 125 mg twice daily or valacyclovir 1 g once daily for 5 days.

Suppressive therapy: for severe and frequent (>6/year) episodes. In immunocompetent—acyclovir 400 mg twice daily. Or famiciclovir 250 mg

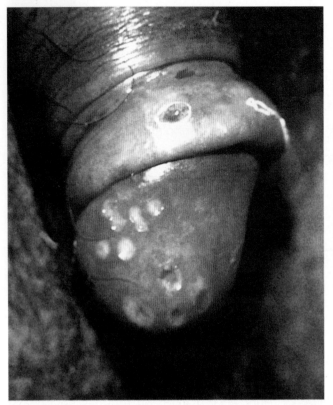

Genital herpes, recurrent: multiple, superficial grouped ulcerations.

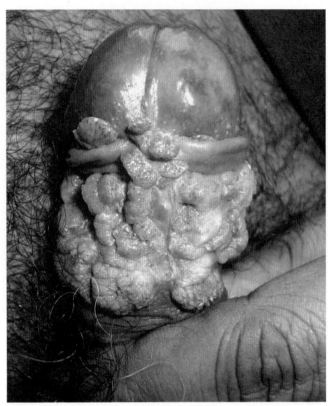

Condyloma acuminata in male.

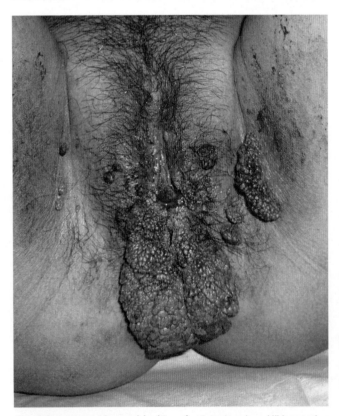

Condyloma acuminata: blocking the introitus in a HIV negative female.

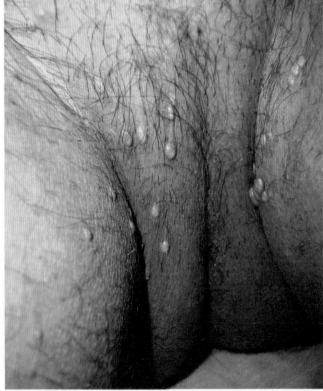

Umblicated pearly white papules of molluscum over inner thighs and perineum.

twice daily or valacyclovir 500 mg once daily for at least one year. In immunocompromised— acyclovir 400–800 mg twice daily. Or famciclovir 250 mg twice daily. Or valacyclovir 500 mg twice daily.

For neonates and HIV-coinfection: acyclovir 5 mg/kg, IV 8 hourly for 7–10 days.

GENITAL WARTS

Common, amongst sexually active population. Caused by human papilloma virus (HPV) particularly HPV 6 and HPV 11. Polymorphic. Several clinical types including papular, common wart, condyloma acuminata and plane wart. Condyloma acuminata term restricted to cauliflower-like warts on moist surfaces. Coronal sulcus, frenulum, prepucial inner surface or urethral meatus, perianal region. And vaginal wall and vulva generally affected. Giant condylomas during pregnancy may interfere with vaginal delivery. Giant and cervical condylomata may be coinfected with high risk HPVs (like 16, 18, 33, etc.), prone to malignant transformation. Common verruca vulgaris type present on the non-moist sites—shaft of penis, vulva.

Treatment

Imiquimod 5% cream treatment of choice. Applied overnight on every alternate day for a period of 12–16 weeks. Podophyllin 25% solution in benzoin tincture (more suitable for warts on moist partially keratinized areas), physician applied strictly to the lesion with the surrounding skin protected by petrolatum. Wash off after 2–4 hours; repeat once a week. Podophyllotoxin, a patient—applied alternative (currently not available in market). If no response in 4–6 weeks, treat with cryotherapy, electric cautery or carbon dioxide laser. Intralesional interferon therapy has variable efficacy. Other therapies include topical cidofovir, sinecatechins (green tea extract), topical trichloro/bichloroacetic acid, cryotherapy. Intralesional immunotherapy with Mw (new name *Mycobacterium indicus pranii*) vaccine quite effective. First dose is immunizing and given intradermally in shoulder, then 2 weekly intralesional injections given till resolution [usually after 3–4 intralesional (I/L) injections].

GENITAL MOLLUSCUM CONTAGIOSUM

Incubation period 2–3 months. By skin to skin contact during sex. Pearly white umblicated monomorphic papules involving pubic/inguinal area, inner thighs, vulva, scrotum (more than penis). May resolve spontaneously or get secondarily infected or eczematized. Treated by extirpation/ curettage, radiofrequency, chemical cautery (TCA/ BCA, silver nitrate), topical retinoic acid.

20

HIV Infection and Acquired Immunodeficiency Syndrome

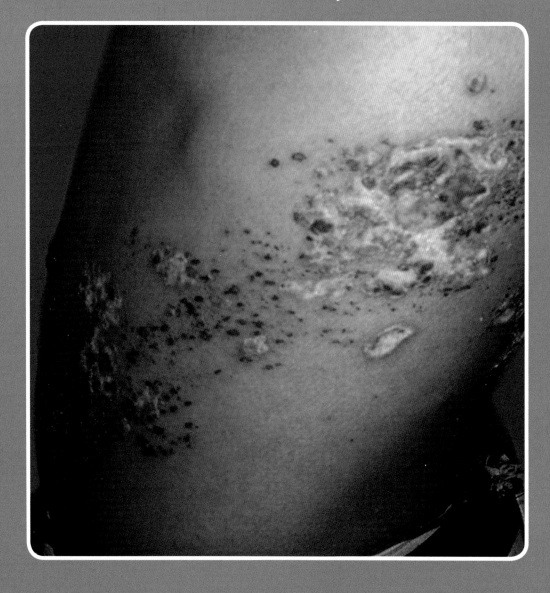

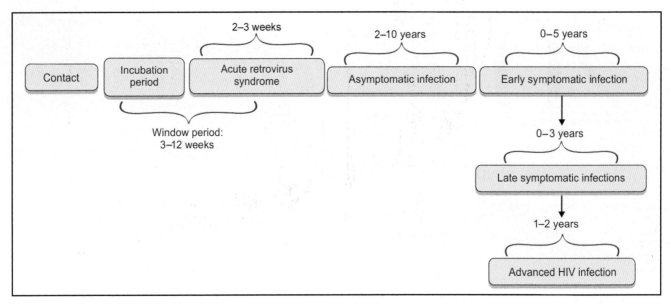

Course and stages of HIV infection.

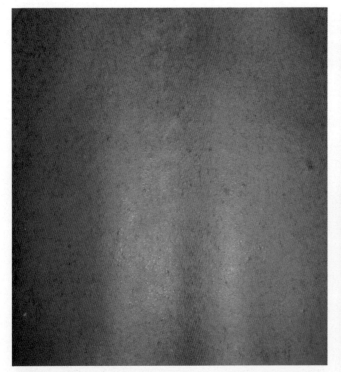

Rash of acute retroviral syndrome: a maculopapular rash is seen in 70% of patients, but is often disregarded.

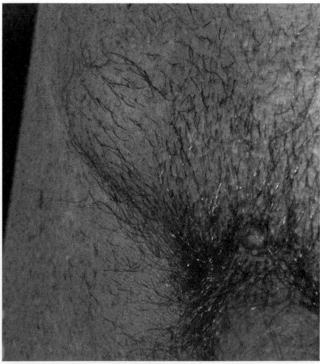

Persistent generalized lymphadenopathy in an HIV-positive patient: enlarged inguinal lymph nodes in a clinically otherwise asymptomatic but serologically HIV-positive patient.

Acquired immunodeficiency syndrome (AIDS) and human immunodeficiency virus (HIV) infection, a major global health problem.

EPIDEMIOLOGY

Geographic Distribution

- Globally, number of people living with HIV and AIDS (PLHA) variable.
- Prevalence of HIV/AIDS in high risk goups higher.

Number of PLHAs and prevalence of HIV infection		
	PLHA in millions	*Prevalence (%)*
Global[1]	34.0 (2011)	0.8
India[2]	2.08 (2011)	0.29

Prevalence of HIV/AIDS in high risk groups	
	Prevalence
Intravenous drug users (IDU)	9.2%
Males having sex with males (MSM)	7.4%
Commercial sex workers	4.9%
STI clinic attendees	2.5%
Antenatal clinic attendees	0.49%

Demographic Distribution

- Prevalence lower in women as compared to men, but susceptibility greater in women.
- Adults more frequently affected than children.

ETIOLOGY

Etiological Agent

Caused by HIV, a lymphotropic enveloped retrovirus.
- **Structure:** spherical, single-stranded, enveloped RNA virus, 120 nm in size. Consists of 2 parts:
  - *Outer envelope:* bilipid membrane; with HIV antigens (glycoproteins[3] gp 120 and gp 41) embedded.
  - *Inner core:*
    - Bounded by 2 layers of protein coat (outer layer of p17 and inner of p24).
    - Core of 2 strands of viral RNA and 3 important viral enzymes, reverse transcriptase (RT), integrase and protease.

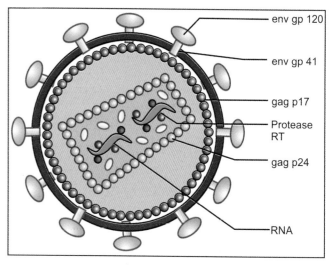

Structure of HIV.

- **Genes and proteins of HIV:**
  - *Major structural genes:*
    - Gag: coding for nuclear proteins p17 and p24
    - Pol: coding for reverse transcriptase (RT), protease and integrase.
    - Env: coding for envelope proteins gp120 and gp41.
  - *Regulatory genes:* rev, tat and nef, and other small accessory genes (vif, vpu, vpr) important for infection.
- **Types:** two types—HIV-1 and HIV-2 with several differences in epidemiology and manifestations.

Differences between HIV-1 and HIV-2		
	HIV-1	*HIV-2*
Prevalence	Higher	Lower
Incubation period	Shorter	Longer
Progression to AIDS	Higher, faster	Lower, slower
Natural history	Clearly defined	Not yet clear/may not have phase of acute retroviral syndrome
Lab diagnosis	Easily diagnosed	Difficult to diagnose
Response to ART	Commonly used drugs effective	Nucleoside molecules and few protease inhibitors virucidal

---

[1]**Globally:** Sub-Saharan Africa and Caribbean region most afflicted.

[2]**In India:** States with high prevalence—Maharashtra, Andhra Pradesh, Karnataka, Tamil Nadu and Manipur.

[3]**Glycoproteins:** Responsible for attachment of virus to CD4 receptors of host cells and subsequent fusion of virus envelope with host cell membrane.

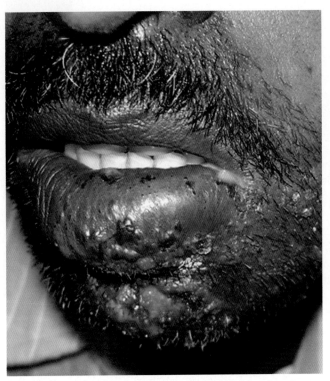

Herpes zoster in an HIV-positive patient: involvement of mandibular division of V cranial nerve. Zoster occurs when CD4+ count < 500/mm^3.

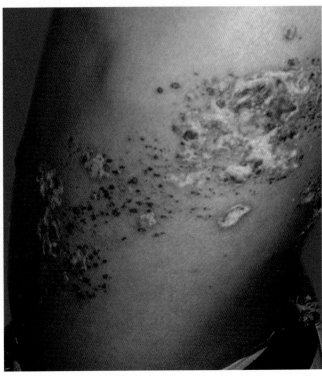

Herpes zoster in an HIV-positive patient: involvement of trunk in dermatomal pattern. Deeper ulcers with necrotic slough a clue to test for underlying HIV infection.

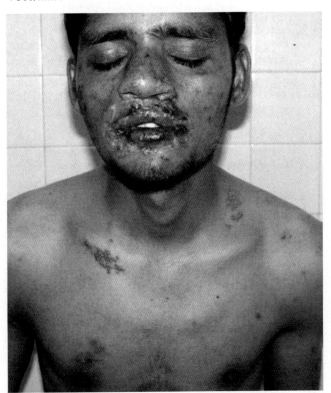

Herpes zoster in an HIV-positive patient: multidermatomal and bilateral involvement with dissemination. Such widespread distribution suggestive of HIV-positive state. Herpes zoster often seen in early symptomatic HIV infection.

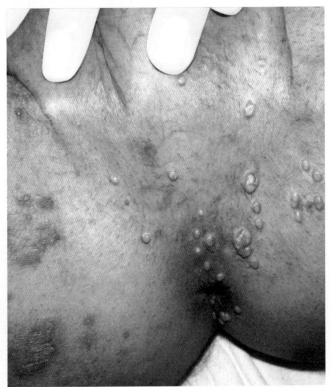

Molluscum contagiosum in an HIV-positive patient: multiple lesions, some large. Multiple lesions occur when CD4 counts < 250/mm^3.

- *HIV 1:* classified into a major or M group. And an outlier or O group. Group M consists of clades (subtypes) A to N. Different geographic distribution of subtypes: India: subtype C, along with subtypes A, B and E. Africa: subtypes A, C and D. Other parts of World: subtype B.
- *HIV 2:* HIV-2 less frequently encountered; initially identified in West Africa; now spread to many parts of Asia, including India.

Transmission

Humans main reservoir of HIV. Transmission from HIV infected person to uninfected person by several routes:

- **Sexual:** unprotected sexual intercourse:
  - *Heterosexual:* risk of transmission higher from female to male (0.5%) *vs* male to female (0.2%). In India, commonest (87.1%) mode of transmission.
  - *Homosexual:* in MSM (risk of transmission, 2%)
- **Vertical:** from HIV positive mother to child, antenatally, perinatally or postnatally (lactation). Risk of transmission 25%. Commonest mode of transmission in India, after hetrosexual exposure.
- **Transfusion:** from infected blood and blood products, transplantation of organ/tissue and through artificial insemination.
- **Use of contaminated needles:** mainly in intravenous drug users.
- **Nosocomial infection:** due to accidental needle stick injury or sharp instrument cuts from an HIV-positive patient. Rare, if universal precautions adopted.
- **No transmission through:** arthropod bites; fomites. Or by physical touch.

Pathogenesis

HIV Replication Cycle

HIV an enveloped retrovirus.[4]

- **Entry into target cells:** HIV capsid (along with HIV RNA and enzymes) enters target cell (CD4+ T cells and macrophages) by:
  - Binding of HIV surface glycoproteins to CD4 receptors on target cells.
  - Fusion of viral envelope with cell membrane of target cells.

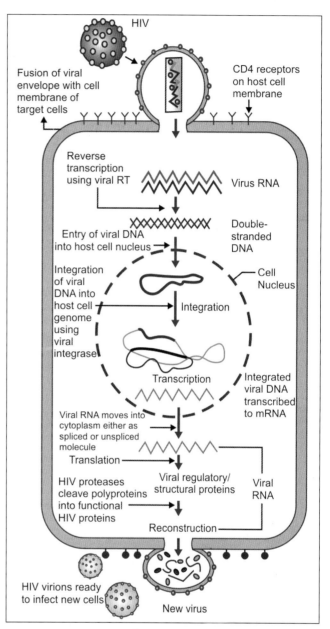

Replication of HIV.

- **Reverse transcription:** RT copies single-stranded RNA genome into a complementary DNA (cDNA) strand.[5] A sense DNA strand is created from this antisense cDNA to form double-stranded viral DNA, which is transported into host cell nucleus.
- **Integration into host cell genome:** on entering host cell nucleus, viral DNA integrated into host cell's genome (using viral enzyme integrase), a step inhibited by integrase inhibitors.

---

[4]**Retroviruses:** So named because of an unusual step in life cycle—synthesis of DNA from RNA template, using enzyme reverse transcriptase.
[5]**Process of reverse transcription:** Extremely error-prone, resulting in mutations—responsible for evasion from host's immune system as also development of drug resistance.

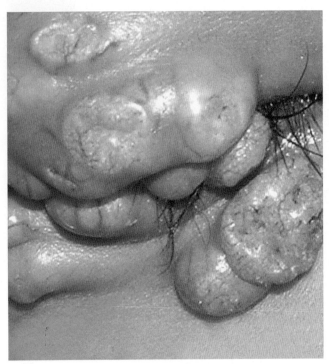

Molluscum contagiosum in an HIV-positive patient: giant, closely aggregated lesions on the face. Giant lesions surrogate marker of low CD4 count (< 50/mm³).

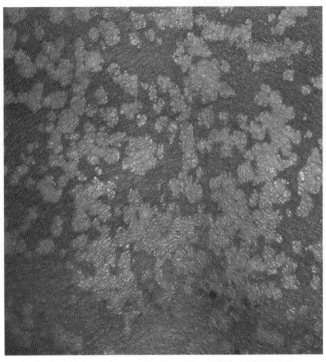

Human papilloma virus infection in an HIV-positive patient: extensive pityriasis versicolor-like lesions, similar to those seen in epidermodysplasia verruciformis.

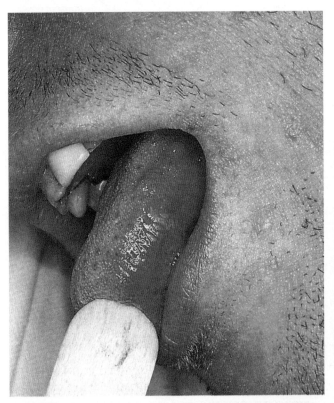

Oral hairy leukoplakia in an HIV-positive patient: due to *Epstein Barr virus*. Manifests as asymptomatic, white plaques with characteristic vertical corrugations on lateral aspect of tongue.

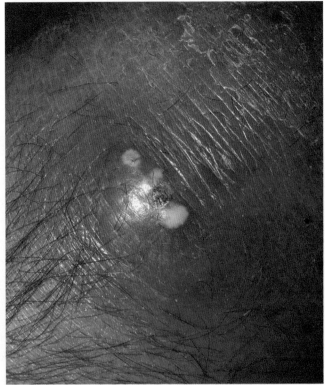

Pyogenic infections in an HIV-positive patient: cutaneous pyogenic (especially *Staphylococcus aureus*) infections common. Sometimes resistant to treatment.

- *Viral replication:* integrated viral DNA may lie dormant (in latent HIV infection). Or replicate (as infection progresses). During viral replication integrated DNA provirus transcribed into mRNA. May be spliced (into smaller pieces) or remain unspliced. Both move into cytoplasm → translated proteins.
  - Spliced viral RNA → translated into regulatory proteins Tat and Rev.
  - Unspliced RNA → translated into structural proteins Gag and Env which help in packaging of new virus particles.
- *Assembly and release:* occurs on plasma membrane of host cell.
  - Components of HIV move towards plasma membrane. And virion buds develop from host cell.
  - Maturation of virion occurs either in forming buds or in the immature virion after it buds off from the host cell.
  - During maturation, HIV proteases cleave polyproteins into individual functional HIV proteins (a step inhibited by protease inhibitors).
  - On maturation, virion able to infect another cell.

Host's Response

- Initially, though some virions are killed, HIV continues to multiply rapidly, infecting more CD4 cells. Antibodies against HIV absent (patient seronegative, albeit falsely) but highly infectious (window period).[6]
- After 3–12 weeks, patient mounts serological response and viral load decreases.
- Clinical manifestations depend on effects on immune system:
  - In early period of immune destruction, clinical latency, *i.e.* no clinical symptoms, but serological positivity, viral load low and CD4+ counts normal.
  - Later, as immunosuppression progresses, patient becomes symptomatic. Viral load increases and CD4+ count decreases.

CLINICAL MANIFESTATIONS

Course

- Primary HIV infection at the end of which acute retroviral syndrome occurs (indicating seroconversion) 2–4 weeks after infection→ 2–10 years of asymptomatic period → symptomatic phases (early, late and advanced) → death in 1–3 years (without ART).

Stages of Disease

- *Acute retroviral syndrome (ARS):*
  - *Incidence:* up to 50–90% develop ARS. Commoner if infection sexually acquired.

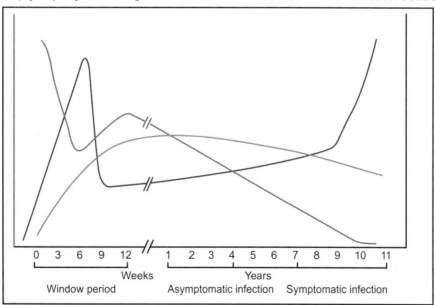

Relationship of HIV load (red), HIV antibodies (green) and CD4 counts (blue) as HIV infection progresses.

---

[6]**Window period:** Variable; shorter for transfusion acquired infection. Diagnosis of HIV infection during window period by detection of p24 antigen. Or using nucleic acid-based assays.

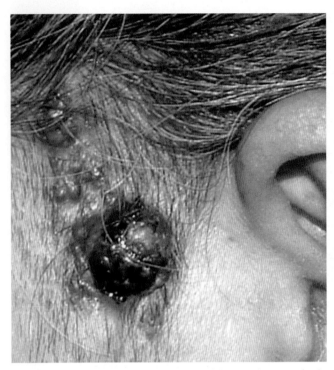

Bacillary angiomatosis in an HIV-positive patient: multiple (sometimes solitary) pyogenic granuloma-like nodules. Local lymphadenopathy frequent.

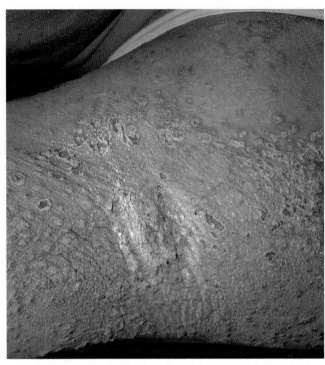

Candidiasis in an HIV-positive patient: most common cutaneous infection. Often severe, extensive and indicative of disease progression.

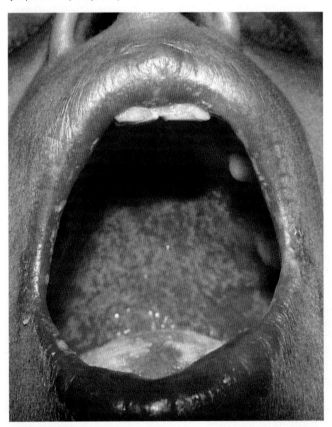

Oral candidiasis in an HIV-positive patient: extensive, recurrent oropharyngeal infections. Associated dysphagia a clue to esophageal involvement, an AIDS defining criteria.

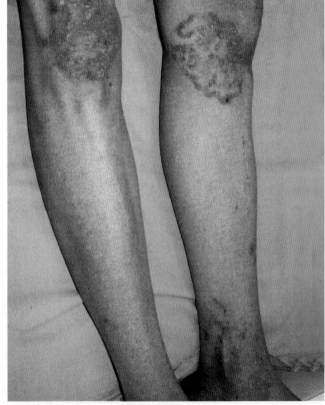

Dermatophyte infection in an HIV-positive patient: tinea corporis, multiple extensive, recurrent lesions.

➤ *Lasts:* 2–3 weeks.
➤ *Manifestations:*
  ▪ Fever, lymphadenopathy, pharyngitis, arthralgia, myalgia, neck stiffness.
  ▪ And in 70%, maculopapular rash and mucosal ulcers.
  ▪ Trunk, palms and soles.
➤ *Treatment:* antiretroviral treatment (ART) given during ARS may ? delay/abort progress to AIDS.

- *Asymptomatic HIV infection:* WHO clinical stage 1.
  ➤ *Incubation period:* 2–10 years.
  ➤ *Lasts:* 2–10 years.
  ➤ *Manifestation:* clinically asymptomatic. But persistent generalized lymphadenopathy often present.

- *Early symptomatic disease:* WHO clinical stage 2.
  ➤ *Lasts:* 0–5 years.
  ➤ *Manifestations:* moderate unexplained weight loss (< 10% of presumed or measured body weight), recurrent respiratory tract infections (sinusitis, tonsillitis, otitis media and pharyngitis). And cutaneous manifestations (herpes zoster, onychomycosis, angular cheilitis, recurrent oral ulcerations, seborrheic dermatitis).

- *Late symptomatic disease:* WHO clinical stage 3.
  ➤ *Lasts:* 0–3 years.
  ➤ *Manifestations:*
    ▪ Constitutional symptoms: progressive. Include unexplained severe weight loss (> 10% of presumed/measured body weight), unexplained chronic diarrhea (> 1 month) and unexplained persistent fever (> 1 month).
    ▪ Infections: persistent oral candidiasis, oral hairy leukoplakia, pulmonary tuberculosis, severe bacterial infections (pneumonia, empyema, pyomyositis, bone/joint infections, meningitis or bacteremia), acute necrotizing ulcerative stomatitis, gingivitis or periodontitis.
    ▪ Hematological manifestations: unexplained anemia (< 8 g/dL), neutropenia (< 0.5×10^9/L), chronic thrombocytopenia (< 50×10^9/L).

- *Advanced HIV:* WHO clinical stage 4.
  ➤ *Lasts:* 1–2 years.
  ➤ *Manifestations:*
    ▪ HIV wasting syndrome.
    ▪ *Infections:* AIDS defining opportunistic infections like *Pneumocystis* pneumoniae, recurrent bacterial pneumonia, chronic herpes simplex infection, *Cytomegalovirus* infection (retinitis or infection of other organs), esophageal candidiasis, extrapulmonary cryptococcosis (including meningitis), disseminated coccidioidomycosis and histoplasmosis, extrapulmonary tuberculosis, disseminated non-tuberculous mycobacterial infections chronic isosporiasis. And cryptosporidiosis, atypical leishmaniasis recurrent non-typhoidal *Salmonella* bacteremia.
    ▪ Neoplasms: Kaposi's sarcoma, lymphoma (cerebral or B-cell non-Hodgkin). Or other solid HIV-associated tumors.
    ▪ Symptomatic HIV-associated nephropathy. Or symptomatic HIV-associated cardiomyopathy. Or neurological changes like HIV encephalopathy, progressive multifocal leukoencephalopathy.

Cutaneous Manifestations

Skin involvement invariable in HIV-infected; generally not life-threatening. Often distinct helping in early recognition of disease and recognizing progression.

Infections

Viral infections

- *Herpes zoster:* initially normal course. Later, multidermatomal involvement, dissemination (involvement of > 3 contiguous dermatomes, > 20 lesions outside initial dermatome or systemic involvement) and hemorrhagic. Also severe postherpetic neuralgia. Always treat with antivirals.
- *Molluscum contagiosum:* initially typical presentation. Later atypical—larger (also giant), aggregated, progressive, persistent. Extragenital lesions (on face) of adult warrants ruling out HIV infection. Also excellent marker of HIV disease progression, number of lesions correlate inversely with CD4 cell count. Treatment response erratic often resistant to standard therapy. May respond to antiretroviral therapy (ART). Topical and systemic cidofovir helpful.

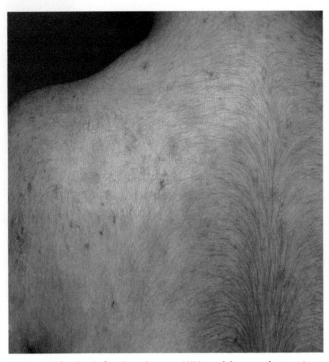

Dermatophytic infection in an HIV-positive patient: tinea incognito. Ill defined lesions with diffuse scaling. Diagnosis confirmed by potassium hydroxide mount which shows innumerable dermatophyte hyphae.

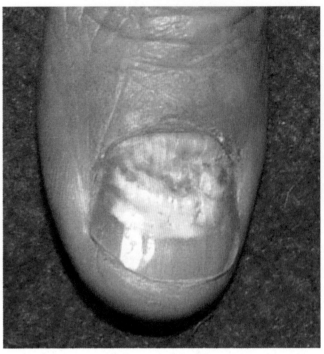

Onychomycosis in an HIV-positive patient: proximal subungual onychomycosis. Characterized by presence of whitish discoloration in proximal nail plate with only minimal thickening of nail. This type of onychomycosis typically present only in an HIV-positive patients.

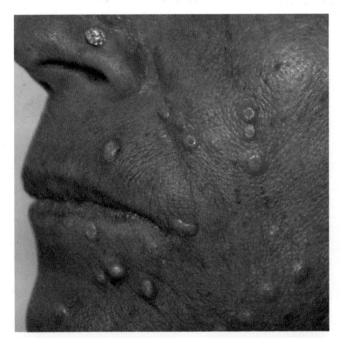

Cryptococcosis in an HIV-positive patient: multiple skin colored papules with umbilication, resembling molluscum contagiosum on the face. Confirmed on biopsy.

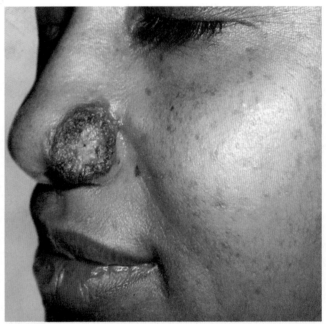

Histoplasmosis: well-defined erythematous scaly nodule which on biopsy revealed histoplasmosis.

- **Human papillomavirus:** normal presentation. Or warts extensive, numerous, exuberant. May present as a pityriasis versicolor—like eruption akin to epidermodysplasia verruciformis.

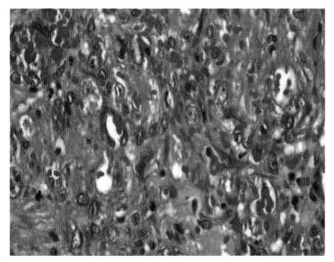

Histopathology of bacillary angiomatosis: *is a reactive vascular proliferation triggered by Bartonella henselae.* Histopathologically shows abundant vessels lined by plump endothelium with clear cytoplasm, mild atypia, and occasional mitotic figures and polymorphs in interstitium.

Greater oncogenic potential. Anogenital lesions exuberant. May contribute to causation of Bowen's disease, erythroplasia of Queyrat and bowenoid papulosis.

- **Oral hairy leukoplakia:** due to *Epstein Barr virus.* Asymptomatic white plaques with characteristic vertical corrugations. On lateral aspect of tongue. May occur even with CD4+ counts > 500/mm^3.

Bacterial infections

- **Pyogenic infections:** cutaneous and systemic pyogenic (especially *Staphylococcus aureus*) infections common. Sometimes resistant to treatment.
- **Tuberculosis:** (And ? leprosy) get reactivated.
- **Bacillary angiomatosis:** *Bartonella henselae* infection. Typical pyogenic granuloma-like papules and nodules. Or Kaposi's sarcoma-like

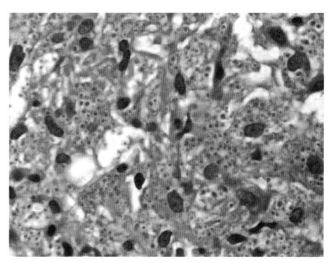

Histopathology of histoplasmosis: presence of intracytoplasmic budding yeast cells in macrophages.
Courtesy: Prof. M. Ramam, Department of Dermatology, AIIMS, New Delhi.

plaques. Occurs when CD4+ counts < 250 mm^3. Responds to erythromycin.

Fungal infections

- **Candidiasis:** most common cutaneous infection. Manifests in oropharynx, esophagus, bronchi, genitalia and nail folds. Severe and recurrent. Indicates progression of HIV disease. Esophageal candidiasis (when CD4 cell count < 100/μL), an AIDS-defining illness.

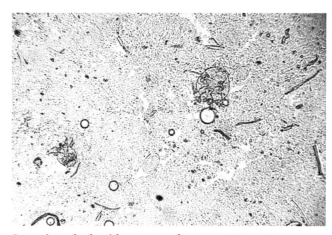

Potassium hydroxide mount: from an HIV-positive patient showing multiple mites.

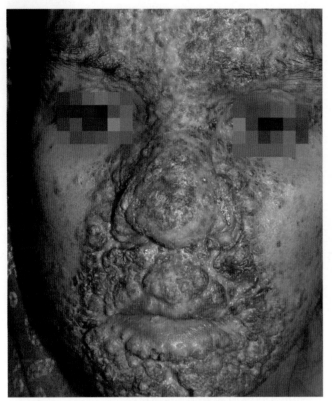

Histoplasmosis in an HIV-positive patient: multiple crusted nodules and plaques. Diagnosis often made histolopathologically.

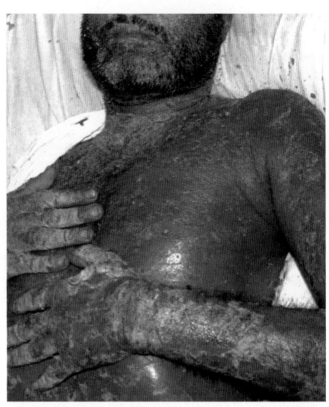

Scabies in an HIV-positive patient: may manifest as classic disease. Or as crusted (Norwegian) scabies presenting as hyperkeratotic, crusted plaques or as erythroderma. Often not diagnosed clinically.

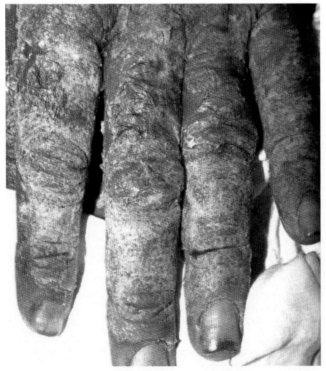

Crusted scabies in an HIV-positive patient: presenting as hyperkeratotic, crusted plaques. Often diagnosed on scraping or biopsy.

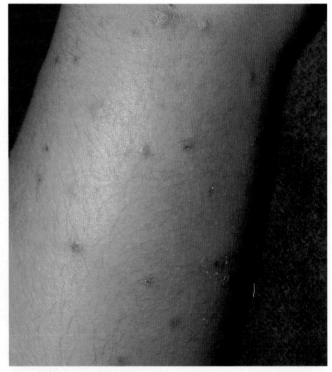

Insect bite hypersensitivity in an HIV-positive patient: excoriated papules on exposed parts-extremities and face. Presence of such lesions in adults warrants HIV testing.

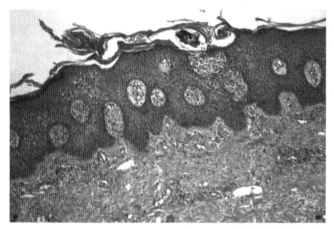

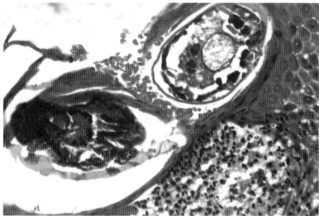

Histopathology of Norwegian scabies: histopathology reveals multiple mites in hyperkeratotic acanthotic epidermis and inflammation in dermis.

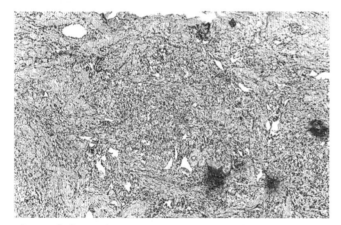

Histopathology of Kaposi's sarcoma: areas of sarcomatous fascicles intermingled with vascular channels.

- **Dermatophytic infections:** Very common. Usually typical lesions. Later chronic, recurrent, extensive. Or tinea incognito.[7]

---

[7]**Tinea incognito:** Does not have classical lesions.

- **Onychomycosis:** usually of proximal subungual type which occurs only in HIV-infected.
- **Deep fungal infections:** disseminated cryptococcosis, and histoplasmosis—develop with CD4 count 50–150/µL.
  - ➢ *Cryptococcosis:* usually presents as papules and nodules. Sometimes umbilicated molluscum contagiosum-like lesions.
  - ➢ *Histoplasmosis:* manifests as umbilicated skin colored, crusted papules and nodules usually on face. Or as cellulitis, panniculitis, palpable purpura and ulcers. Relapses common, even after adequate antifungal therapy.

Infestations

- **Leishmaniasis:** with progress of HIV disease, florid cutaneous or visceral leishamaniasis may develop. Relapses frequent.
- **Scabies:** in advanced HIV disease, pruritus subtle. Or severe. May present with classical disease. Or Norwegian (crusted) scabies or erythroderma. Diagnosed often on potassium hydroxide mount. Or on biopsy. Response to conventional therapy with permethrin/ivermectin adequate.
- **Insect bite hypersensitivity:** initially seasonal, later persistent; excoriated papules on exposed sites. Such lesions, especially if extensive and persistent and in adults warrant HIV testing.

Non-infectious Cutaneous Manifestations

Skin rashes

- Several types described in ARS.
- Also a manifestation of drug reaction, which are more frequent in HIV-infected.

Seborrheic dermatitis

- Most common cutaneous manifestation in HIV infected.
- May be mild-moderate. Or florid and extensive with intense erythema, thick scales and involving unusual sites. And extensive.
- Responds to antiretroviral therapy.

Eosinophilic folliculitis

- In spectrum of pruritic papular eruption of HIV disease.
- Etiology unknown. Seen with low CD4 counts.
- Severely itchy, chronic follicular papules and pustules.

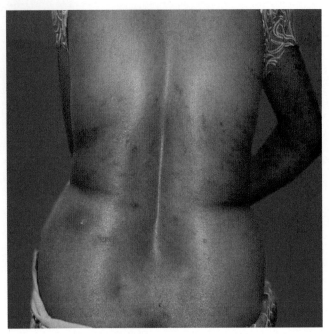

Insect bite hypersensitivity: exposed area on waist involved with excoriated erythematous papules with sparing of area covered by garments. Lesions may be persistent and extensive.

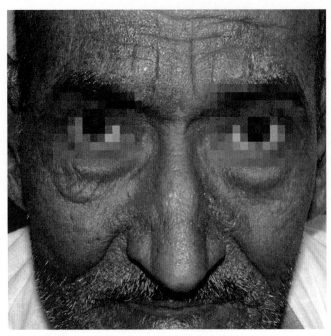

Seborrheic dermatitis in an HIV-positive patient: erythematous plaques with greasy scales on the eyebrows and nasolabial folds. Sudden onset of extensive lesions in elderly warrants ruling out underlying HIV infection.

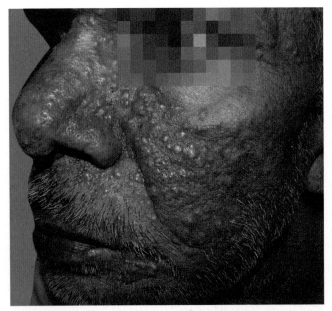

Eosinophilic folliculitis in an HIV-positive patient: severely itchy, chronic follicular papules and pustules on the face. Eosinophilic folliculitis in the spectrum of pruritic papular eruption of HIV disease.

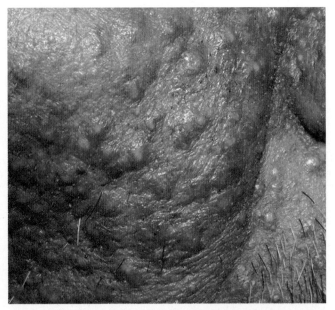

Eosinophilic folliculitis in an HIV-positive patient: severely itchy, chronic follicular papules and pustules in neck, upper trunk and face. Treated with topical steroids and phototherapy.

- Upper trunk, head and neck.
- Responds to topical steroids and phototherapy.

Psoriasis

- Can present as extensive lesions. Or as atypical lesions.
- Difficult to treat. May need oral retinoids/phototherapy (methotrexate avoided as immunosuppressive).

Reiter's syndrome

- Post chlamydial or salmonella infections
- Mucocutaneous lesions: rupioid/pustular lesions, keratoderma blenorrhagicum, circinate balanitis, oral lesions.
- Extracutaneous lesions: severe, often mutilating sacroiliitis and lower limb arthritis. And eye involvement.
- Often resistant to treatment.

Kaposi's sarcoma

- Probably due to human herpes virus 8 which is sexually cotransmitted; most frequently seen in HIV infection acquired homosexually.
- Single or multiple. Asymptomatic brown to dusky red-purple macules or plaques. On ankles and shins, face, trunk and mucosae involved.
- Treatment includes radiofrequency desiccation, mechanical curettage, excision, interferon therapy, radiotherapy and chemotherapy.

Others

Xerosis and acquired ichthyosis common. Long eyelashes (trichomegaly) and photosensitivity reported.

HIV and STIs

Effect of STIs on HIV

- **STIs associated with genital ulcerations:** amplified transmission of HIV 10-fold, due to epithelial breach, concentration of inflammatory cells (like CD4 cells which are target cells for HIV) in genital mucosa.
- **STIs associated with discharges:** amplified transmission of HIV 4-fold due to microfissures in epithelium, concentration of inflammatory cells (like CD4 cells which are target cells for HIV) in genital mucosa.

Effect of HIV on STIs

- **Syphilis:**
  - Usually manifestation and course of syphilis in HIV unaltered, especially if no immune depletion. So also serological and therapeutic response.
  - Less frequently atypical presentation. Include:
    - Chancre: slow healing of chancre, multiple chancres, phagedenic lesions and large painful ulcers.
    - Secondary syphilis: lues maligna.
    - Neurosyphilis: rapid progress to neurosyphilis even in secondary stage. More frequent occurrence.
    - Serology: aberrant response. So other tests (dark ground microscopy, biopsy) needed.
- **Chancroid:** in early HIV infection course similar. With immunosuppression atypical features seen:
  - Atypical ulcers: more in number, larger, extragenital lesions.
  - Reduced response of chancroid to therapy, so single dose regimens avoided.
- **Lymphogranuloma venereum:** no effect generally noted.
- **Donovanosis:** in early HIV-infection course similar. Treatment regimens same as in non-HIV individual. But treatment failure and slower response. Then consider adding parenteral aminoglycosides.
- **Genital herpes:**
  - In early HIV infection, course similar. Later, prolonged and severe episodes of genital, perianal or oral herpes. Chronic non-healing ulcers, lasting more than a month and with herpetiform margins in perianal area characteristic of GH in HIV infected.
  - Lesions atypical—verrucous plaques, chronic non healing ulcers, pseudogranulomatous herpes.
  - Increased asymptomatic shedding.
- **Anogenital warts (AGW):**
  - AGW more frequent in HIV-positive.
  - More numerous lesions, extensive involvement and larger nodules. Also multiple clinical types.
  - Higher prevalance of carcinoma *in situ* in cervix, vulva and anal canal. So regular monitoring of these areas.

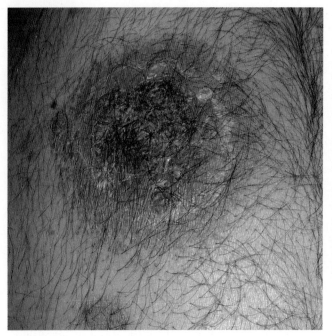

Psoriasis in an HIV-positive patient: can present as extensive lesions. Or as atypical lesions with intense erythema.

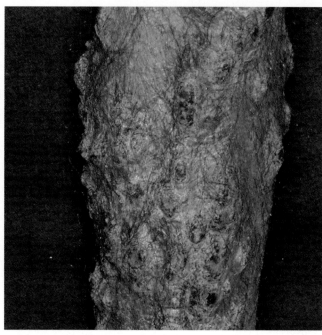

Reiter's syndrome in an HIV-positive patient: hyperkeratotic lesions some conical resembling a limpet-the so called rupioid lesions. Many of have a central cupping, similar to an oyster shell.

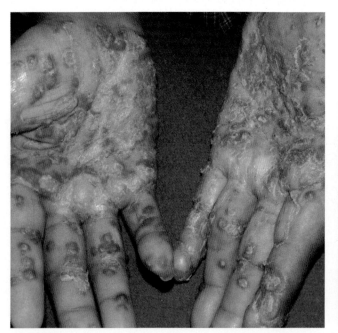

Keratoderma blenorrhagicum in an HIV-positive patient: erythematous hyperkeratotic plaques on palms (and soles).

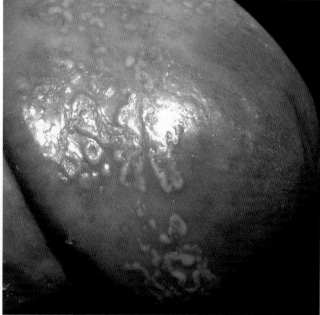

Circinate balanitis in an HIV-positive patient: moist annular plaques with serpiginous margin.

Diagnosis of HIV infection	
Serological tests	*Virological tests*

• Screening tests:
  – ELISA
  – EIA
• Supplemental:
  – Western blot
  – Immunofluorescence
  – Line immunoassay
	• Viral RNA
	• p24 antigen
	• Viral culture

Laboratory tests for diagnosis of HIV infected patients in different clinical stages				
Clinical stage	*HIV serology*	*P24 antigen assay*	*PCR*	*Plasma viral load*
Window period	–	–/+	+	++
Asymptomatic HIV infection	+	–/+	+	–/+
Early and late symptomatic infection	+	+	+	+
Advanced HIV	+	++	+	+++

➤ More resistant to treatment. And more recurrences.
- *Molluscum contagiosum:*
  ➤ MC more frequent and numerous in HIV.
  ➤ Atypical lesions—giant lesions, verrucous indurated plaques.
  ➤ Resistance to conventional therapy. Response improves once ART started.
- *Candidal genital tract infection:*
  ➤ Increased prevalence.
    ▪ Also of non-albicans candidal infection.
    ▪ Increased severity and extent.

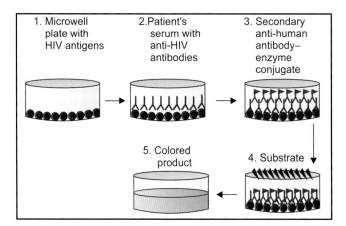

Principle of EIA.

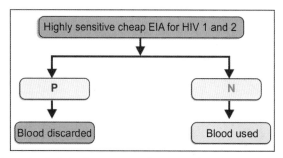

HIV serological testing strategy for screening donors.

- Fluconazole prophylaxis often recommended. But sometimes resistant to treatment.
- *Non-gonococcal genital tract infections:* probably no alteration.
- *Bacterial vaginosis:* clinical presentation of bacterial vaginosis in HIV negative and positive patients probably similar.
- *T. vaginalis:* probably no change.

DIAGNOSIS

Tests for Diagnosis of HIV Infection

Several tests available. And different tests used for different stages due to varying senstivity.
- *Serological tests:* tests to detect antibodies against HIV.
- *Virological tests:* tests to detect components of HIV.

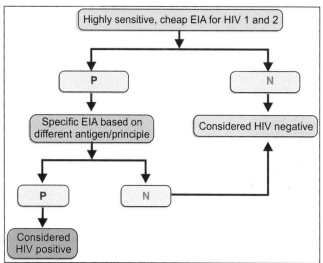

HIV serological testing strategy for diagnosis of HIV for serosurveillance.

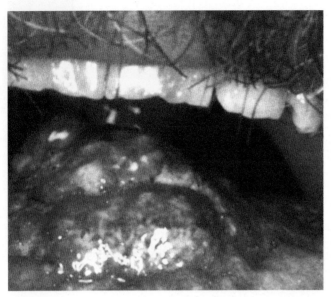

Kaposi's sarcoma in an HIV-positive patient: intraoral lesion manifesting as single dusky erythematous-violaceus plaques. Other sites of predilection include ankles, shins, face and trunk.

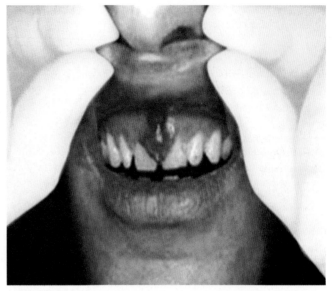

Kaposi's sarcoma in an HIV-positive patient: manifests as a dusky violaceus plaques. Kaposi's sarcoma in HIV-infected can occur both with CD4 counts > 300/mm³ (with a longer median survival) and also in advanced HIV infection (with a shorter median survival). May respond to HAART. Or may need treatment with cryotherapy (if few lesions) or radiotherapy/chemotherapy if extensive.

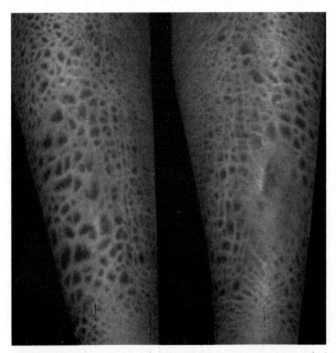

Acquired ichthyosis in an HIV-positive patient: lesions of acquired ichthyosis resemble ichthyosis vulgaris. Appearance of ichthyosis in later life warrants search for an underlying disease including an HIV infection. Ichthyosis in HIV-infected generally occurs in advanced HIV infection.

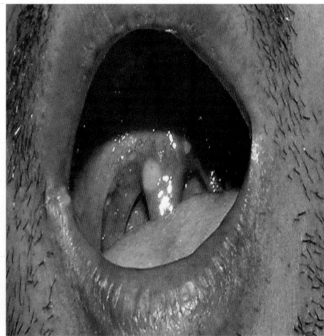

Oral aphthae: ulcers with central necrotic slough and halo of erythema. Occur when CD4+ count < 100/mm³.

Serological Tests

Two types of serological tests for HIV infection:
- Screening tests.
- Supplemental test.

Screening tests

- *Features:* rapid, inexpensive. Highly sensitive, may not be very specific (i.e. false positives

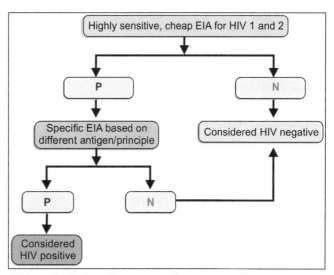

HIV serological testing strategy for serosurveillance.

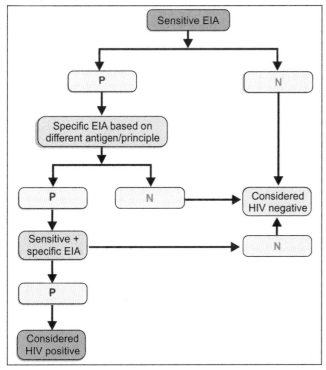

HIV serological testing strategy for diagnosis of HIV infection in asymptomatic patients.

occur), so are presumptive and not confirmatory tests.
- *Types:* of 2 types:
  - *Lab-based tests:* include ELISA or EIA. Are the most frequently used tests.
  - *Point of care tests:* available at point of contact of physician and patient. Most use color change (immunochromatographic assays) or particle agglutination. Some do not require blood samples as can be done on saliva (oraquick and orasure) or urine.
- *Indications and interpretation of screening tests:*
  - *Screening donors:*

- Is unlinked, anonymous sampling, without pretest counseling because patient not informed about HIV status.
- Uses single, highly sensitive, reliable, cheap enzyme immunoassay (EIA) for HIV-1 and HIV-2.
- Positive samples discarded; negative samples used.
  - *Serosurveillance:* epidemiologically for sentinel serosurveillance:
    - Is unlinked, anonymous sampling, so pretest counseling not needed.
    - Samples tested 1st with highly sensitive, reliable, cheap EIA for HIV-1 and HIV-2.
    - Positive samples need confirmation by a specific EIA based on another antigen; negative samples considered negative.
  - *Diagnosis of HIV infection:* pretest counseling mandatory. And strategy used depends on whether patient is asymptomatic or symptomatic.
    - If asymptomatic: samples 1st tested with sensitive EIA; if positive→ Repeat tested with 2nd specific EIA (based on a different antigen or principle). If positive, further confirmed with 3rd (both specific and sensitive) EIA. Negative samples from 2nd test considered negative.
    - If symptomatic: samples 1st tested with highly sensitive, reliable, cheap EIA for HIV-1 and HIV-2. Positive samples need confirmation by a specific EIA based on another antigen; negative samples considered negative.

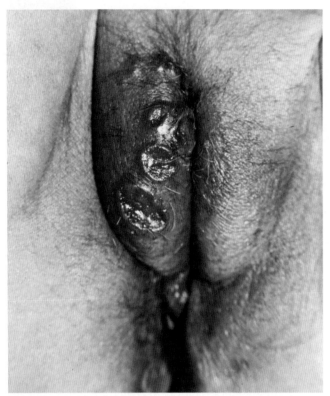

Syphilis in an HIV-positive patient: multiple chancres. Many raised indurated ulcers with regular margins and clean base.

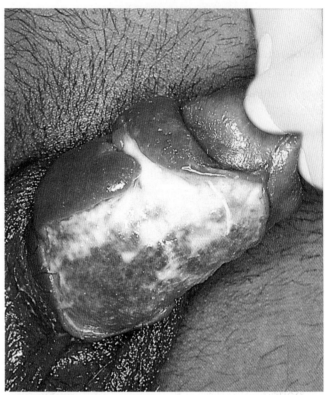

Chancroid in an HIV-positive patient: phagedenic variant: most of the shaft of penis involved.

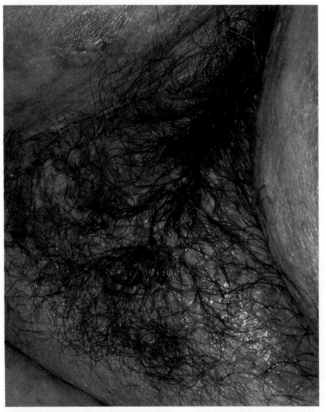

Genital herpes in an HIV-positive patient: extensive polycyclic lesions extending from genital area onto lower abdomen.

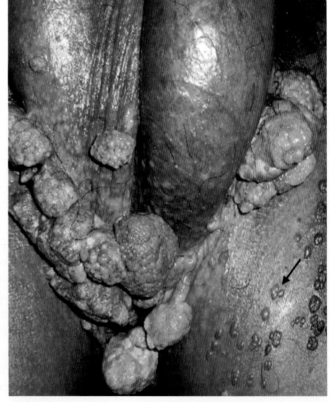

Anogenital warts in an HIV-positive patient: large lesions of condyloma acuminata and smaller lesions of bowenoid papulosis (marked).

Supplemental tests

- Done to validate the positive tests of screening.
- Two types available:
  - Western blot (WB) assay.
  - Immunofluorescence test.
- Are expensive (Western blot) and difficult to interpret (both). So replaced by combination of 2 or > EIAs (using different principles/antigens, one highly sensitive, 2nd highly specific) now used instead of ELISA-WB combination as more reliable and less expensive.

Virological Tests

Confirmatory tests, as detect HIV antigens. So positive even in window period in seronegative patients. And confirm presence of virus in a seropositive (or serologically equivocal) patient.

Detection of viral RNA

- 1st test to become positive, so short window period (median 17 days). Expensive and resource intensive.
- Uses polymerase chain reaction (PCR). And real time PCR. Can be used to determine viral load (expressed as number of RNA copies/mL).

Detection of HIV specific core antigen (p24)

- Useful in:
  - Window period: p24 detectable earlier than seropositivity in 30% of patients.
  - Diagnosis of HIV infection in newborn: Because just presence of antibodies in new-born often due to transplacental transfer of maternal antibodies.
  - Detection of HIV in CSF.

- Test sometimes falsely negative, if antigen complexed with p24 antibody; overcome by preliminary acid hydrolysis of serum sample.

Viral Culture

- Not routinely done as resource intensive and not safe. And takes 4–8 weeks for reporting.
- But is 100% specific. And sensitivity depends on stage of infection.

Other Tests

- **Tests to monitor progress of HIV infection:**
  - Viral load.
  - CD4 counts.
- **Tests to rule out:**
  - Opportunistic infections.
  - Development of neoplasia.
- **Tests to monitor side effects of drugs:** since drugs often toxic base line and follow-up hematological and biochemical tests needed.

Treatment

Treatment encompasses counseling (always and repeatedly), prescribing (often providing) antiretroviral treatment (ART) when indicated, and managing complications including opportunistic infections and neoplasia.

Counseling

- In HIV and AIDS counseling a core element of holistic management.
- **Objectives:** 2 objectives
  - Prevention of HIV transmission: spread of HIV hugely curtailed by behavior change—safe

Classification of ART						
NRTI	NtRTI	NNRTI	Protease inhibitor	Fusion inhibitor	Integrase inhibitor	CCR-5 inhibitor
Zidovudine (AZT)*	Tenofovir (TDF)*	Nevirapine (NVP)*	Indinavir (INV)*	Enfuvirtide (T-20)	Raltegravir	Maraviroc
Didanosine (ddI)*		Efavirenz (EFV)*	Ritonavir (RTV)*			
Zalcitabine (ddC)*		Delaviridine (DLV)	Saquinavir (SQV)*			
Stavudine (d4T)*		Etravirine	Nelfinavir (NFV)*			
Lamivudine (3TC)*			Lopinavir (LPV)*			
Abacavir (ABC)*			Atazanavir (ATV)*			
Emtricitabine (FTC)			Darunavir			
*Available in developing countries						

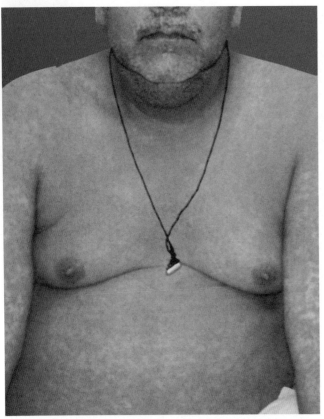

Morbilliform eruption: generalized erythematous, maculopapular eruption due to nevirapine. Similar rash can develop with abacavir.

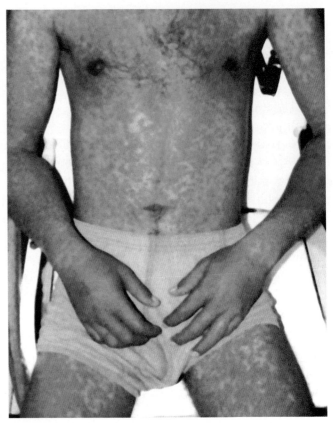

Drug hypersensitivity reaction: generalized erythematous maculopapular eruption with peripheral edema due to nevirapine. Abacavir can also cause similar reactions.

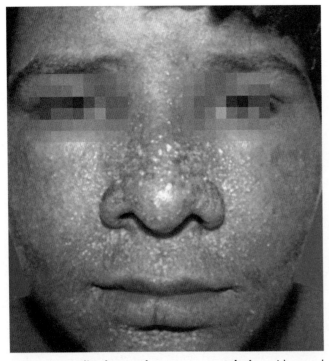

Acute generalized exanthematous pustulosis: widespread eruption of sterile pustules due to nelfinavir.

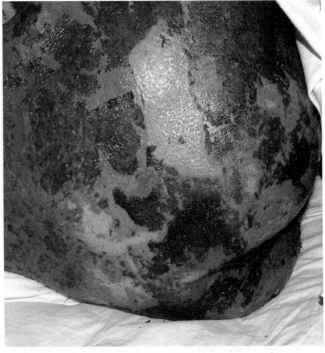

Toxic epidermal necrolysis: large areas of sheets of dusky red skin which denude to reveal erosions. Due to nevirapine can also develop with abacavir.

sexual practices including consistent and correct use of condoms, avoiding casual sex and intravenous drug use.

> *Supporting of those afflicted directly and indirectly by HIV:*

● **Types:**

> *Pre-test counseling:* involves providing basic information on HIV/AIDS. And risk assessment of those being HIV tested.

> *Post-test counseling:* depends on result:

▪ If negative: basic knowledge on HIV reiterated to assist client to adopt behaviors that reduce future risk of getting infected. A repeat test is recommended after 12 weeks.

▪ If positive test: client assisted to cope with result. And helped to access treatment and care. And supported to disclose HIV status to partner.

NACO 2007 guidelines for starting ART (modified by 2011 memorandum)		
Clinical scenario (WHO clinical stage)	CD4 test not available	CD4 test available
Asymptomatic (1)	Do not treat	Treat if CD4 < 350 cells/mm^3
Mild symptoms (2)	Do not treat	
Advanced symptoms (3)	Treat	Treat irrespective of CD4 count
Severe/advanced symptoms (4)	Treat	

▪ Follow-up counseling: to re-emphasize adoption of safe behaviors to prevent transmission of HIV infection. And assists in establishing linkages and referrals to services for care and support including ART, nutrition, home-based care and legal support.

WHO 2013 guidelines for starting ART in HIV-positive patients	
Population	Recommendation
Adults and adolescents (≥ 10 years)	**Initiate ART if CD4 cell count ≤500 cells/mm^3** • As a priority, initiate ART in all individuals with severe/advanced HIV disease (WHO clinical stage 3 or 4) or CD4 count ≤350 cells/mm^3 **Initiate ART regardless of WHO clinical stage or CD4 cell count** • Active TB disease • HBV coinfection with severe chronic liver disease • Pregnant and breastfeeding women with HIV • HIV-positive individual in a serodiscordant partnership (to reduce HIV transmission risk)
Children ≥5 years old	**Initiate ART if CD4 cell count ≤500 cells/mm^3** • As a priority, initiate ART in all children with severe/advanced HIV disease (WHO clinical stage 3 or 4) or CD4 count ≥350 cells/mm^3 **Initiate ART regardless of CD4 cell count** • WHO clinical stage 3 or 4 • Active TB disease
Children 1–5 years old	**Initiate ART in all regardless of WHO clinical stage or CD4 cell count** • As a priority, initiate ART in all HIV-infected children 1–2 years old or with severe/advanced HIV disease (WHO clinical stage 3 or 4) or with CD4 count ≤750 cells/mm^3 or <25%, whichever is lower
Infant <1 years old	Initial ART in all infants regardless of WHO clinical stage or CD4 cell count

WHO 2013 ART guidelines; Source: *apps.who.int/iris/bitstream/10665/85321/1/9789241505727_eng.pdf*

Which antiretroviral therapy to start when		
Target population	WHO, 2013 guidelines	NACO, 2007 guidelines
HIV + ARV-naive adults and adolescents	TDF + 3TC (or FTC) + EFV	3TC + AZT/ d4T + NVP/EFV
HIV + pregnant women	TDF + 3TC (or FTC) + EFV	AZT + 3TC + NVP
HIV/TB coinfection	TDF + 3TC (or FTC) + EFV	AZT/D4T+ 3TC+EFV/NVP
HIV/HBV coinfection	TDF + 3TC (or FTC) + EFV	AZT/+ 3TC+EFV/NVP

Abbreviations: 3TC: lamivudine; ARV: antiretroviral (drug); AZT: zidovudine; d4t: stavudine; EFV: efavirenz; FTC: emtricitabine; NVP: nevirapine; TDF: tenofovir disoproxil fumarate

Antiretroviral Therapy

Antiretroviral Drugs

● **Objective of therapy:** antiretroviral treatment (ART) suppresses disease, does not eradicate virus. So reduces morbidity and mortality but does not cure.

● **Classification:** ART broadly classified by phase of retrovirus life-cycle inhibited:

> *Reverse transcriptase inhibitors:*

▪ Nucleoside reverse transcriptase inhibitors (NRTI): compete with natural deoxynucleotides[8] for incorporation into viral DNA

[8]**NRTIs:** Are analogs of naturally occurring deoxynucleotides which are needed to synthesize HIV DNA.

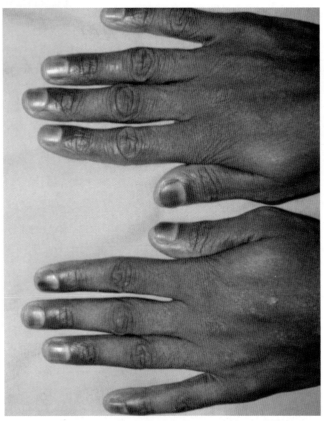

Nail pigmentation: bluish-black nail pigmentation due to zidovudine. Pigmentation of nail may appear as early as 1 month after inititation of zidovudine.

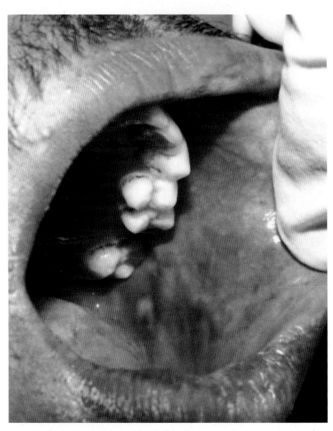

Mucosal pigmentation: bluish-black mucosal pigmentation due to zidovudine. Zidovudine typically causes pigmentation of lateral aspect of tongue.

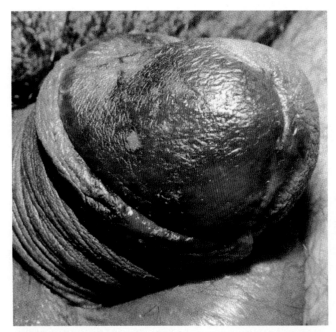

Fixed drug eruption on glans: well-defined erythematous plaque on the glans which developed after taking cotrimaxozole for prophylaxis for pneumocytis pneumonia.

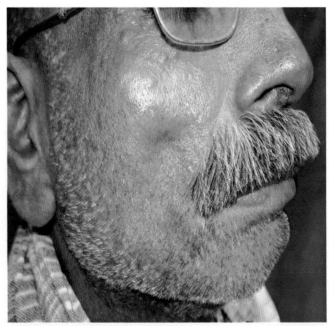

Facial lipoatrophy: irreversible loss of subcutaneous fat began 6 months after starting therapy with zidovudine (also seen with stavudine).

chain but form defective DNA which cannot extend DNA chain resulting in chain termination.

- Nucleotide reverse transcriptase inhibitors (NtRTI): act as NRTI.
- Non-nucleoside reverse transcriptase inhibitors (NNRTI): act as non-competitive inhibitors of reverse transcriptase (by binding to it).
  - ➢ *Protease inhibitors (PI):* inhibit protease which cleaves polyproteins for final assembly of new HIV virions.
  - ➢ *Fusion inhibitors (FI):* prevents fusion of viral envelope with cell membrane of target cells.
  - ➢ *Integrase inhibitors (II):* inhibit enzyme integrase, which integrates HIV DNA into infected cell DNA.
- **Side effects:** several side effects described with ART. Common ones include:
  - ➢ *Zidovudine (AZT):* anemia, (hemoglobin monitoring recommended) and lipoatrophy.
  - ➢ *Stavudine (d4T):* peripheral neuropathy, lipodystrophy, dyslipidemia lactic acidosis.
  - ➢ *Lamivudine (3TC):* relatively safe, but drug most prone to HIV developing resistance.
  - ➢ *Tenofovir* (TDF): nephropathy (so renal function monitoring).
  - ➢ *Nevirapine (NVP):* drug eruptions (maculopapular eruptions, Steven-Johnson syndrome-toxic epidermal necrolysis), hepatotoxicity.
  - ➢ *Efavirenz (EFV):* gastrointestinal side effects, hepatotoxicity, nephrotoxicity.? Safety in pregnancy.
  - ➢ *Abacavir (ABC):* severe hypersensitivity reaction not uncommon.
  - ➢ *Protease inhibitors:* dyslipidemia (high total and LDL cholestrol, decreased HDL cholestrol and elevated triglycerides).

Indications

ART to be initiated only if indicated, not only on basis of presence of HIV infection.

Drug Regimens

- ART given as Highly Active Antiretroviral Therapy (HAART), a combination of 3 drugs:

Monitoring of HAART

Real challenge to monitor efficacy of ART because of immunological and virological discordancy. And to diagnose resistance to initiate. 2nd line therapy.
- **Viral load estimation.**
  - ➢ Most sensitive marker of efficacy. But resource intensive.
  - ➢ Recommended to measure every 3–6 months.
  - ➢ Expressed as RNA copies.
- **Surrogate markers:** used individually or in combination but poorly sensitive.
  - ➢ Clinical improvement.
  - ➢ CD4 counts.

Drugs for Opportunistic Infections

Various regimens recommended for prophylaxis and therapy of opportunistic infections.

Management of opportunistic infections in HIV patients			
	Treatment (daily)	Prophylaxis	
Infections		Indications	Drug regimen (daily)
Pneumocystis jiroveci	TMP (15 mg/kg) + SMZ* (75 mg/kg) × 3 weeks	CD4+ < 200/mm³	TMP (2.5 mg/kg) + SMZ (12.5 mg/kg)
Toxoplasma encephalitis	Sulfadiazine (4–8 g) + Pyrimethamine (200–400 mg) × 6 weeks	Toxoplasma seropositive CD4+ < 100/mm³	Sulfadiazine (2-4 g) + Pyrimethamine (100 mg)
Herpes simplex virus	Acyclovir 400 mg × 5 times × 2 weeks	> 6 recurrences/year	Acyclovir 400 mg bid
Herpes zoster	Acyclovir 800 mg × 5 times × 2 weeks		
M. tuberculosis	Standard therapy. Look for MDR tuberculosis. ATT initiated before HAART		
Candidiasis	Fluconazole 100–200 mg daily × 3 weeks		Fluconazole 150 mg weekly

*TMP-SMZ: trimethoprim-sulfamethoxazole

21

Miscellaneous and Rare Dermatoses

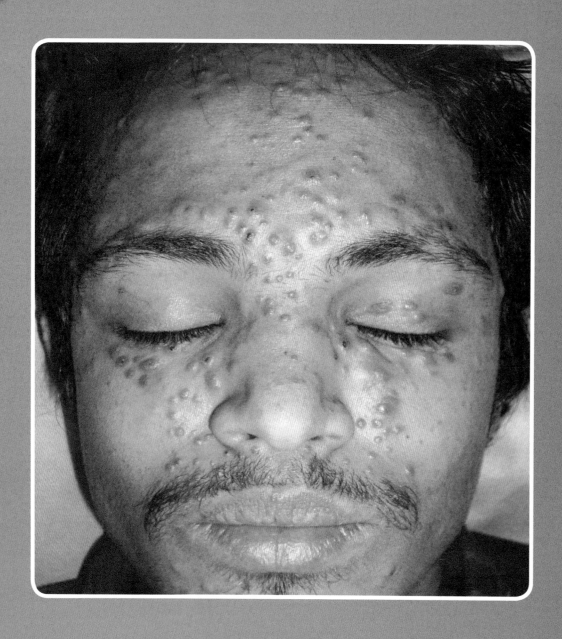

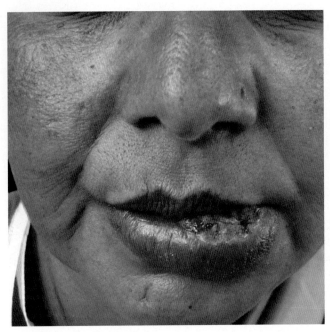

Orofacial granulomatosis: asymmetric thickening of the lower lip with ulceration over its inner aspect.

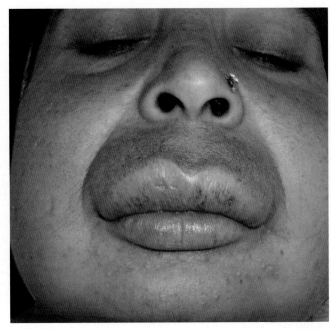

Orofacial granulomatosis: massive upper lip swelling, mild lower lip swelling and diffuse indurated swelling over lower face.

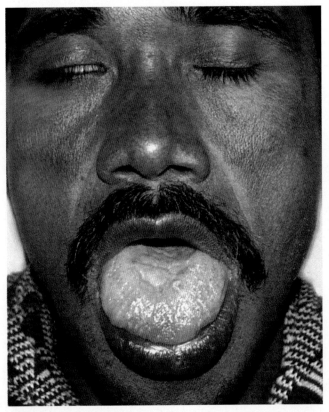

Melkersson Rosenthal syndrome: triad of facial palsy (right side), furrowed tongue and labial swelling.

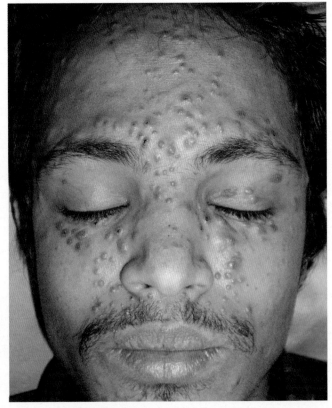

Lupus miliaris disseminatus faciei: inflammatory papules and nodules in centrofacial distribution. Prominent eyelid lesions.

GRANULOMATOUS DISORDERS

Orofacial Granulomatosus

Persistent or recurrent lip swelling, oral ulcers and other oral mucosal findings, in the absence of identifiable cause. Uncertain etiology. May be an early presentation of known entities. Thought of as variant of mucosal Crohn's or sarcoidosis.

Clinical Manifestations

Persistent or recurrent lip swelling, oral ulcers, gingival hyperplasia, facial swelling, facial nerve palsy, fissured tongue, etc. May present with a combination of one or more features. Isolated upper lip swelling referred to as granulomatous cheilitis. Association with GIT Crohn's uncertain. Melkersson Rosenthal syndrome is a triad of oro-facial edema, facial nerve palsy and furrowed tongue. Orofacial edema: lips-diffuse, doughy swelling. Facial nerve palsy, unilateral/bilateral, partial/complete, lower motor neuron type. May develop before, after or simultaneously with lip swelling.

Diagnosis

Work up to rule out Crohn's disease of GI tract and sarcoidosis. Confirmation comes from histopathology. It shows some chronic inflammation and non-caseating granulomas.

Treatment

None proven completely effective. Based on literature, topical or systemic glucocorticoids, oral clofazimine, thalidomide and azathioprine have been tried.

Lupus Miliaris Disseminatus Faciei (Acne Agminata)

Etiology unknown. Not a tuberculide. Unclassified. Variant of granulomatous rosacea. Or termed FIGURE (facial idiopathic granulomas with regressive evolution). Common in Asians; young adults. Copper or yellow-brown papules, inflammatory nodules; sometimes pustules may be seen. Commonly on face—cheeks, nose, eyelids, ear rim, forehead, chin. Neck may be involved.

Latter site seems to have nodular/cystic lesions more commonly. Rarely in axillae. May show apple-jelly nodules on diascopy. Resolve spontaneously in 1–3 years, residual pitted scarring. Centrofacial distribution.

Histopathology

Granulomas with caseation. Sometimes oriented around follicles.

Treatment

Doxycycline, dapsone, isotretinoin and sometimes oral steroids. Laser resurfacing, dermabrasion, chemical peel for residual scars.

Foreign Body Granuloma

Granulomatous reaction to foreign bodies, two types. Non-allergic (more common)—to surgical sutures, wood, talc, spines, etc. Allergic—to inorganic material like beryllium, zirconium, dyes used in tattoos (more with red dyes). Distinction between the two based on history and less so on histopathology. Non-allergic type shows multinucealte giant cells phagocytosis the material and less inflammation including lymphocytes and plasma cells. Allergic type shows more inflammation, may contain neutrophils as well and phagocytic giant cells less common. Granulomas more compact in allergic type.

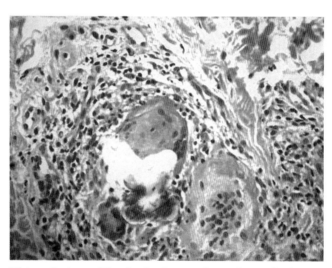

Histopathology of foreign body granuloma: foreign body type giant cells (nuclei located in the center of cell), one of which is engulfing calcified material (deep purple amorphous substance).

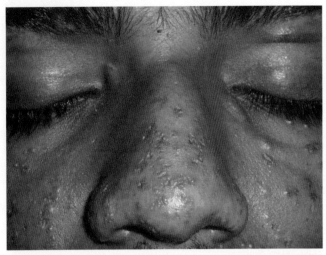

Lupus miliaris disseminatus faciei: lesions on nose and cheeks subsiding with irregular pitted scars.

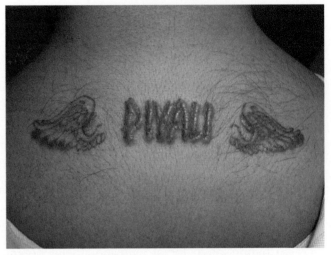

Foreign body granuloma: due to black dye in tattoo.

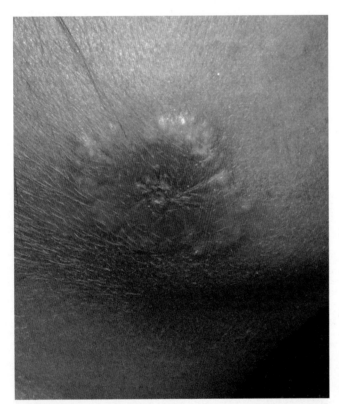

Sweet's syndrome: edematous, erythematous plaque on cheek with pseudovesicular appearance (note tiny pustules) at the margins.

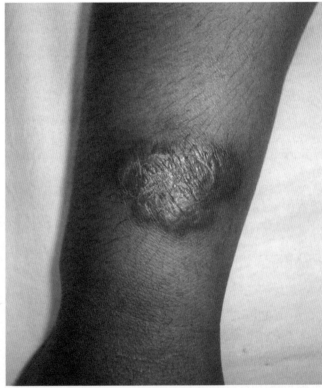

Sweet's syndrome: shiny erythematous plaque with slightly bosselated surface.

Clinical classification of neutrophilic dermatosis	
Clinical lesion	*Types*
Papules and plaques	Sweet's syndrome
	Neutrophilic eccrine hidradenitis (NEH)
	Erythema elevatum diutinum
	Neutrophilic rheumatoid dermatitis
	Pyoderma gangrenosum–Granulomatous type
Non-follicular flat pustules	Subcorneal pustular dermatosis
	IgA pemphigus
	Pustular-bullous pyoderma gangrenosum
	Atypical SS
Nodules, abscesses, and ulcerations	Pyoderma gangrenosum
	Behçet's syndrome
	Neutrophilic panniculitis
	Aseptic abscesses

Diagnostic criteria for sweet syndrome	
Classical[a]	*Drug-induced[b]*
1. Abrupt onset of painful erythematous plaques or nodules	A. Abrupt onset of painful erythematous plaques or nodules
2. Histopathological evidence of a dense neutrophilic infiltrate without evidence of leukocytoclastic vasculitis	B. Histopathological evidence of a dense neutrophilic infiltrate without evidence of leukocytoclastic vasculitis
3. Pyrexia >38°C	C. Pyrexia >38°C
4. Association with an underlying hematologic or visceral malignancy, inflammatory disease, or pregnancy, OR preceded by an upper respiratory or gastrointestinal infection or vaccination	D. Temporal relationship between drug ingestion and clinical presentation, OR temporally-related recurrence after oral challenge
5. Excellent response to treatment with systemic corticosteroids or potassium iodide	E. Temporally-related resolution of lesions after drug withdrawal or treatment with systemic corticosteroids
6. Abnormal laboratory values at presentation (three of four): erythrocyte sedimentation rate >20 mm/hr; positive C-reactive protein; >8,000 leukocytes; >70% neutrophils	

a. The presence of both major criteria (1 and 2), and two of the four minor criteria (3, 4, 5, and 6) is required in order to establish the diagnosis of classical Sweet's syndrome; the patients with malignancy-associated Sweet's syndrome are included with the patients with classical Sweet's syndrome in this list of diagnostic criteria.
b. All five criteria (A, B, C, D, and E) are required for the diagnosis of drug-induced Sweet's syndrome.

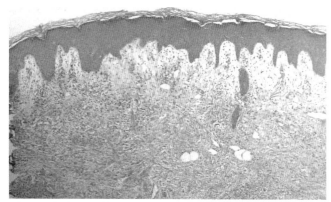

Histopathology of sweet syndrome: marked papillary dermal edema (pale, hypocellular area vis a vis reticular dermis), pandermal perivascular and interstitial nuetrophilic infiltrate.

Treatment

Removal/excision of the foreign material. Topical/intralesional steroids may help.

NEUTROPHILIC DERMATOSES

Sweet's Syndrome (Acute Febrile Neutrophilic Dermatosis)

Probably hypersensitivity reaction to infectious or tumor antigen. Three clinical types—idiopathic or classic, malignancy associated, and drug induced. Multiple, painful, sharply demarcated

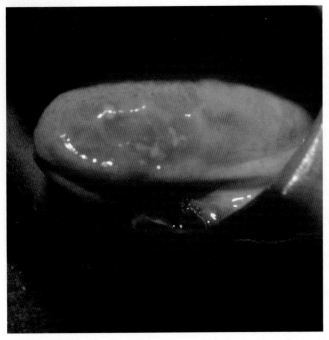

Sweet's syndrome: tiny, grouped necroted ulcers with polygonal margins (herpetiform) over the side of tongue.

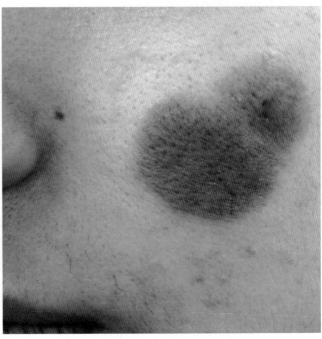

Granuloma faciale: solitary reddish brown plaque on cheek, follicular accentuation and telangiectasias seen over the plaque.

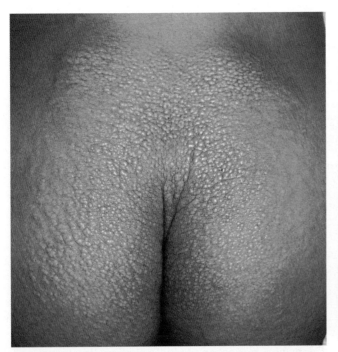

Scleromyxedema: grouped waxy papules over lower back and gluteal area, many showing linear configuration.

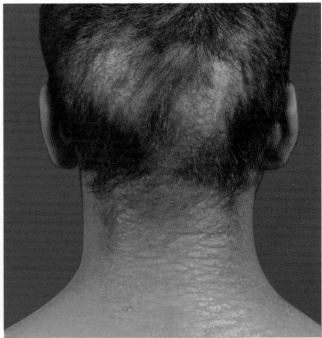

Scleromyxedema: waxy papules and plaques over nape of neck and upper back. Patchy hair loss over occipital scalp secondary to papular lesions is seen.

erythematous papules coalescing to form plaques and nodules with a mamillated surface—giving look of pseudovesicles. Face, neck and upper extremities. Associated high fever, constitutional symptoms. Leukocytosis. Recurrences common.

Histopathology: Papillary dermal edema and dense dermal neutrophilic infiltrate admixed with lymphocytes and eosinophils. No vasculitis.

Treatment

Systemic steroids. Also potassium iodide, colchicine, dapsone, clofazimine and cyclosporine.

Granuloma Faciale

Rare. Unknown etiology. Technically a form of localized fibrosing eosinophilic vasculitis. Asymptomatic solitary papule, plaque or nodule. Skin colored to erythematous/brownish lesions with follicular accentuation (peau d' orange appearance). Often central telangiectasias seen.

Classification of cutaneous mucinoses

Primary
- *Diffuse (degenerative-inflammatory mucinoses)*
  - Generalized myxedema
  - Pretibial myxedema
  - Lichen myxedematosus (papular mucinosis, scleromyxedema)
  - Acral persistent papular mucinosis
  - Cutaneous papular mucinosis of infancy
  - Self-healing papular cutaneous mucinosis; juvenile and adult
  - Hereditary progressive mucinous histiocytosis
  - Reticular erythematous mucinosis (plaque-like mucinosis
  - Scleredema
- *Follicular forms*
  - Follicular mucinosis (alopecia mucinosa)
  - Urticaria-like follicular mucinosis
- *Focal (neoplastic-hamartomatous mucinoses)*
  - Cutaneous focal mucinosis
  - Mucous (myxoid) cyst
  - Mucinous nevus

Secondary
- Papular and nodular mucinosis associated with lupus erythematosus
- Collagen vascular diseases (especially dermatomyositis, lupus erythematosus)
- Malignant atrophic papulosis (Degos' syndrome)
- Papular mucinosis in i-tryptophan-induced eosinophilia-myalgia syndrome
- Papular mucinosis of the toxic oil syndrome
- Mucinosis accompanying mesenchymal and neural tumors

Most commonly on face—cheeks, preauricular area, eyelids, forehead. Multiple lesions may occur on trunk or extremities.

Histopathology

Usually dense mixed inflammatory infiltrate in upper dermis with a thin sub-epidermal grenz zone. Infiltrate rich in eosinophils, neutrophils and lymphocytes. May be denser around blood vessels and appendages. Some fibrosis in chronic lesions.

Treatment

Primarily topical/intralesional steroids. Destructive therapies like cryotherapy, laser may be used with success. Topical tacrolimus may help.

CUTANEOUS MUCINOSES

Group of disorders characterized by dermal mucin deposition.

Scleromyxedema

Rare, generalized type of lichen myxedematosus. Waxy, skin colored papules arranged linearly. Surrounding skin may also be infiltrated. Erythema and edema sometimes also there. Occasional binding down of skin as in scleroderma. Common sites—face, neck, upper trunk and thighs. Alopecia rarely reported-eyebrows, axilla, more rarely scalp.

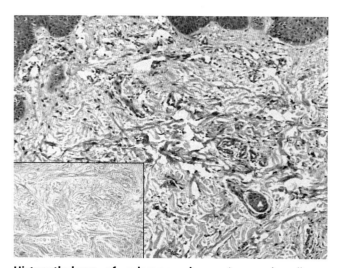

Histopathology of scleromyxedema: increased collagen deposition in upper dermis, mild lymphocytic infiltrate. Inset— abundant bright blue dermal mucin (alcian blue-PAS stain).

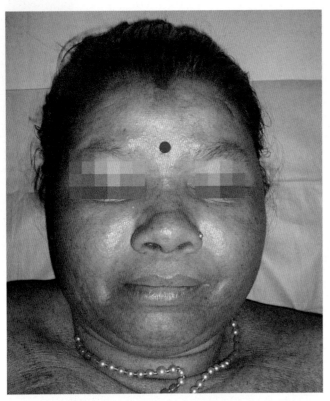

Scleromyxedema: facial plethora and infiltration.

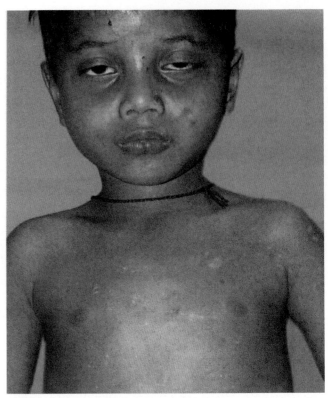

Scleredema: woody-hard, taut, induration of skin of face, neck and upper trunk. Note shiny appearance.

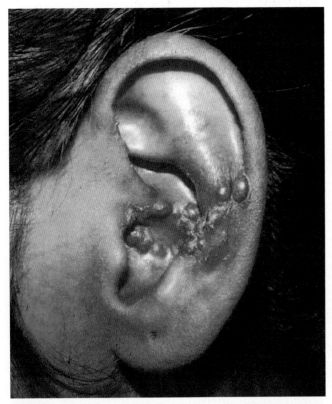

Angiolymphoid hyperplasia: asymptomatic, erythematous papules and nodules on pinna—a characteristic site.

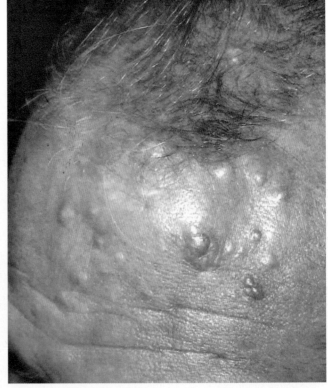

Angiolymphoid hyperplasia: deep seated swelling over the frontal scalp. Reddish papules and nodules over and around the swellings.

Subcutaneous nodules also recently reported. Associated underlying paraproteinemia in 80–90% cases. Cases without paraproteinemia labelled atypical.

Histopathology

Triad of fibroblast proliferation, collagen deposition and abundant dermal mucin (upper and mid reticular).

Treatment

Difficult and disappointing, variable clinical response. Systemic steroids and immunosuppressants like cyclophosphamide, melphalan (more commonly used) may help but have serious toxicities over long term use. Anecdotally isotretinoin tried. Other but expensive alternatives—plasmapharesis, intravenous immunoglobulins and stem cell transplantation.

Scleredema

Rare. Sudden onset symmetric induration of skin usually preceded by prodrome of fever, body aches. Onset from neck, upper back and shoulders, progress to face and arms later. Abnormality only felt on palpation, otherwise skin appears normal. Difficulty in mouth and eye closure, joint movement, rarely dysphagia may occur. Four types: idiopathic, poststreptococcal, type II diabetes-associated and paraproteinemia-associated.

Histopathology

Square shaped biopsy (normal tapering shape lost due to diffuse dermal thickening). Thick dermis with widely seperated collagen bundles. Empty spaces contain mucin that stain positive with alcian blue.

Treatment

Streptococcal-associated cases self-limiting, resolve over months to years. Diabetes associated: refractory to therapy. Paraproteinemia-associated: extracorporeal photopheresis. PUVA therapy and cyclosporine effective in some. Physiotherapy to prevent limitation in movement in all.

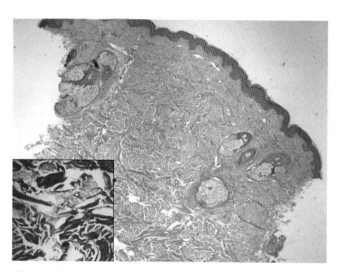

Histopathology of scleredema: square shaped biopsy, thickened collagen bundles with spaces between the bundles. Inset— abundant bright blue mucin (alcian blue-PAS stain)

CUTANEOUS PSEUDOLYMPHOMAS

Skin disorders that mimic lymphomas histopathologically in form of dense lymphoid aggregates.

Classification of cutaneous pseudolymphomas	
Subtype	Predominant cell type
Cutaneous lymphoid hyperplasia	B and T cell
Angiolymphoid hyperplasia with eosinophilia	B and T cell
Kimura's disease	B and T cell
Jessner's lymphocytic infiltrate	T cell
Lymphomatoid contact dermatitis	T cell
Lymphomatoid drug eruption	T cell
Pseudomycosis fungoides	T cell
Castleman disease	B and T cell

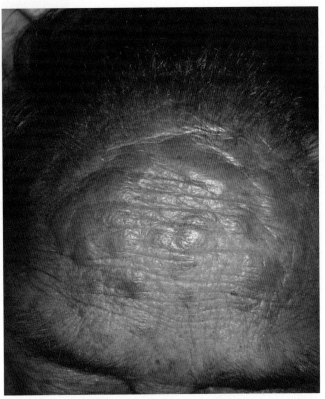

Cutaneous lymphoid hyperplasia: erythematous nodules grouped over forehead.

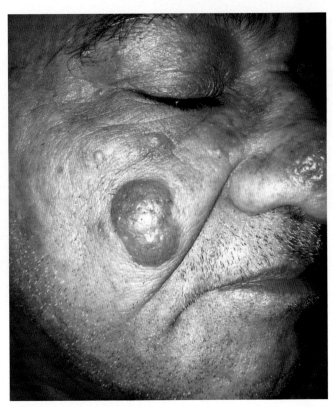

Cutaneous lymphoid hyperplasia: erythematous shiny nodules over cheek and nose.

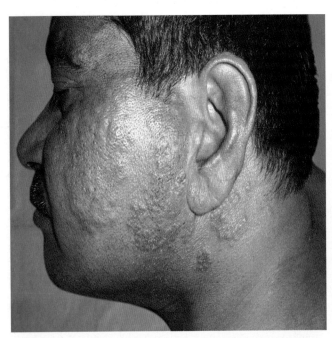

Jessner's lymphocytic infiltrate: erythematous plaques with confluent papules at the periphery, many showing annular configuration.

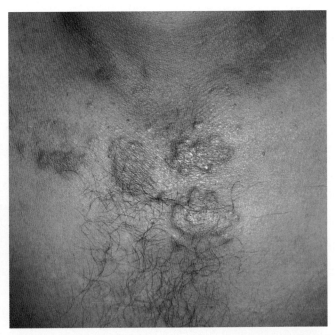

Jessner's lymphocytic infiltrate: erythematous plaques over 'V' area of upper chest.

Angiolymphoid Hyperplasia with Eosinophilia (ALHE, Epithelioid Hemangioma, Pseudopyogenic Granuloma)

Etiology unknown. Probably, a reactive proliferative disorder of blood vessels. More common in females. Often symptomatic-pruritus, bleeding on minor trauma or of aesthetic concern. Lesions red to pink colored papules and nodules. Scalp, face and ears. Peripheral eosinophilia frequent.

Histopathology

Dilated vascular channels, lined by plump, vacuolated endothelial cells which resemble epithelioid cells. Perivascular moderate to dense nodular infiltrate of lymphocytes, eosinophils and plasma cells. Variable vascular and lymphoid components; some have more vascular and some have more lymphoid findings.

Treatment

Difficult, recurrent condition. Medical therapies usually fail. Topical/Intralesional steroids may give symptomatic relief. Electrosurgery, lasers, cryosurgery, radiotherapy tried with some success. Complete surgical excision treatment of choice if feasible. Recently intralesional radiofrequency described with good relief in solitary lesion.

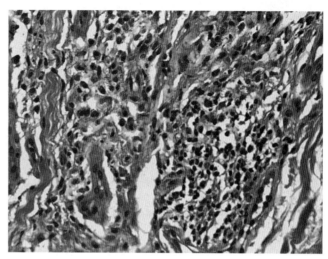

Histopathology of angiolymphoid hyperplasia with eosinophilia: numerous capillaries with slit like lumen lined by plump endothelial cells. Nodular aggregate of lymphocytes and numerous eosinophils.

Cutaneous Lymphoid Hyperplasia (Syn—Lymphocytoma Cutis, Spiegler Fendt Sarcoid)

Hypersensitivity response to various stimuli like insect bite, vaccination, gold body piercing, tattoos, etc.

Clinical Manifestation

Mildly firm to firm solitary nodule or tumor, occasionally papules or plaques. Sometimes

Clinicopathological features	Kimura's disease	Angiolymphoid hyperplasia with eosinophilia
Age of onset	Younger age	Old people
Duration of disease	Longer	Shorter
Clinical appearance	Deep seated large soft tissue mass	Multiple small dermal papular or nodular eruptions
Overlying skin	Normal	Normal or ulcerated
Blood eosinophilia	++	+/-
Lymphadenopathy	+/-	+/-
Elevated serum IgE	+/-	-
Blood vessels	Thin walled	Thick walled and concentric
Plump, histiocytoid endothelial cells	-	++
Lymphoid follicles with active germinal centers	+	+/-
Folliculolysis by eosinophils and lymphocytes	++	-
Fibrosis	+	-

Difference between Kimura's disease and ALHE

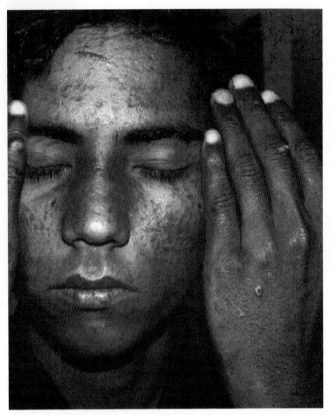

Reactive perforating collagenosis: mildly atrophic linear scars on face with keratotic umblicated papules on dorsa of hands.

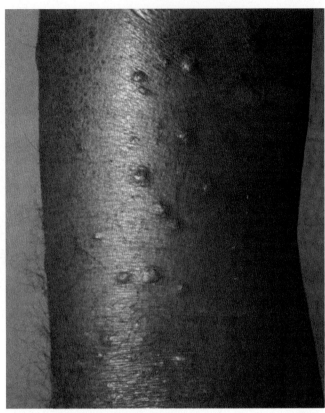

Acquired perforating dermatosis: keratotic papules with central plugs in a post renal transplant patient.

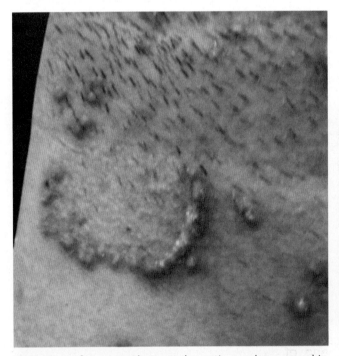

Elastosis perforans serpigenosa: keratotic papules arranged in serpigenous and arcuate manner on neck

Courtesy: Dr Geeti Khullar, Department of Dermatology, PGI Chandigarh.

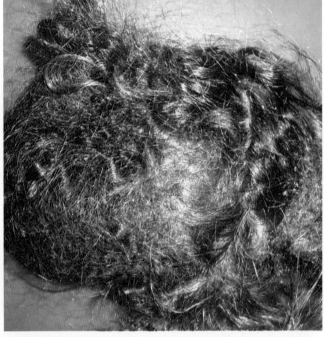

Plica polonica: scalp hair entangled into multiple plaits and an irreversible mass.

clustered lesions in a region or, rarely, widely scattered. Color varies from reddish brown to reddish purple. Scaling and ulceration absent. Involvement of particular body sites (earlobe, nipple, scrotum) common.

Histopathology

Dense, nodular, mixed cell infiltrates (lymphocytes, eosinophils, plasma cells) with lymphoid follicles. Infiltrate is 'top heavy'.

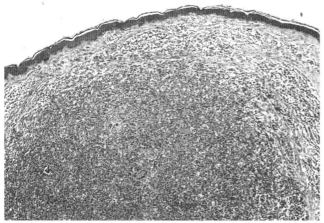

Histopathology of cutaneous lymphoid hyperplasia: dense nodular lymphoid aggregate in dermis sparing the epidermis (grenz zone).

Courtesy: Dr Sudheer Arava, Assistant Professor of Pathology, AIIMS, New Delhi.

Treatment

Resolve spontaneously in several months or years. If persistent or patient complaints, topical/ intralesional steroids, electrosurgery, cryosurgery done.

Jessner's Lymphocytic Infiltrate

Thought to be due to sunexposure. Asymptomatic non-scaly, erythematous papules, plaques and, less commonly, nodules most commonly over head, neck and upper back. Annular plaques with central clearing also observed. Individual lesions last several weeks to months. Few sites involved.

Histopathology

Superficial and deep, primarily perivascular and sometimes periappendageal lymphocytic infiltrate.

Treatment

Spontaneous resolution without scarring in months to years. Moderate success with topical/ intralesional steroids, oral hydroxychloroquine, oral antibiotics.

PERFORATING DISORDERS

Disorders characterized by transepidermal extrusion (perforation) of dermal material. Previously several entities were kept and differentiation was tried on the basis of clinical features and histopathology. Now, all acquired disorders are classified under 'acquired perforating dermatosis' and if serpiginous, under 'acquired elastosis perforans serpiginosa' (acquired EPS). Some variants that are heritable include reactive perforating collagenosis, EPS and Flegel's disease.

Intense pruritus in acquired dermatosis. Mostly occur on extensors on lower and upper extremities. Umblicated papules with central white keratinous crust, may become hyperkeratotic nodules (esp. in Kyrle's disease). In EPS, the papules are form a serpiginous border with annular or arcuate configuration.

Lesions subside with scarring over months. These disorders most often associated with diabetes mellitus, chronic kidney disease and hemodialysis.

Reactive Perforating Collagenosis

Autosomal recessive or dominant. Characterized by transepithelial elimination of altered collagen. First decade. Asymptomatic pinhead-sized umblicated keratotic papules on dorsa of hands, forearms and face. Resolve spontaneously in 3–4 weeks, leaving a thin varioliform scar or hypopigmentation. Koebnerization seen.

Histopathology

Cup-shaped depression in epidermis filled with parakeratotic keratin, collagen and inflammatory debris. Basophilic collagen at the papillary dermal end of the perforation. In perforating folliculitis, collagen comes out through follicular ostium. In EPS, elastin is extruded.

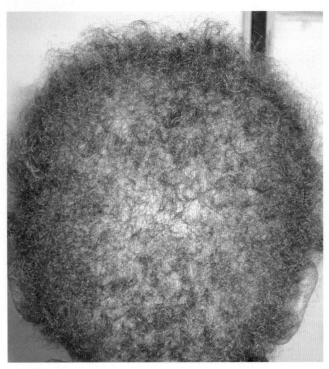

Trichorrhexis nodosa: curly, easily breakable scalp hair.

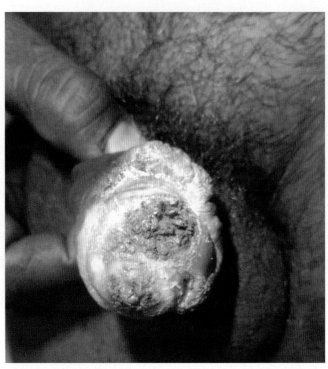

Pseudoepitheliomatous keratotic amd micaceous balanitis: firm hyperkeratotic plaque on glans penis (surrounding the urethral meatus). Adherent 'mica-like' scales seen at periphery of the verrucous part.

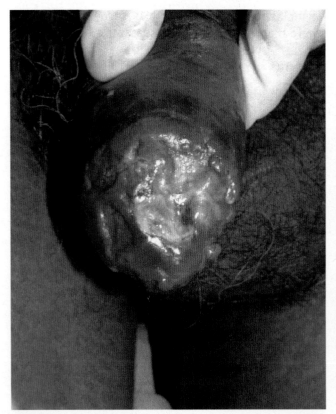

Papulonecrotic tuberculide of glans: necrotic ulcer with bridging scars on the glans.

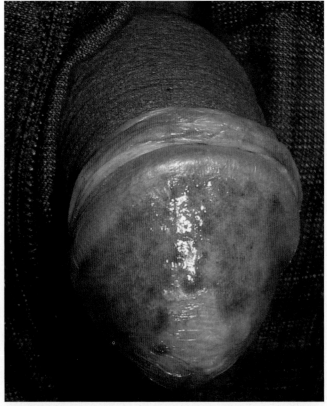

Zoon's balanitis: solitary glistening red plaque over the dorsum of glans penis. Telangiectasias visible over the plaque ('cayenne pepper spots')

Treatment

If underlying disease present, control of that improves pruritus and perforating process. Otherwise treatment relied on keratolytics like urea-lactic acid combinations, topical retinoids, oral doxycycline, UVB, PUVA, etc.

RARE HAIR DISORDERS

Plica Polonica (Syn—Plica Neuropathica)

Rare, acquired condition, sudden onset. Scalp hair is compacted into irregularly twisted, irreversibly entangled plaits and matted mass. More likely in longer hair. Initially thought to be associated with psychiatric disorders but currently this association seems spurious/by chance. Multi-factorial causation (primarily thought to be due to physical factors)—physical: mechanical action, temperature, electrostatic forces, hair elasticity, density and coiling; chemical: detergents, creams, gels, perms; behavioral: neglected personal hygiene. Treatment is shaving of entagled hair. Organic solvents may be used to dismantle the mass. Some reports mention no recurrence after shaving.

Trichorrhexis Nodosa

Nodes of hair showing cuticle bulge and longitudinal fissure giving an appearance of a 'splayed paint brush'. Response of the hair shaft to injury and thus can be seen in normal hair also. Some hereditary conditions showing this finding—Argininosuccinic aciduria, citrullinemia, Menkes syndrome, trichothiodystrophy.

It can also be acquired:

- **Proximal:** repeated chemical or hot comb straightening
- **Distal:** excessive brushing, back combing, sporadic use of permanent waves.

Treatment

- Might improve as the patient grows up. Avoid aggressive hair grooming practices such as excessive back combing, tight pony tails, use of hair waves or straighteners.

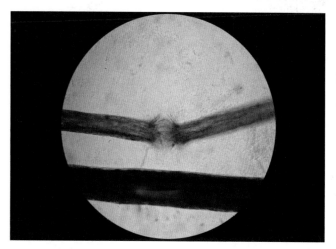

Trichorrhexis nodosa, hair mount: hair shaft partially broken in the center with few interconnecting strands remaining ('splayed paint brush' appearance)

MISCELLANEOUS DISEASES INVOLVING GENITALIA

Pseudoepitheliomatous Keratotic and Micaceous Balanitis of Civatte (PKMB)

Rare penile disorder. Intermediate between benign and malignant disease—tendency to show delayed malignant potential but usually benign at baseline. Etiology uncertain, may be response to chronic low grade infection in background of phimosis. Role of human papilloma virus not defined.

More in elderly adults who undergo late circumcision for phimosis. Verrucous firm plaque over penis with 'mica-like' adherent scales. Intermittently sheds, only to reform. Usually asymptomatic, fissuring and maceration may occur. Long-term follow-up essential to monitor natural course and detect malignant change at the earliest.

Histopathology

Pseudoepitheliomatous hyperplasia. Lower epidermal atypical changes may be seen.

Treatment

Resistant to treatment. Partial remission irrespective of therapy used (unless completely excised). Topical 5-fluorouracil, podophyllin

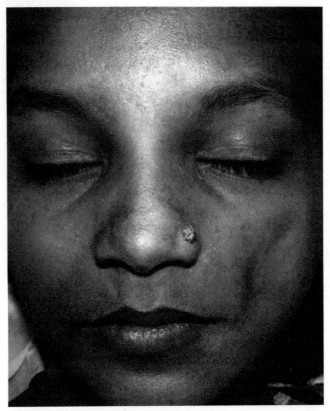

Parry Romberg syndrome: hemifacial atrophy without binding down of the overlying skin.

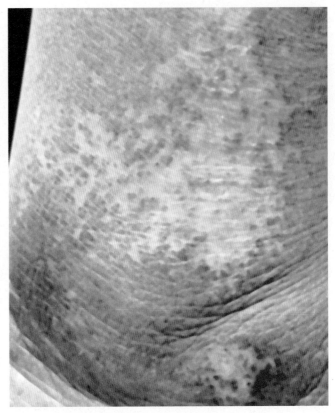

Atrophie blanche: irregular porcelain white atrophic scars, studded with red papules (dilated capillaries).

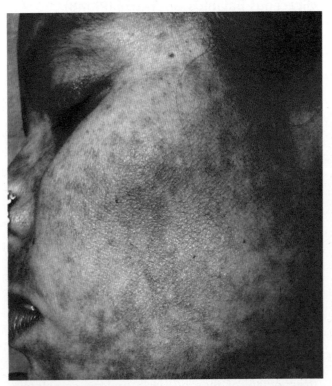

Exogenous ochronosis: violaceous blotchy/reticulate pigmentation over the cheek and forehead. Note, the epidermal wrinkling and shininess, suggestive of triple combination induced atrophy.

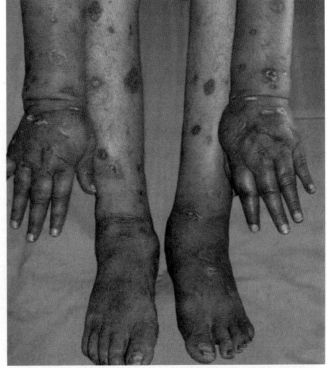

Pentazocine abuse: multiple crusted ulcers along veins with non-pitting edema of hands (puffy-hand syndrome).

resin used with some success, imiquimod off-late used. Destructive therapies like cryosurgery, radiotherapy and surgical excision useful.

Papulonecrotic Tuberculide of the Glans

Rare. Tender, necrotizing papules on glans. Heal with characteristic bridging scars. *Tuberculin test:* positive. Systemic focus of tuberculosis often present.

Histopathology

Tuberculoid granulomatous infiltrate with necrosis. Granulomatous vasculitis occasional.

Treatment

Antitubercular therapy.

Zoon's Balanitis (Plasma Cell Balanitis)

Seen in uncircumcised, middle aged to elderly males. Asymptomatic. Usually solitary, glazed erythematous plaque over the glans penis with minute red spots caller 'cayenne pepper spots'. May be multiple or extending to subpreputial skin. Close clinical differentials include erythroplasia of Queyrat and mucosal bowen's disease. Biopsy should be done if suspicion of these entities high.

Histopathology

Atrophic epidermis with lozenge shaped keratinocytes in suprabasal part. Dermal moderate to dense infiltrate with predominant plasma cells and lymphocytes.

Treatment

Topical steroids, tacrolimus, electrosurgical or laser ablation. Circumcision curative.

OTHER MISCELLANEOUS DERMATOSES

Parry Romberg Syndrome

Etiology unknown. More common in females. Slowly, progressive hemifacial atrophy, usually of left side. Muscular atrophy and bone loss can occur over a period of several years. Associated with seizures and trigeminal neuralgia.

Treatment

None available to prevent progress of disease. Systemic steroids tried without much success. Reconstructive surgery (using muscle or bone grafts), once disease static.

Atrophie Blanche (Syn—White Atrophy)

Result of healing of chronic ulcers and leaving scars over lower legs and feet. Commonest site being around the malleoli. Asymptomatic atrophic porcelain white scars with intervening capillaries visible as red dots. Intermitten superficial ulcers develop which are painful. Common association with chronic venous incompetence. Other causes include scleroderma, vasculitides, lupus erythematosus, cryoglobulinemia, polycythemia and leukemia.

Histopathology

Atrophic epidermis, dermal sclerosis with proliferating capillaries.

Treatment

No effective treatment. Antiplatelet agents tried with some success.

Exogenous Ochronosis

Long-term side-effect of topical hydroquinone use/abuse for hyperpigmentary disorders. Most prominently secondary to inadvertent use of hydroquinone based preparations for melasma. Mechanism of action is possibly by inhibition of enzyme homogentisic acid oxidase (as quinones are known to inhibit the enzyme), followed by deposition of homogentisate in dermal connective tissue leading to localized ochronosis. Clinically, asymptomatic, blue-black pigmentation develops over background of primary pigmentary disorder for which hydroquinone was being used. Common sites cheeks, sides and back of neck. More common in dark skin types. Pigmentation usually irregular and mottled or reticulate. Rarely papules may appear in advanced cases.

Histopathology

Yellow to light brown, round or ovoid amorphous pigment deposits occur in papillary dermis. No systemic deposition.

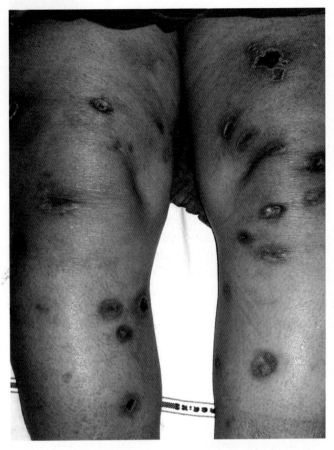

Pentazocine abuse: multiple crusted ulcers along veins of lower limbs.

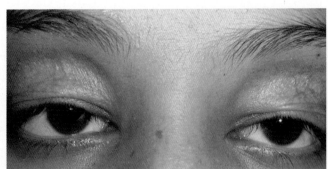

Blepharochalasis: laxity, atrophy and wrinkling of bilateral upper eyelids.

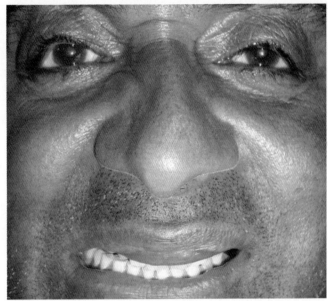

Ascher syndrome: laxity of bilateral upper eyelids along with laxity and duplication of upper lip mucosa (Note upper incisors and canine teeth are hidden by a upper lip mucosal extension).

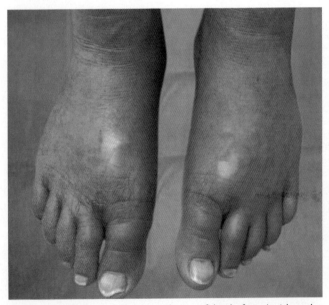

Erythromelalgia: prominent redness of both feet (evident by area of blanching produced by pressure from thumb).

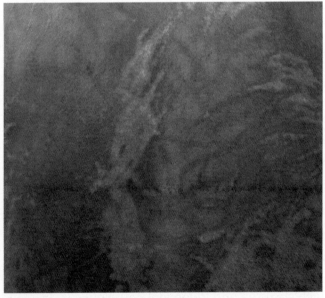

Flagellate pigmentation: caused by bleomycin.

Treatment

Stopping usage of hydroquinone based creams. Pigmentation may subside partially over a period of time, but never completely. Q-switched alexandrite laser has shown encouraging results.

Pentazocine Induced Ulcers

Pentazocine, a common analgesic. Has agonist-antagonist action on opioid receptors. On repeated use produces tolerance, psychological and physical dependence with abuse potential. Can be administered orally or parenterally— intramuscular, subcutaneous or intravenous. Repeated injections leads to localized fibrosis. Occlusion of veins or lymphatics produces non-pitting edema of hands, known as 'puffy-hand syndrome'. Irregular deep ulcers along veins with surrounding hyperpigmentation and woody induration conspicuous. Patient indifferent to his illness. Presence of pentazocine in urine confirms recent abuse.

Treatment

Difficult. Patient denies abuse. Psychiatric assistance essential. Ulcers gradually heal spontaneously.

Blepharochalasis

Rare disorder of eyelid. Mostly acquired or autosomal dominant. Cause unknown.

Onset around puberty, recurrent transient attacks of asymptomatic eyelid swelling (mainly upper), subside in few days. Followed by wrinkling, laxity and atrophy of eyelids. Gives appearance of premature aging (laxity of eyelids normal with advanced age). May be associated with generalized cutis laxa, Ehler Danlos syndrome. Ascher's syndrome is association of blepharochalasis and upper lip enlargement and mucosal doubling. Treatment is surgical correction/plastic repair of sagging eyelid.

Erythromelalgia

Disorder of abnormal vascular response to heat. Painful red extremities with sensation of burning and vasodilatation.

Three types—type 1 with thrombocythemia, type 2 congenital and type 3 with inflammatory vascular disorders.

Pain and redness on exposure to warmth and more on keeping the legs in dependant position. Important association with myeloproliferative disorders.

Treatment

No effective treatment. Antiplatelet agents like aspirin and clopidogrel may relieve pain. Neuropathic pain treatments may help. Limb elevation important.

Bleomycin Induced Flagellate Pigmentation

Bleomycin, an anticancer drug used in cancers cervix, uterus, head and neck, testicle, penis and in lymphomas. Characteristic flagellate linear hyperpigmentation in 20–30%. Upper trunk and limbs. Dose dependent (usually after 90–285 mg) and reversible.

Meningococcemia

Dissemination of *Neisseria meningitidis* (encapsulated Gram negative diplococcus) into bloodstream. Petechial, purpuric, bullous or hemorrhagic lesions with central necrosis. High fever, meningeal symptoms, disseminated intravascular coagulation may develop. Gram's stain and culture from skin lesions shows organisms.

Treatment

Medical emergency. Prompt and aggressive anti-microbial therapy (penicillin. Or cephalosporin). Chemoprophylaxis during epidemics (rifampin/ciprofloxacin). And vaccination of susceptible contacts.

Ainhum (Dactylolysis Spontanea)

Autoamputation of fifth toe due to constricting band- probably due to abnormal blood supply. Common in blacks. *Pseudoainhum:* annular constriction of digits secondary to hereditary I non-hereditary diseases like leprosy.

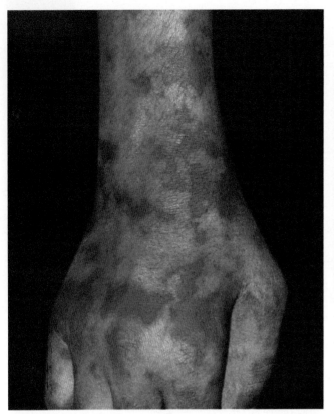

Meningococcemia: widespread purpuric lesions.

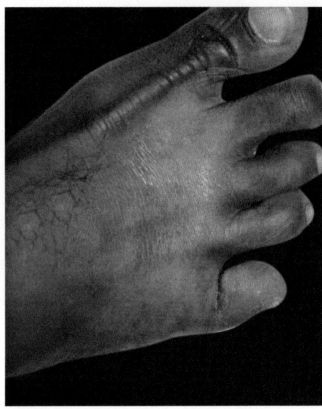

Ainhum: spontaneous painful amputation of fifth toe.

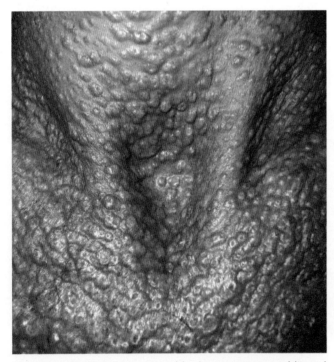

Muir Torre syndrome: innumerable discrete greasy umblicated papules (sebaceous adenomas) over the neck and chest.

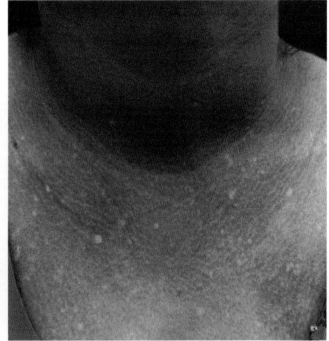

Amyloidosis cutis dyschromica: rippled hyperpigmentation over photo-exposed area of chest. Punctate hypopgimented macules also present.

Treatment

Early stage: topical salicylic acid ointment and intralesional steroid. *Late stage:* surgical amputation. Antibiotics for secondary infections.

Muir Torre Syndrome

Rare syndromic association between skin neoplasia (sebaceous adenomas, sebaceous carcinomas, keratoacanthoma) with internal malignancies (colorectal, small bowel, endometrial or urothelial). Autosomal dominant inheritance, defect in MSH2 and MLH1 genes. Associated with HNPCC (hereditary non-polyposis colorectal cancer). Skin lesions precede or succeed internal malignancy. Sebaceous adenomas appear as raised umblicated paules or nodules. In MTS, trunk more commonly involved. Sebaceous carcinomas involve eyelids commonly.

Histopathology

Multilobular, lobules well-defined, variable numbers of small, basophilic, sebaceous matrix cells peripherally and larger mature sebaceous cells.

Treatment

Mainly preventive. Screening for internal malignancy in view of large number of truncal sebaceous tumors. Oral isotretinoin (@0.8 mg/kg/day) may prevent development of cutaneous malignancy.

AMYLOIDOSIS CUTIS DYSCHROMICA

Familial pigmentary disorder of unknown cause and pathogenesis.

Characterized by reticular hyperpigmentation studded with punctate hypopigmented macules distributed extensively, onset usually before puberty, no or little itch, and focal papillary dermal amyloid deposition. Rarely papules may also occur. Considered as differential diagnosis for reticulate pigmentary disorders and dyschromatotic disorders.

Treatment

No definitive treatment available. Photo-protection, topical keratolytics, CO_2 laser, oral retinoids may help.

22

Therapeutics in Dermatology

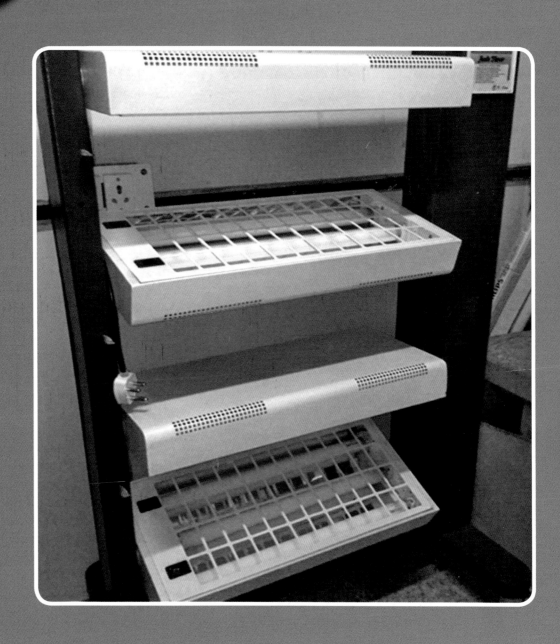

Dermatologic therapy—unique in several ways. Apart from systemic medications, skin disorders are treatable with topical applications, intralesional administration and physical modalities—each one with its own merits and demerits.

Topical therapy assures direct application of active ingredient(s) at the diseased site, in appropriate concentrations and suitable formulations. Messy, at times unacceptable, but relatively non-toxic. Intralesional therapy introduces drug into the depth of skin—often painful and difficult to administer. Systemic therapy, non-messy and mostly standardized—useful in extensive disease or topically inaccessible sites. Toxicity depends on individual drug.

TOPICAL THERAPY

Consists of local application of an active substance dispersed, dissolved or suspended in a base (vehicle). Choice of active ingredient and vehicle extremely and perhaps equally important.

VEHICLES

Choice determined by acuteness of condition, site of diseased area, solubility/dispersibility of active ingredient and local and environmental factors.

Lotions

Clear Lotions

Aqueous solution of active substances. Useful for exudative and crusted, vesiculobullous and pustular lesions. Also useful in hairy and intertriginous areas. Spirituous (alcoholic) clear lotions are called *tinctures*—incorporate lipophilic active substances for topical use.

Lotions used as—*compresses* or *wet dressings:* soaked pads wrapped around localized diseased areas. Or as *soaks:* the limb or a part of limb immersed in the solution. Or *baths:* for extensive scaly dermatoses—psoriasis, exfoliative dermatitis, ichthyosis—a major part or the whole body immersed in the bath. Active substance incorporated could be silver nitrate, aluminum acetate (Burrow's solution) or potassium permanganate—astringents and oxidizing agents.

Shake Lotions

Consists of powder(s) suspended, with the help of suspending agent, in water; useful for acute, non-exudative conditions; unsuitable for hairy regions or folds of the skin. Evaporation of water cools skin leaves suspended protective powder on surface. Additional active substances could be dissolved or suspended. Calamine lotion—a common shake lotion.

Emulsions/Creams/Gels

A system of two *immiscible liquids*—oil and water. One phase suspended with the help of an emulsifier in the other—outer or continuous phase, as small droplets. Water in oil (w/o) emulsions—cold creams. Oil in water (o/w) emulsions—vanishing creams. *Gel*—a semisolid emulsion that liquefies on contact with skin.

Emulsification helped by emulsifying agents—long chain molecules with one hydrophobic pole and other hydrophilic; some additives destabilize emulsions. Emulsions cause cooling. Also help penetration of hydrophilic as well as lipophilic substances.

Ointments

Consist of base of animal and plant fats. Or mineral greases (petroleum or paraffin, lanolin, waxes). Or synthetic fats (polyethylene glycols). Ointments keep active agents in contact with the skin for long periods—enhancing penetration. Useful for treating dry skin, hyperkeratotic and scaly dermatoses. Unsuitable for acute exudative conditions—may produce maceration and increase inflammation.

Pastes

Consist of insoluble powders in high concentrations (up to 50%) in an ointment base. Semi-solid, stiff preparations. Difficult to remove. Have anti-inflammatory, cooling and protective effect. And a drying and absorbing effect—so useful in exudative conditions (*c.f.* ointments). Help to retain active principle on to localized areas for long periods. Suitable for ulcers. Or thick lichenified plaques.

Powders

Consist of micronized and dispersed granular particles. Promote drying by increasing evaporation of water from skin surface. Used with benefit in exudative lesions.

In decreasing order of acuteness of inflammation, the bases may be selected in the following order:
Clear lotions—shake lotions—creams pastes —ointments.

ACTIVE SUBSTANCES

May have specific, quasi-specific or symptomatic action. Commonly employed active substances are the following as mentioned below.

Antibacterial Agents

Wide choice—from soaps and antiseptics to antibiotics. Soaps act by being anionic detergents; potassium permanganate and hydrogen peroxide by being oxidizing agents; antibiotics by bacteriostatic or bactericidal actions. Commonly used antibacterials are: *triphenylmethane dyes* (0.5–2% brilliant green and 0.5–1% gentian violet), 3% *hydrogen peroxide*, 0.5–2% *silver nitrate*; 10% *hexachlorophene*. Commonly used topical antibiotics—neomycin, polymyxin band bacitracin. Lotion, gel or cream bases preferred. Ointments avoided as they cause occlusion—hence spread infection. Agents such as nitrofurazone, penicillin, sulphonamides, streptomycin and salicylanilides best avoided because of their potential to sensitize.

Mupirocin, 2% ointment or cream and *fusidic acid* 2% cream have various indications. Mupirocin bactericidal. Spectrum-staphylococcal species and beta hemolytic streptococci. Increasing resistance amongst methicillin resistant *Staphylococcus aureus* effective in impetigo, folliculitis and infected eczema. Not to be used for prolonged periods—results in development of resistance. Fusidic acid bacteriostatic but broader spectrum of activity-all bacteria as in case of mupirocin plus MRSA, neisseria and bacteroides. Can penetrate intact skin and crusts. Useful in furuncles, impetigo. Also erythrasma.
New antibiotics-nadifloxacin 1% cream and retapamulin 1% ointment. Nadifloxacin bactericidal, used for treatment of acne but also for infections. Broad spectrum activity—Gram positive, MRSA, Gram negative and anaerobic bacteria. No cross resistance with other quinolones. Retapamulin bacteriostatic. Spectrum—Gram positives, MRSA, propionibacterium acnes, anaerobes. Used for impetigo and secondarily infected eczema.

Antifungal Agents

Several agents. Some specific for dermatophytic or candidal infections, others cover both as well as *Pityrosporum orbiculare* (pityriasis versicolor). Advisable to use all topical antifungal agents for 2–3 weeks after clinical and mycological cure.

- *Azoles:* Broad spectrum fungistatic agents— inhibit growth through action on cell wall. Effective against dermatophytes, candida and *P orbiculare*. Also effective in erythrasma. Miconazole nitrate 2%, clotrimazole 1%, econazole 1% and ketoconazole 2%. Newer congeners-sertaconazole 2% cream and luliconazole 1% cream. Sertaconazole has greater reservoir effect in startum corneum than older azoles. Good activity against tinea, candida and also Gram positive bacteria. Luliconazole 1% cream. Once a day therapy for 2 weeks for tinea cruris, corporis and pedis. Advantage of single application.

- *Allylamines and benzylamines:* Terbinafine 1%, naftifine 1% and butenafine 1%. Fungicidal agents—inhibit squalene epoxidase. Effective against dermatophytes, pityrosporum and candida (*c.f.* oral terbinafine effective only against dermatophytes).

- *Others:* *Tolnaftate* 1%: effective against dermatophytes but not against candida. *Haloprogin:* 1% cream/solution: effective against dermatophytes and *P orbiculare* and possibly candida. *Ciclopirox olamine* 1% cream: broad spectrum fungistatic agent effective against dermatophytes, candida and *P orbiculare*. Also available as 8% nail lacquer. *Amorolifine* 5% nail lacquer. Both nail lacquers effective as monotherapy for distal onychomycosis and superficial white onychomycosis. Also as adjuvant therapy with systemic antifungal agents. Amorolfine now available as 0.25% cream, used as once a day application for tinea. *Nystatin, amphotericin B* and *gentian violet* creams or lotions effective against candida only. *Selenium sulphide* (1.25–2.5%) effective in pityriasis versicolor.

Whitfield's ointment (6% benzoic acid and 3% salicylic acid) combines fungistatic and keratolytic action. Now obsolete.

Antiviral Agents

Idoxuridine (5-iodo 2-deoxyuridine; IDU): 0.1–0.5%, useful in herpetic keratitis. For herpes genitalis, 5–15% IDU with dimethylsulfoxide (DMSO) applied early in course of disease shortens the duration of attack in some patients. Allergic contact dermatitis may occur.

- *Acyclovir:* 5% cream; virostatic-inhibits DNA synthesis through activation of thymidine kinase. Topical application gives only symptomatic relief and perhaps shortens the course. Not very useful.
- *Podophyllin resin:* 10–25% in compound tincture of benzoin. Cytotoxic effect; useful in anogenital warts, as physician-applied therapy. Adjoining skin should be protected with petrolatum. *Podophyllotoxin* (0.5%)—patient-applied therapy, twice daily for 3 consecutive days a week. Both can cause irritation. Not be used in pregnancy.
- *Imiquimod:* 5% cream; an immunomodulator. Used in anogenital warts, molluscum contagiosum. Thrice a week; wash after 6–10 hours after application. Available as single use sachets.
- *5-flurouracil:* 5% cream; cytotoxic agent. Used more frequently for treating solar keratoses, Bowen's disease and some basal cell carcinomas.
- *Sinecatechin:* 15% ointment; reduces expression of human papilloma virus oncoproteins E6 and E7. FDA approved for external anogenital warts.
- *Cidofovir:* 1% gel; inhibits viral polymerases. Broad spectrum activity, used in resistant genital herpes, resistant molluscum contagiosum, anogenital warts.

Antiparasitic Agents

- *Permethrin:* 1% cream, lotion. Treatment of choice in pediculosis capitis–safe, has residual effect. 5%—used for scabies. Safe in children. May be used in pregnant women.
- *Gamma benzene hexachloride* (GBH): 1% cream or lotion. Effective against scabies, pediculosis pubis and capitis. Toxic. Not to be used in children <5 years and pregnant women.
- *Benzyl benzoate:* 25% emulsion. Effective against scabies. Less so against pediculosis pubis and capitis.
- *Crotamiton:* 10% lotion or cream. Effective in scabies. Also mild antipruritic. Useful in children.
- *DDT:* 5% powder—for disinfection of clothes in pediculosis corporis.
- *Spinosad:* 0.9% suspension-for pediculosis capitis. Found to be more effective than permethrin 1%.
- *Benzyl alcohol:* 5% lotion-pediculosis capitis.
- *Ivermectin:* 0.5% lotion-pedicluosis capitis. Also used as oral preparation for scabies (@200 µg/kg, 2 doses 2 weeks apart).

Anti-inflammatory Agents

Topical corticosteroids—most potent anti-inflammatory preparations. Tars, shake lotions, emollients such as oils and creams—moderate anti-inflammatory agents. Topical calcineurin inhibitors also commonly used, efficacy equivalent to lower-mid potent steroid.

- *Corticosteroids:* Choice of corticosteroid depends upon acuteness of inflammation, site(s) affected, age, expected duration of use and cost of preparation. Available as creams, ointments, lotions or gels. Concentration and potency of corticosteroids varies widely. Steroids dispensed in ointment base generally more potent than same concentration in cream base. Occlusion and combination with keratolytics enhance absorption and improve effectiveness. Combination with antibiotics and other antibacterials and/or antifungals available. Combination with tars may, however, disturb pharmaceutical stability.

The following preparations are commonly available for therapy (in decreasing order of potency).

Classification of some common topical steroids according to potency

S.No	Potency	Examples	Preparation
1	Superpotent	**Clobetasol propionate 0.05%**	**Oint/Cr** Oint/Cr
		Halobetasol propionate 0.05%	Oint
		Betamethasone dipropionate 0.05%	
2	Potent	Betamethasone dipropionate 0.05%	**Cr**
		Fluocinonide 0.05%	Oint
		Mometasone furoate 0.1%	Oint
3	Upper midstrength	Betamethasone dipropionate 0.05%	**Lotion**
		Fluticasone propionate 0.005%	Oint
		Triamcinolone acetonide 0.1%	Oint

Side effects: Local atrophy of the skin and striae distensae (particularly in the folds of skin). Prolonged use of potent fluorinated corticosteroid preparations on the face may result in perioral dermatitis; and in children systemic toxicity due to efficient percutaneous absorption. Pustular psoriasis—after withdrawal in patients of psoriasis. Under occlusion, may cause folliculitis. Indian skin tolerates topical corticosteroids rather well.

- *Topical calcineurin inhibitors:* Most preferred anti-inflammtory agents for facial application or long term use, because of good safety profile. Bind to calcineurin, inhibit synthesis of interleukin 2, effectively inhibiting activation and proliferation of T lymphocytes. Tacrolimus 0.03 and 0.1% ointments; and Pimecrolimus 1% cream.

Indications similar except pimecrolimus preferred over facial lesions, expensive and safer in infants. Common indications of tacrolimus-atopic dermatitis, vitiligo, psoriasis, lichen planus, rosacea, morphea/lichen sclerosus. Common indications of pimecrolimus-vitiligo, psoriasis, lichen planus, atopic dermatitis, lichen sclerosus. Side effects include local irritation, burning, local infections (viral, fungal). Therapy under occlusion may provide enhanced effect.

Keratolytic Agents

Act by dehiscing or removing keratin:

- *Hydroxy acids:* alpha (glycolic acid, lactic acid, pyruvic acid), beta (slaicylic acid). Act by dissolving demosomal junctions, causing desquamation. Long term use leads to thickening of dermis. Glycolic acid (20–70%) and salicyclic acid (2–10%) used commonly in chemical peels for pigmentary disorders and acne scars. Higher concentrations of salicylic acid used for corns and callosities.
- *Urea 20–40%:* as aqueous solution or ointment base, dissolves hydrogen bonds and epidermal keratin.
- *Resorcinol:* a phenol derivative, occasionally employed in 1% concentration in acne preparations.
- *Retinoic acid:* 0.025, 0.05 and 0.1%, is a weak keratolytic agent.

Keratoplastic Agents

Restore abnormal keratinization process to normalcy. Useful in psoriasis and subacute eczemas. Several agents available:

- *Tars:* distillation products of organic substances. Crude coal tar supposed to be therapeutically superior to wood tars, bituminous tars and petroleum tars. Active constituent(s) unknown. Exact mode of action ill-understood. Weak phototoxic action; UVA and/or UVB perhaps augment its therapeutic value. Crude coal tar, coal tar solution (liquor carbonis detergens) or ichthammol can be incorporated into ointments, creams, shampoos, in concentrations varying between 1 and 10%. Side effects-staining of clothes, follicultis, erythema, contact dermatitis, etc. Liposomal preparations available, reduce irritation and staining side effects.
- *Anthralin (1,8 dihydroxyanthranol):* a synthetic substance prepared from anthracene. Useful in psoriasis. Mode of action uncertain. Applied locally as a paste in concentrations of 0.5–1% and washed off after 4–6 hours to prevent irritation. 'Short contact' therapy involves application of 2–5% for 12–2 hours. Claimed

to give better results and cause less irritation. Disadvantages: irritates skin and stains clothes. Inactivation of dithranol zinc paste—prevented by addition of salicylic acid.

- **Retinoic acid (vitamin A acid, tretinoin):** has 'regulatory' effect on epidermal cell differentiation. Most often used in acne in concentrations of 0.025, 0.05%, or 0.1%. Comedonic acne responds best. Also useful in Darier's disease, verrucous epidermal nevi, ichthyosiform dermatoses and palmoplantar keratoderma. Therapeutic value in psoriasis debatable. Contraindicated in pregnancy.

Depigmenting Agents

- **Hydroquinone (2–5%):** has antityrosinase activity and toxic effect on melanocytes. An effective and safe remedy in treatment of melasma.
- **Monobenzyl ether of hydroquinone (MBH):** a melanocyte poison, could result in mottled depigmentation—often irreversible. MBH 20%, however, profitably employed in the treatment of residual pigmented areas in widespread vitiligo to achieve uniform white color. May need maintenance applications especially on photo-exposed areas. However, difficult to procure.
- **Azelaic acid (10–20% cream):** proven useful but mechanism uncertain. Possibly by inhibiting microbial respiratory chain (useful as anti-acne medication) and inhibits tyrosinase (anti-melasma medication).
- **Kojic acid 2% cream:** moderately effective in pigmentation disorders. Mechanism same as azelaic acid. Arbutin 3% questionable efficacy.

Antipruritic Agents

Relieve itching by a variety of mechanisms: by blocking the nerve impulses as with local anesthetics, chloretone (1–2%) and phenol (1–2%). Or by change of itch to some other sensation—cold as with menthol (0.01–1%) and calamine lotion (cooling by evaporation)—or warmth as with camphor (1–2%). Or by ill-understood mechanisms as in case of corticosteroids. Antipruritics can be incorporated in lotions, creams, ointments or pastes. Phenol avoided on extensive surfaces since percutaneous absorption can result in nephrotoxicity. Local anesthetics and local antihistamines, good antipruritics but have a high contact sensitizing potential and so should not be used. Crotamiton (10%) is a good antipruritic, besides being scabicidal.

Sunscreens

Protect from light. Two broad categories recognized: *organic* (earlier designated as chemical) sunscreens. Or *inorganic* (earlier designated as physical) sunscreens.

- **Organic sunscreens:** act by absorption of specific wavebands of light. Para-aminobenzoic acid (PABA) or one of its esters absorbs UVB <320 nm). Only infrequently used now due to sensitizing potential. Benzophenones absorb UV and partially visible light. Dibenzoylmethanes (*e.g.* avobenzone) absorb UVA while cinnamates are UVB absorbers.
- **Inorganic sunscreens:** act by physically deflecting light and thus acting as barriers (sun blocks). Titanium dioxide, zinc oxide, kaolin, talc deflect light or simply impose a physical barrier. Effect not restricted to any specific waveband, though shorter wavelengths get scattered better. Also widely used in cosmetics.
- **SPF:** is a measure of protection provided by sunscreen (primarily against UVB). It is given by the ratio of the minimum erythema dose (MED) of the skin protected by sun screen to MED of the unprotected skin. Being a ratio, it has no unit.

Astringents

Precipitate surface proteins and reduce oozing. Useful in exudative conditions. Liquor aluminum acetate 0.52%; silver nitrate 0.05–2%.

Caustics

Act by chemical destruction of lesions; useful in removal of growths, xanthelasma, warts, Bowen's disease. Phenol 80% w/v solution of water and trichloroacetic acid are potent caustics. High concentrations of silver nitrate (10–20%) or low concentrations of trichloroacetic acid (5%) are mild caustics and used for destruction of epidermis or exuberant granulation tissue.

Ingenol Mebutate

Available as 0.15% gel. Causes mitochodrial swelling in dysplastic keratinocytes and cell death due to necrosis. FDA approved as 2–3 day treatment of actinic keratosis (once a day application).

INTRALESIONAL THERAPY

Involves deposition of active medicaments in suitable (mostly aqueous) vehicle with a dental syringe and fine needle or with a dermojet injector. Permits placement of high concentrations of drug at the site of disease. Slow release and sustained therapeutic effect additional advantages. Corticosteroids are the most frequently used intralesional preparations; triamcinolone acetonide and diacetate preferred because of small particle size and lack of crystal growth on storage. Useful in keloids, lichen simplex chronicus, hypertrophic lichen planus, discoid lupus erythematous and alopecia areata. Principal toxic effect: local atrophy and hypopigmentation. Several vaccines used for extensive cutaneous warts as inralesional agents-BCG, MMR, Mw. Intralesional bleomycin used for keloids, periungual warts. Intralesional 5-FU given for keloids/hypertrophic scars.

SYSTEMIC THERAPY

Indicated in situations where diseased area is not accessible to topical therapy—deep seated. Or widespread disease. Or the disease has a systemic component.

Antibacterial Agents

Chiefly antibiotics. Indicated in deep seated infections. Or when wide spread.
- *Streptococcal infections:* erysipelas, cellulitis, extensive impetigo contagiosa. Use penicillins—procaine penicillin injections daily. Or macrolides—erythromycin or azithromycin. For recurrent cellulitis—benzathine penicillin once in 3 weeks for several courses. All penicillins given after testing for allergy.
- *Staphylococcal infections:* furuncles, carbuncles, deep folliculitis. Preferably use antistaphylococcal antibioticscloxacillin or flucloxacillin. Patients with staphylococcal

scaled skin syndrome (SSSS) need aggressive, often parenteral antibiotics (cloxacillin. Or other penicillins in combination with β lactamase inhibitors—clavulanic acid or sulbactum) because of systemic toxemia. Other antibiotics such as tetracyclines or gentamycin infrequently used in pyodermas. Doxycycline—used in treatment of several sexually transmitted diseases. Tetracycline including minocycline used, for prolonged periods, in treatment of acne. As also in several unrelated conditions like bullous pemphigoid (tetracycline and niacinamide) and sarcoidosis (minocycline).

Antifungal Agents

Indicated in *Tinea capitis, Tinea barbae, Tinea unguium*, or widespread tinea corporis. And in systemic or deep mycotic infections.
- *Terbinafine:* an allylamine; fungicidal inhibits squalene epoxidase. Now the drug of choice for dermatophytic infection. Oral preparation ineffective in pityriasis versicolor and candidal infection (*c.f.* topical preparation). Given as daily doses, 250 mg daily for 2–12 weeks—the longer duration being for *Tinea unguium*. Pulsed schedule of terbinafine not as effective in *T. unguium*. Terbinafine useful in sporotrichosis and chromoblastomycosis.
- *Itraconazole:* a triazole; broad spectrum fungistatic agent—inhibits synthesis of ergosterol. Effective against dermatophytes, candida and *P. orbiculare*. Also effective against several deep fungal infections—aspergilli, histoplasma. Dose: onychomycosis—200 mg BD for 1 week every month, for 2–3 months. *T. capitis* (pediatric dose)— 3–5 mg/kg/daily—4–6 weeks. *For others*—200 mg daily for 1–2 weeks. Several drug interactions: antacids—reduce absorption; cisapride-causes sudden death; statins–rhabdomyolysis.
- *Fluconazole:* a triazole; broad spectrum fungistatic agent—inhibits synthesis of ergosterol. Effective against dermatophytes, candida and *P. orbiculare*. Also effective against several deep fungal infections—aspergillus, histoplasma, *Cryptococcus*. Dose: *dermatophytic infection*–150 mg once a week for 2–8 weeks. *Onychomycosis*—150–300 mg

weekly for 15–18 weeks. *Candidiasis and pityriasis versicolor*–150 mg single dose. Weekly dose useful in recurrent infections.

- **Ketoconazole:** a water soluble imidazole. Well absorbed orally (*c.f.* miconazole). Effective against dermatophytes, candida, *Cryptococcus* and coccidioidomyces but used infrequently due to hepatotoxicity. Dose: 200–400 mg/day.
- **Griseofulvin:** a penicillium derived fungistatic antibiotic effective against only dermatophytic species. With availability of other drugs, no longer a drug of choice. Dose: 10 mg/kg/day, preferably given, for better absorption, after a fatty meal. Length of treatment depends upon site of infection. Thus for *T. corporis*, 3–4 weeks and for *T. capitis* 6–8 weeks. *T. unguium* takes 3–6 months for finger nails and 6-18 months for toe nails. Drug interactions seen with barbiturates and coumarin anticogulants. Toxicity generally mild-headaches, gastrointestinal upsets; occasionally severe: photosensitivity, precipitation of porphyria cutanea tarda or acute intermittent porphyria and systemic lupus erythematosus. Resistance to drug uncommon.
- **Nystatin:** a polyene antibiotic. Not absorbed from the gut. Oral administration useful in buccal, esophageal or intestinal candidiasis and in cutaneous or other forms of candidiasis. Tablets of 500,000 units or oral suspension containing 100,000 units per ml given 3–4 times a day. Of little value in the treatment of systemic candidiasis.
- **Amphotericin B:** a polyene antibiotic effective against number of deep mycotic infections. Administered intravenously (absorption by oral route poor) in gradually increasing doses. Start with 1–5 mg/day and raise up to 0.65 mg/kg/day. Several side effects, including serious ones: headaches, chills, hemolytic anemia, phlebitis, anorexia, impaired renal function—reversible or permanent and fatal.
- **Flucytosine:** 5-fluorocytosine. Antifungal activity additive to that of amphotericin B. Mild to moderate toxicity-anemia, leukopenia, headaches, hallucinations and vertigo.
- **Potassium iodide:** almost specific for sporotrichosis and subcutaneous phycomycosis. Start with 5 drops of saturated solution,

administered in fruit juice, thrice daily and gradually build it up to 15 drops three times a day or till signs of iodism (lacrymation, epiphora) appear.

Antileprosy Therapy

For purpose of therapy, leprosy patients classified into paucibacil/ary (less than 6 lesions and 2 nerve trunks) or multibacillary (more than 5 lesions and 1 nerve trunk):

- **Dapsone (diaminodiphenyl sulphone, DDS):** primary drug in all but dapsone-resistant forms of leprosy. Bacteriostatic. Dose: 1–2 mg/kg/day administered as a single daily oral dose. Given for 6 months in paucibacillary and 1 year (or more in highly bacillated patients) in multibacillary leprosy. Hemolytic anemia, a universal but mild side effect. Serious toxicity rare—includes psychosis, hepatitis.
- **Rifampicin:** highly bactericidal morphological index (MI) and perhaps viability of bacteria reduced to zero within 4 weeks. Dose: single supervised 600 mg (or 450 mg for patients weighing 45 kg or less) once a month for 6 months in paucibacillary and for 1 year (or more in highly bacillated patients) in multibacillary leprosy. Empty stomach aids absorption. Always warn patient regarding changed color of urine. Hepatotoxic, nephrotoxic and causes 'flu-like' syndrome.
- **Clofazimine:** a fat soluble imino-phenazine compound. Bacteriostatic and anti-inflammatory. Employed in addition to rifampicin and dapsone in MDT of multibacillary leprosy. Dose: 50 mg/day unsupervised and 300 mg once a month under supervision given for 12 months (or longer in highly bacillated patients). Useful also in the treatment of type II reactions in leprosy; dose: 200–300 mg/day. Toxicity: reddish discoloration of skin and ichthyosiform change; skin discoloration may be objectionable and unacceptable.

All medicines started concurrently and discontinued after stipulated periods. Patients followed up for 2 years in paucibacillary and 5 years in multibacillary disease. In dapsone resistant cases, several alternatives available: minocycline, ofloxacin and clarithromycin.

- **Treatment of reactions in leprosy:** non-steroidal anti-inflammatory agents (NSAIDs) useful in mild to moderate type I or type II reactions. In severe type I reactions, corticosteroids may be used, particularly in impending nerve palsies. In type II reactions, corticosteroids better avoided, as patients are likely to become steroid-dependent. Use thalidomide instead—is almost as good. Notoriously teratogenic, hence avoided in females of child-bearing age. Intradermal Mw vaccine may be used as adjunct in the management of type II lepra reaction.

Antileishmanial Agents

Several choices available; none entirely satisfactory. Pentavalent antimonial, sodium stibogluconate, 330 mg/mL (equivalent to 100 mg of pentavalent antimony). Dose: 10 mg/kg/day. Average course: 6–10 injections for cutaneous leishmaniasis and 90–120 injections for post kala azar dermal leishmaniasis. Reasonable results. Rifampicin, metronidazole give inconsistent results. Ketoconazole 200–400 mg single daily dose, seems a promising alternative or additive. Systemic and local chloroquine therapy needs further evaluation. Miltefosine, 2.5 mg/kg/day for 28 days—a promising new oral therapy.

Corticosteroids

Revolutionary drugs in dermatologic therapeutics. Widely used in variety of dermatoses with high morbidity or high mortality. Often a life saving measure. *Common indications:* autoimmune bullous diseases (pemphigus, pemphigoid), collagen vascular diseases (systemic lupus erythematosus, dermatomyositis, systemic sclerosis). Or disseminated or severe dermatitis (air borne contact dermatitis). Or angioedema associated with respiratory symptoms. Or cutaneous T cell lymphoma. Or severe drug eruptions. Role of corticosteroids in Stevens Johnsons syndrome and toxic epidermal necrolysis is controversial-many patients receive systemic steroids. Use in psoriasis (except impetigo herpetiformis) and atopic dermatitis is best avoided. *Action:* anti-inflammatory, immuno-suppressive, antipruritic, keratoplastic or other ill-understood mechanisms.

Dose: varies depending on the nature, extent and severity of disease. Alternate day therapy preferred (patient's condition permitting) when long term corticosteroid treatment is required. Large parenteral or oral bolus 'pulse' therapy indicated in conditions needing long term therapy. Possibly induces remission faster; toxic effects similar, maybe less. Immunosuppressives, such as cyclophosphamide , methotrexate or azathioprine may be used as adjuvants- steroid sparing. *Adverse effects:* multiple and sometimes serious. *Cutaneous:* acne, hypertrichosis, striae, susceptibility to pyococcal or fungal infections. *Systemic:* hypertension, diabetes, reactivation of tuberculosis.

Immunosuppressive and Cytotoxic Agents

Used generally in psoriasis, pemphigus, mycosis fungoides and histiocytosis. Different modes of action; used alone. Or in combinations. May have steroid sparing effect. Some of the commonly used ones are:

- **Methotrexate:** an antimitotic agent. Acts by substrate competition for dihydrofolate reductase. Useful in erythrodermic, pustular, extensive plaque psoriasis and psoriatic arthropathy. Also used as an adjuvant to corticosteroids in pemphigus and dermatomyositis. Dose: 0.2–0.4 mg/kg once a week. Toxicity: bone-marrow depression, hepatocellular damage and cirrhosis, mucosal ulcerations, gastrointestinal haemorrhages. A close watch on liver functions required; periodic liver biopsies needed once the cumulative dose exceeds 1.5 g. Concomitant therapy with folic acid reduces toxicity.
- **Azathioprine:** a 6-mercaptopurine derivative. Used in pemphigus, systemic lupus erythematosus, air borne contact dermatitis and allergic vasculitis. Also an adjuvant in dermatomyositis and pyoderma gangrenosum. Dose: 3 mg/kg/day. Toxicity: bone-marrow depression, hepatocellular damage and infections.
- **Cyclophosphamide:** an alkylating agent. Used in mycosis fungoides, pemphigus and mUltisystem histiocytosis. Dose: 5–10 mg/kg bolus dose monthly followed by more conservative

daily dose of 1–2 mg/kg/day. Toxicity: alopecia (anagen effluvium), bonemarrow depression, liver damage, hemorrhagic cystitis. Regular monitoring with blood counts and urine examination.

- **Mycophenolate Mofetil:** It is a prodrug, inhibits inosine monophosphate dehydrogenase reducing purine synthesis and eventually decreased T and B lymphocytes. Dosage is 25–50 mg/kg/day, higher dose required for antibody mediated diseases. Not FDA approved for any dermatological indication, but may be used wherever steroid sparing effect is needed. Commonly associated GI intolerance.

- **Cyclosporine:** Works by inhibiting calcineurin, resulting in stoppage of IL-2 synthesis and effectively, inhibition of T cell activation and proliferation. Approved use in psoriasis and atopic dermatitis. Widely used wherever steroid sparing effect required. Dosage 2.5–5 mg/kg/day. Step up regimen in stable cases and step down used in crisis or widespread disease. Common side effects hypertension, hyperkalemia, deranged renal function (urea, creatinine) and dyslipidemias. Not to be co-administred with phototherapy as risk of cutaneous malignancy may increase.

- **Vinca alkaloids:** vincristine and vinblastine. Used intravenously in the treatment of mycosis fungoides and histiocytosis. Dose: vinblastine: 0.1 mg/kg/week with a weekly increment of 0.05 mg until a remission is induced or leukopenic response (commonest toxicity) is caused. Vincristine: 0.015–0.05 mg/kg or 2 mg/ sqm. Toxicity: neuropathy.

Biological Agents

Substances derived from living organisms. Of several types: fusion proteins (alefacept, etanercept, abatacept), monoclonal antibodies (infliximab, adalimumab, rituximab, ustekinumab), recombinant cytokines (Il-4, IL-10, IL-11, etc.) and immunotoxins (denileukin deftitox). Classification and indications of common biologics given in Table.

Agents Causing Pigmentation

- **Psoralens (+ UVA = PUVA):** Three chemicals: 5-methoxypsoralen, 8-methoxypsoralen and trimethoxypsoralen. All act as pigmentogenic agents through their phototoxic potential, hence need UVA (action spectrum of 320–400 nm with peak at 360 nm) following application/ ingestion. Improvement occurs with perifollicular pigmentation in most but not all patients. Non-hairy regions slow to repigment. Also effective in psoriasis due to antimitotic potential because of formation of photoadducts of psolarens with DNA.

Classification and indications of common biologics used in dermatology		
Target molecule	**Agent**	**Use**
	Inflixiab	Psoriasis, psoriatic arthiritis
	Adalimumab,	
TNF α antogonists	Etanercept	Psoriatic arthritis, rheumatoid arthritis, ankylosing spondylitis
	Golimumab	
	Certolizumab	Rheumatoid arthritis, Crohn's disease
T cell activation inhibitors	Alefacept, Abatacept	Psoriasis, rheumatoid arthritis
Anti IL 12/23 antibodies	Ustekinumab	Psoriasis
IL-17/IL-17R inhibitors	Secukinumab, Ixekizumab, Brodalumab	Under trial
Anti CD20	Rituximab	B-cell lymphomas, Pemphigus, connective tissue diseases (LE, dermatomyositis)
Anti IgE	Omalizumab	Asthma, atopicdermatitis, chronic urticaria

- **Systemic therapy:** used for treatment of extensive vitiligo, psoriasis, atopic dermatitis and plaque stage of mycosis fungoides. 8-methoxypsoralen (0.6 mg/kg) ingested on alternate days—daily treatment causes cumulative phototoxicity. Followed 1–2 hours later, by gradually increasing exposures to sunlight (PUVA sol) or to UVA sourced from special chambers. *Topical therapy:* useful in treatment of localised lesions of vitiligo and palmoplantar psoriasis. Psora len cream, ointment or alcoholic solution is applied, on alternate days, followed 30 minutes later, by gradually increasing exposures to sunlight or UVA. Side effects include mild to severe phototoxicity.

PRESCRIPTIONS FOR COMMON DERMATOSES

Superficial Bacterial Infections

- Remove crusts with soap and water washes. Or weak Condy's lotion (1 in 8000–10,000 potassium permanganate aqueous solution) compresses or soaks.
- Topical creams (not ointments) containing an antibiotic such as mupirocin or fucidic acid.
- For widespread infection: use systemic antibiotics like erythromycin (has advantage of covering both *Staphylococcus* and *Streptococcus*.
- If staphylococcal infection suspected: preferably use a penicillinase-resistant penicillin, such as cloxacillin or flucloxacillin
- In staphylococcal scalded skin syndrome (SSSS), aggressive treatment, often with parenteral antibiotics (cloxacillin. Or other penicillins in combination with β lactamase inhibitors—clavulanic acid or sulbactum) are used.

Deep Bacterial Infections

- Remove slough/crusts with 3–5% hydrogen peroxide or weak potassium permanganate solution.
- Appropriate supportive treatment such as rest and analgesics should be given.
- Simple furuncles—treated with moist or dry heat. Fluctuant furuncles or those 'pointing' and carbuncles need to be carefully incised and drained.
- Ampicillin + clavulanic acid. Or cloxacillin (2 g/day) in divided doses orally. Parenteral therapy may be needed in case of multiple carbuncles and if patient debilitated or immunosuppressed. To be continued for at least 2–3 days after subsidence of inflammation.

Dermatophytic Infections

Tinea cruris/extensive T. corporis/T. faciei: any of the following used:
- **Allylamines:** terbinafine 1%, naftifine 1%. Applied for 1–2 weeks.
- **Imidazole preparations:** miconazole nitrate 2%, clotrimazole 1%, econazole 1%, ketoconazole, 2%. Applied twice a day for 4 weeks.
- **Tolnaftate 1%:** Applied twice a day for 4 weeks.
- **Haloprogin 1%:** Applied twice a day for 4 weeks.

Extensive T. corporis/recurrent T. cruris/T.pedis: any of the following used:
- Terbinafine: 250 mg daily for 2 weeks.
- Itraconazole 200–400 mg daily for 1–2 weeks.

T. capitis: depending on type:
- Non-inflammatory variety: terbinafine: 3–5 mg/kg mg daily for 6 weeks.
- Inflammatory variety: itraconazole 5–10 mg/kg daily for 6 weeks.

T. ungiuim/onychomycosis: any of the following used:
- Terbinafine: 250 mg daily for 8 (finger nails)–12 (toe nails) weeks.
- Itraconazole 200 mg daily for 1 week every month for 12 weeks.
- When distal 1/2 of single nail plate involved: topical amorolfine 5% lacquer once a week or ciclopirox olamine 8% lacquer daily for 6–9 months.

In all types of dermatophytic infection, the area should be kept dry. In case of recurrent infection, look for a reservoir of infection e.g., *T. ungiuim.*

Pityriasis Versicolor

- Almost all topical anti-dermatophytic applications are effective. Alternatively 2.5% selenium sulphide suspension may be used—apply at the time of bath, leave for 5–10 minutes and rinse off. Or apply once or twice a week at bed time and wash off the following morning. Frequent or prolonged applications may cause local irritation.

- Keep body dry.

Candidal Infections

- *For localized infections:* imidazole preparations: miconazole nitrate 2%, clotrimazole 1%, econazole 1%, ketoconazole, 2%. Applied twice a day for 4 weeks. Or nystatin cream or powder (100,000 units/g).
- *For recurrent/extensive infections:* oral treatment with itraconazole 200 mg daily for 1 week; fluconazole 150 mg once a week for 2 weeks. In recurrent/extensive infections—rule out diabetes mellitus. Or an immunosuppressed state.
- Keep area dry.

Scabies

Any of the following may be used:

- *Permethrin 5% cream:* single application for 8–12 hours, after bath. Can be used in children (including neonates) and pregnant women.
- *Gamma benzene hexachloride 1% lotion/ cream:* single application of 8–12 hours, after bath—but not hot water bath. Do not use in children below 5 years of age. Nor in pregnant women.
- *Benzyl benzoate 10–25% emulsion:* 3 applications at intervals of 8–12 hours. Lower concentration in children and pregnant women.
- *Crotamiton 10%:* twice daily application for 1 week. Preferred treatment in children.
- *For pruritis:* antihistamines to be given for 1–2 weeks, as itching persists for several days. Crotamiton can also be prescribed for the same period.
- *For nodular and eczematised lesions:* topical steroid in addition.
- *For secondary infection:* a course of systemic antibiotics—azithromycin for 3 days.

Following instructions: should be carefully adhered to:

- All medications to be applied, after soap and water scrub bath, all over the body, below the neck. Special care to be given to genitals and subungual region.
- In case a bath is taken, re-apply medication soon after.
- Routine washing or cleaning of personal garments and bed clothes. Expose to sunlight for 4–8 hours before laundering.
- All members of the family to be treated—even those asymptomatic—at the same time.

Pediculosis

Pediculosis capitis

- *Any of the following may be used:*
  - ➤ Permethrin 1% lotion left on the scalp for 8–12 hours is the treatment of choice because of its safety profile and residual effect. Or shampoo left on, for 5–10 minutes.
  - ➤ Gamma benzene hexachloride 1%, rubbed thoroughly and left overnight under a shower cap; followed by shampoo; repeated after 7–10 days. Alternatively, the hair may be washed with gamma benzene hexachloride shampoo, to be repeated, if necessary, after a week.
  - ➤ Malathion 0.5% applied for 12 hours. Has residual effect which prevents reinfection for 6 weeks.
- *All close contacts:* to be treated at the same time. And combs and head wear treated with lysol or pediculocidal agents.

Pediculosis pubis

Single or two weekly applications of one of the above preparations. Important to treat sexual partners. *If eye brows/lashes involved:* apply white petrolatum and remove nits and adult individually.

Pediculous corporis

Important: improvement in personal hygiene-regular soap and water baths. Disinfestation of clothes with 10% DDT powder. Or gamma benzene hexachloride. Or simply hot iron.

Acute Exudative Dermatitis

- Condy's lotion compresses/soaks/bath 2–3 times a day.
- Topical application of 1% aluminium acetate or silver nitrate—both are astringents and so reduce exudation.

- Topical application of betamethasone 17-valerate. Or fluocinolone acetonide. Or clobetasol propionate. Or any other appropriate corticosteroid cream or gel (with antibiotic combination, if lesions are infected), twice a day. If potent steroid used, substitute with less potent ones as improvement occurs.
- Systemic antihistamines, 2–3 times a day to control itching; antihistamines do not alter the course of the disease.
- If generalized/extensive: short course of systemic corticosteroids, daily dose (20–40 mg of prednisolone equivalent).

Acute Non-exudative Dermatitis

- Treatment similar to exudative dermatitis except omit steps (i) and (ii).
- As inflammation subsides, potent topical corticosteroids substituted with midpotency and later low potency corticosteroids or by cold cream or shake lotions such as calamine lotion.

Chronic/Lichenified Dermatitis

- Topical application of betamethasone 17-valerate or fluocinolone acetonide or another potent steroid ointment preferably under occlusive dressing (unsuitable for hot, humid climates!!). Or betamethasone or fluocinolone acetonide with 10–20% urea or 3% salicylic acid in cream base.
- Systemic antihistamines, if required, to control itching. For all eczemas, avoid scratching.
- *Special situations:* in stasis eczema, keep foot elevated. In napkin dermatitis, keep area dry and aerated. Avoid occlusive napkins.

Mild-moderate Acne

- Wash face with soap, 3–4 times a day—enough to render it dry and non-oily.
- Retinoic acid 0.025 or 0.05%, gel or cream. Apply locally small quantities—enough to lightly cover the face, at bed time. Wash off in the morning.
- Benzoyl peroxide 2, 5 or 10% cream or lotion twice a day;

- Erythromycin lotion 1% for local application 2–3 times a day.
- Clindamycin lotion 1% for local use 2–3 times a day.

Severe Acne: Nodulocystic Variety and Acne Conglobata

- Systemic tetracycline 500 mg–1 g/day for several days or weeks, depending on response; along with a topical agent—retinoic acid or benzoyl peroxide.
- *Isotretinoin:* now drug of choice. 0.5–1 mg/kg/day, given after the heaviest meal of the day for a period of 12-16 weeks. In females: rule out pregnancy (potential teratogenic); as also advise contraception beginning 1 month prior to onset of therapy and for 3 months after stopping treatment. Side effects: all patients complain of dryness of skin and cheilitis—self limiting. Monitor at baseline and bimonthly particularly for derangements of lipid profile and liver functions. Initial flare seen in a few patients is self-limiting—if severe control with short course of corticisteroids.

Psoriasis

Topical therapy for patients with localized disease and systemic for patient with extensive disease. Phototherapy and photochemotherapy important modalities of treatment.

Psoriasis involving < 10% body surface area (BSA)

Use any of the following:
- Coal tar preparation: apply at night and wash next morning. Exposure to sunlight may improve efficacy.

Crude coal tar	10
Salicylic acid	5
Yellow soft paraffin to make	100
Dithranol	0.1–0.5
Yellow soft paraffin	100

Apply under cover and wash off after 4 hours. Reduce concentration or duration of application, if irritation occurs. Or try 'short contact' therapy with 2–5% anthralin and washing off after V2 hour.

Psoriasis of scalp: betamethasone dipropionate lotion. Or a steroid foam preparation to be used at night. Shampoo next morning.

Psoriasis involving 10–50% BSA

Phototherapy/photochemotherapy treatment of choice. Phototherapy involves irradiation of skin with *sunlamps* that emit UVB, while photochemotherapy (PUVA) involves administration of psoralen, followed 2–3 hrs later, by exposure to black light lamps (that emit UVA). Or sunlight (PUVA sol). All exposure to be made after application of an emollient to reduce scattering of light. Indicated in patients not responding to tar/anthralin therapy. Or not wanting or tolerating these 'messy' medications

Psoriasis involving >50% BSA, Erythrodermic and Pustular Variants

Any of the following may be used:
- Methotrexate drug of choice. Weekly doses- 7.5–22.5 mg given with daily doses of folic acid (5 mg). Response dramatic in pustular psoriasis less in plaque variants. Causes mucositis. Suppresses bone marrow and hepatotoxic; so baseline and initially fortnightly monitoring of liver function and hematological parameters. Later less frequently (once a month. And later once in 3 months). Some drug interactions important— aspirin, sulphonamides and tetracyclines. Do not use in pregnant/lactating women and HIV-positive patients.
- Aromatic retinoid, acitretin, (1 mg/kg/ day) for several weeks. Given in patients who cannot be given methotrexate—HIV-positive patients and those who have anemia. Response dramatic in pustular psoriasis less in plaque variants. In females: rule out pregnancy (potential teratogenic); as also advise contraception beginning 1 month prior to onset of therapy and for 24 months after stopping treatment. Side-effects: all patients complain of dryness of skin and chielitis—self limiting. Monitor at baseline and bimonthly particularly for derangements of lipid profile and liver functions.
- Methotrexate and acitretin can be combined with phototherapy/photochemotherapy. Always use an emollient.

- Cyclosporine can also be used (@2.5–5 mg/ kg/day). Usually given as step down regimen-started at full dose (5 mg/kg/day), gradually tapered to 2.5 mg/kg/day over several weeks, followed by either maintanence dose or stopping and switching over to conventional therapies. Not recommended to combined with phototherapy or methotrexate. Monitor for deranged renal function, dyselectrolytemia, hypertension and dyslipidemia.
- Care, often inpatient, required in patients with erythroderma or pustular psoriasis.

Vitiligo

Localized lesions need topical, while widespread lesions (or those where topical application may be hazardous, e.g. near the eyes) need systemic psora len therapy followed by exposure to UVA or sunlight. Rapidly progressive lesions need, to be treated with oral corticosteroids.
- ***Topical PUVA:*** Use 8-methoxypsoralen 0.25–1% lotion or cream: Apply locally (as such. Or diluted with rectified spirit or cream base. Or with a topical corticosteroid preparation) on alternate days, followed V2 hour later by exposure to gradually increasing doses of sunlight. Or UVA. Start with 1/2–1 minute of light exposure and increase by 30 seconds every week or fortnight till a faint pink color appears 24 hours after sunlight exposure.
- ***Systemic PUVA:*** Psoralen (0.6 mg/kg) given, as 8-methoxypsoralen or trimethylpsoralen, on alternate days after meals and exposed 2–3 hours later to gradually increasing doses of sunlight (or UVA). Start with 2–5 minutes (or 1–2 J/cm^2 of UVA) and add increments of 1–2 minutes (or 0.5 J/cm^2) every week till a faint pink erythema appears 24 hours after exposure. 5-methoxypsoralen also used—better tolerated. Side effects: nausea, discomfort. Phototoxicity: can be minimized by reducing duration of sun exposure or dose of UVA.
- ***Corticosteroids:*** Given in patients with rapidly progressive vitiligo. Can be given as daily dose for initial period of therapy (4–6 weeks). Or preferably as weekly bolus dose—conveniently termed as oral mini pulse. Always monitor patient for side effects.

- Immunosuppressants like cyclophosphamide, azathioprine may be used as steroid sparing agents or stand alone therapies in progressive vitiligo.

Hyperpigmentary Disorders

Melasma

- *To reduce pigmentation:* can prescribe any of the following applications at night
  - Hydroquinone cream 2–5% for local application at bed time.
  - Combination of: hydroquinone 2% retinoic acid 0.025–0.05% and hydrocortisone/mometasone
  - Azelaic acid 10–20%
  - Kojic acid 2%
- *To protect from sunlight:* preferable to avoid sun exposure between 11 AM and 2 PM. Use of umbrellas, broad brimmed hats.
- *Sunscreens:* all sunscreens need to be applied several times (at least 3 times a day—usually at 8 AM, 12 noon and 4 PM. Several options available:
  - Organic sunscreens
  - Inorganic sunscreens

Lichen Planus Pigmentosus

- Vitamin A 50,000–100,000 units/day for 2 weeks followed by a gap of 2 weeks; the courses may be repeated for 6–8 times. Oral isotretinoin (0.3–0.5 mg/kg/day) has been used off late with encouraging results.

FORMULATIONS OF HISTORICAL VALUE!!

Chemical	Conc/Proportion
i. Calamine lotion	
Calamine*	15
Zinc oxide	5
Bentonite**	3
Sodium citrate	0.5
Glycerine	5
Aqua	to make 100

*Calamine is zinc carbonate with ferric oxide as a coloring agent.
**Bentonite is a suspending agent.

ii. Calamine liniment	
Calamine	15
Peanut oil	50
Calcium hydroxide	to make 100
iii. Simple ointment B.P.	
Wool fat	5
Hard paraffin	5
Cetostearyl alcohol	5
White or yellow soft paraffin	85
iv. Lanolin (hydrous wool fat) B.P.	
Wool fat (anhydrous lanolin)	70 g
Purified water	30 mL
v. Oily cream B.P.	
Wool alcohol ointment	50
Purified water	50
vi. Emulsifying ointment	
Emulsifying wax	30
White soft paraffin	50
Liquid paraffin	20
vii. Compound zinc paste (zinc paste) B.P.	
Zinc oxide, finely sifted	25
Starch, finely sifted	25
White soft paraffin	50
viii. Zinc-salicylic acid paste (Lassar's paste) B.P.	
Zinc oxide, finely sifted	24
Salicylic acid, finely sifted	2
Starch, finely sifted	24
White soft paraffin	50
ix. Salicylic acid ointment B.P.	
Salicylic acid	2
Wool alcohol ointment	98
x. Coal tar solution (Liq. picis carbon is) B.P.	
Prepared coal tar	20
Quillaia (coarse powder)	10
Alcohol (90%) to make	100
xi. Lotio alba	
Potassium sulphurata	5
Zinc sulfate	1
Resorcinol	1
Rectified spirit	10
Water to make	100

23

Diagnostic and Therapeutic Photomedicine

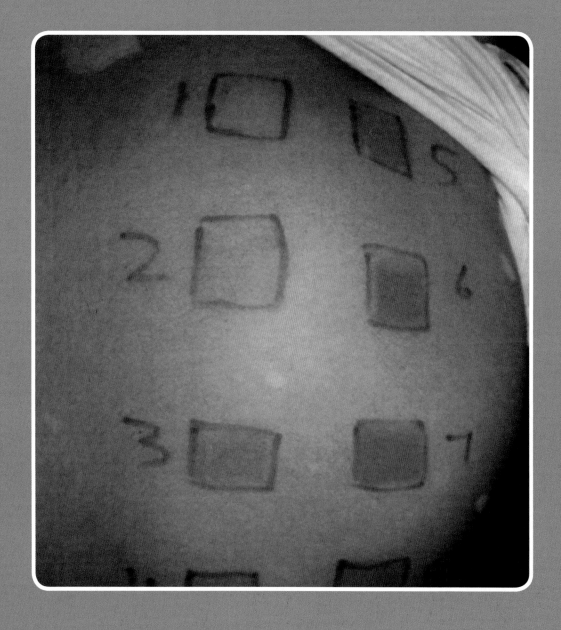

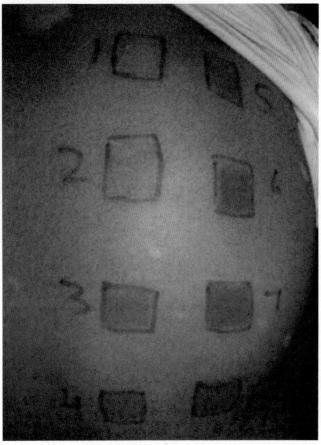

Determination of minimal erythemogenic dose (MED) for narrow band UVB therapy of vitiligo; MED seen in window 2.

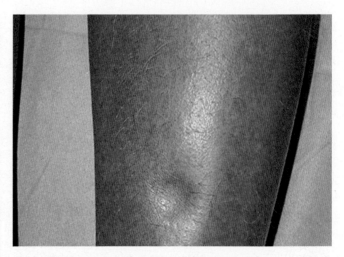

Phototoxicity: marked erythema and edema (shown by pitting) over the shins in a patient on oral PUVA.

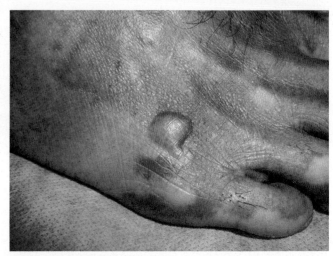

Phototoxicity: blistering and marked erythema over vitiligo patch in patient on oral PUVA sol.

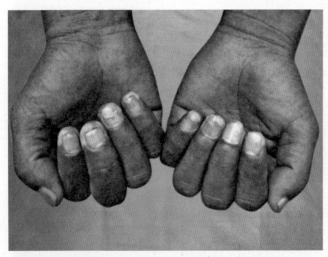

Chronic phototoxicity: photo-oncholysis in patient on long-term PUVA therapy.

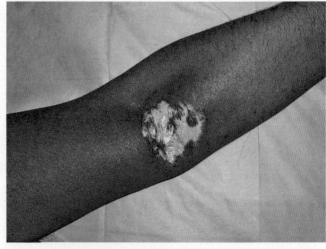

Chronic phototoxicity: thickening and scaling over a vitiligo patch after long-term oral PUVA treatment.

Photomedicine, study of and application of interaction of ultraviolet light (UVL) and visible light (VL) with human tissue. Result—complex biologic effects with beneficial or harmful consequences.

DIAGNOSTIC PHOTOMEDICINE

Photopatch Test

For diagnosis of photoallergic contact dermatitis; irradiation of antigen applied on skin with UVA because most photoallergens for which information is available react to UVA. Another reason-lower wavelengths even if allergen shows strong adsorption, the dosage required to produce photoallergy will be greater than the normal sunburn response.

Method: two identical strips of allergens placed on patient's back: control and test strip. Contact sensitivity determined at 48 hours. Overall, PUVA therapy chambers are convenient, especially hand and foot panel mounted vertically on wall. One side (test) irradiated with 5–10 J/cm^2 of UVA (in skin types 1 to 3, MED should be calculated and then UVA at 50% of MED given), second (control) side kept covered during irradiation. Read after another 48 hours for photoallergy. Control—negative; test side—positive indicates photoallergy to that antigen.

Phototesting

Exposure of the skin to incremental doses of UV or visible radiation followed by recording of skin responses. Uses:
- *Diagnostic:* in suspected photosensitivity, calculation of minimal erythema dose (MED), photoprovocation.
- *Therapeutic:* MED/minimal phototoxic dose (MPD) calculation for appropriate phototherapy/photochemotherapy.

- *Others:* monitoring of disease activity and response to treatment, check efficacy of sunscreens.
- *Method:* ideal, but very expensive, equipment is irradiation monochromator. Practically, NBUVB, PUVA chambers and slide projector (as source of visible light) may be used. Application of a UV opaque template with several apertures (mostly over back) able to be covered or uncovered in turn and different doses are achieved for each uncovered site. Increments of 40% (or square root of 2) are given in a geometric progression. Erythema checked after irradiation and again after 24 hours for UVB. For UVA, erythema checked after 48–72 hours. Positive reaction is taken as erythema covering all 4 corners of the square template. MED values found in Indian studies-BBUVB (10–61 mJ/ cm^2); NBUVB (500–1100 mJ/ cm^2); for UVA, MED has not been achieved till date. Amongst idiopathic photodermatoses, MED is lowered in following: actinic prurigo (mainly to UVA), hydroa vacciniforme (mainly to UVA) and chronic actinic dermatitis (UVB>UVA>visible).

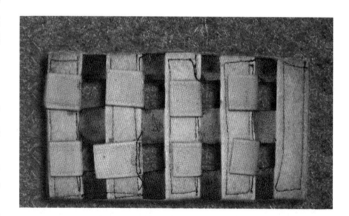

Phototesting template: opaque template with coverable windows.

Interpretation of photopatch test		
Reading at unexposed site	*Reading at UVA exposed site*	*Interpretation*
—	—	No allergy
—	++	Photoallergy
+	+	Contact allergy
+	++	Contact allergy with photoaggravation

RESPONSE TO ORAL PUVA THERAPY IN GENERALIZED VITILIGO

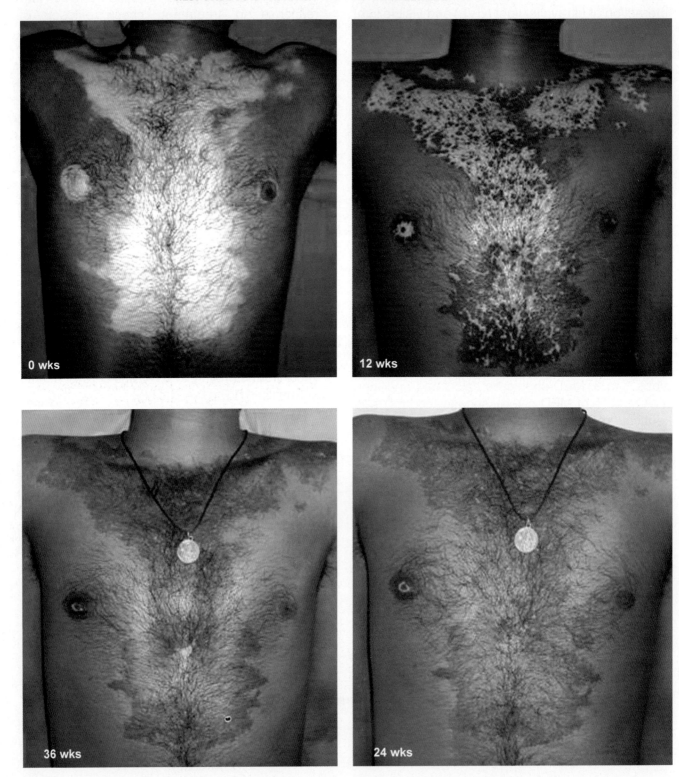

WOOD'S LAMP

Variety of photopatch test series allergens are used to detect the culprit allergen like sunscreen chemicals, antibacterials, fragrance ingredients, miscellaneous compounds etc. Photopatch positivity is seen (often with multiple antigens) in patients with chronic actinic dermatitis.

Wood's lamp emits UVL between 320 and 400 nm, peak at 365 nm.

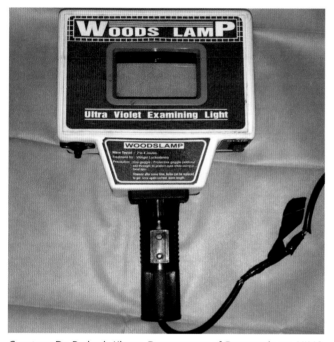

Courtesy: Dr. Prakash Khute, Department of Dermatology, AIIMS, New Delhi.

Applications: diagnosis of superficial fungal infections (tinea capitis, pityriasis versicolor), bacterial infections (Pseudomonas infections, erythrasma). Detection of porphyrins (teeth, urine, stool, red blood cells and blister fluid) fluorescence under Wood's light, diagnostic. Also for pigmentary disorders (vitiligo, ash leaf macules in white skin)—color variation enhanced. Also used to decide judge level of melasma: if margins are sharp and accentuate with wood's lamp, it is epidermal melasma; if margins are faded and do not accentuate, it is mixed or dermal melasma. Currently this is not a reliable method and also the concept of dermal melasma itself is questionable.

THERAPEUTIC PHOTOMEDICINE

Principle

Phototherapy (using UVB-290–320 nm; UVA1-340–400 nm) and photochemotherapy (using psoralens with UVA, 320–400 nm, so termed PUVA) well-established treatment modalities in dermatology. Main use in psoriasis and vitiligo. Application broadened in recent years. Mechanism of action shown in table. Further, the mechanisms common to both UVA and UVB include-increased regulatory T-cells and reduced effector T-cells, locally increased levels of IL-10, decreased keratinocyte expression of CD-54 (ICAM-1) which reduces T-cell binding to keratinocytes. These

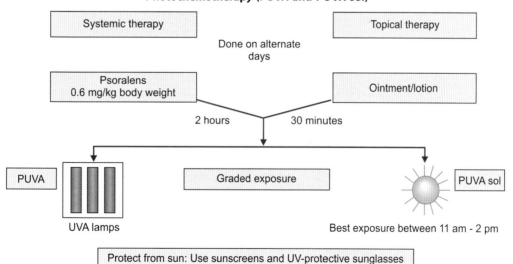

lead to improvement in T-cell mediated diseases like psoriasis, atopic dermatitis, cutaneous T-cell lymphoma, etc. T-cell apoptosis has been demonstrated for UVA1 in atopic dermatitis and NBUVB in psoriasis. Exact mechanisms in vitiligo unknown but findings include-activation of follicular melanocytes, increased number, hypertrophy, melanization and migration of melanocytes. Other UVA1 and PUVA mechanisms-activation of matrix metalloproteinases useful in sclerotic diseases and apoptosis of mast cells and stabilization of mast cell membrane useful in mastocytosis.

Erythema, a limiting factor in therapeutic photomedicine. Graded as EO (no erythema), E1 (minimally perceptible erythema: faint pink), E2 (marked erythema: red), E3 (fiery red erythema with edema), E4 (fiery red erythema with edema and blistering). E1 should not be exceeded. Pigmented patients do not develop perceptible erythema—instead, complain of hotness and tightness of skin.

Minimal erythemogenic dose (MED): dose of UVB required to produce E1 grade erythema, 24 hours after exposure.

Minimal phototoxic dose (MPD): dose of UVA required to produce E1 reaction after ingestion of psoralens, 48 hours after exposure.

UVB Phototherapy

UVB light, 290–320 nm; narrow band UVB (NB-UVB), 311 +/- 2 nm. BBUVB not used any more for risk of cutaneous malignancy, burns, pigmentation.

Method: determine MED before starting treatment. Start with 70% of MED. Increase dose by 10–20% at each sitting, till E1 achieved treatment usually administered 2–3 days per week. In India, the usual dosing followed is: starting at 250–500 mj/cm^2 (commonly 280–300 mj/cm^2) and increasing it by 20% every sitting up to maximum of 1.2–2 J/cm^2, depending on the patient's tolerance. Therapy given on 2–3 days per week (usually alternate days).

Indications: psoriasis (chronic plaque type): NB-UVB phototherapeutic modality of choice. As effective as PUVA therapy, does not require psoralens, safe in pregnancy and children, circumvents need for photoprotection (for eyes). Effectively used in combination with tar (Goeckerman regimen). Or dithranol (Ingram regimen). Vitiligo, atopic dermatitis, lichen planus, pityriasis lichenoides et varioliformis acuta (PLEVA), pityriasis lichenoides chronica (PLC), pityriasis rosea and uremic pruritus, granuloma annulare, etc.

Mechanism of action of phototherapy/ photochemotherapy	
UVA	*UVB*
Reaches up to mid to lower dermis	Reaches up to superficial dermis
Less efficient than UVB in forming pyrimidine dimers	Pyrimidine dimers, 6,4 pyrimidine-pyrimidine photoproducts
Reactive oxygen intermediates damage DNA, lipids, structural and non-structural proteins and organelles such as mitochondria	Conversion of trans- to cis-urocanic acid which mediates cutaneous immunosuppression
Psoralen compounds intercalate with DNA causing termination of replication	Conversion of tryptophan into a complex compound which activates the prostaglandin E2 pathway
Psoralens augment singlet oxygen production which activates arachidonic acid pathway	Reactive oxygen intermediates which cause DNA, lipid peroxidation, stimulates cytokine production

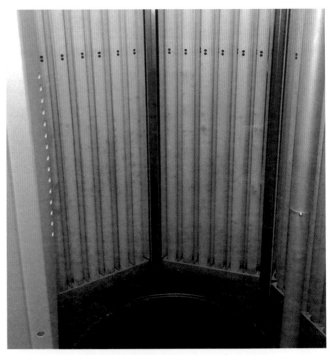
Whole body narrow band UVB phototherapy chamber.

Photochemotherapy

Exposure to UVA light following use of psoralens, topical or systemic. Psoralens (natural or synthetic —tricyclic furocoumarins) bind to DNA base pairs, producing cross-linking within the double helix strand, on UVA exposure. Results in suppression of DNA synthesis and cell division.

PUVA

Method: systemic, psoralens (8-methoxypsoralen at 0.4–0.6 mg/kg, trimethylpsoralen at 0.6–1.2 mg/kg and 5-methoxypsoralen at 1.2–1.8 mg/kg) administered 1 Y2-2 hours before UVA exposure, in especially designed chambers fitted with fluorescent tubes. Systemic psoralens generally prescribed when disease extent is >10% body surface area. Topical, psoralens applied locally (solution, ointment, cream or bath) Yz hour before UVA exposure. For both-starting dose of UVA, 70%

of MPD. In Indian scenario or darker skin types, MPD not calculated. PUVA is started at the UVA dose of 1.5–2 J/cm^2 and increased by 0.25–0.5 J/cm^2 on every third sitting, this effectively means 1 increment every week. Treatment prescribed on alternate days (or less frequently) to prevent cumulative phototoxicity.

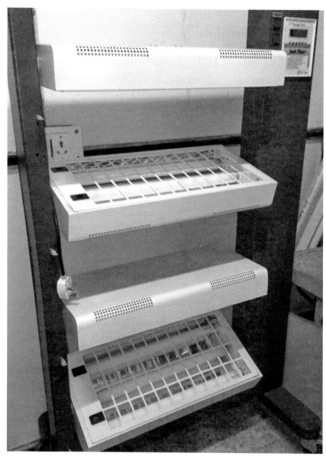

Hand and foot UVA machine.

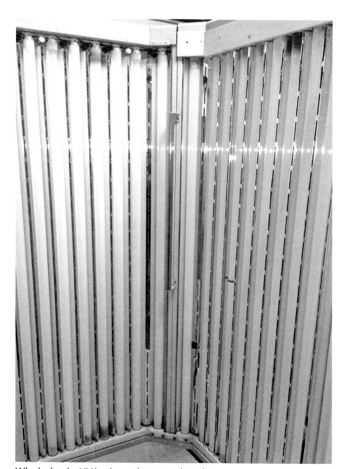

Whole body UVA phototherapy chamber.

Indications: Psoriasis: in extensive chronic plaque psoriasis. Best avoided in unstable form-generalized pustular and erythrodermic psoriasis.

Mycosis fungoides (CTCL): used in patch and plaque stage. Vitiligo: response better on face than on limbs and trunk. Other indications: atopic dermatitis, lichen planus, PLEVA, PLC, prurigo nodularis, polymorphic light eruption solar urticaria, chronic actinic dermatitis, morphea, chronic graft versus host disease, generalized granuloma annulare, Langerhan's cell histiocytosis and mastocytosis.

Contraindications: pregnancy, children (< 12-years), photosensitivity, severe cardiac, hepatic or renal disease, history of skin cancers, aphakia or cataracts and immunosuppressed states.

Complications: systemic PUVA—nausea, phototoxicity (pruritus, erythema, edema and blistering), skin thickening and scaling (esp in vitiligo patches which tend to become plaques with chronic exposure), prematurely aged skin and cutaneous malignancies (no risk reported in skin types 4–6, no Indian reports till date) and cataracts. Topical PUVA: phototoxicity, photoallergic contact dermatitis, hyperpigmentation, rarely hypertrichosis.

PUVA sol (psoralens + solar exposure)

Method: Direct sunlight used instead of UVA chamber. Systemic therapy, affected parts exposed to direct sunlight (best between 11 AM and 2 PM), 2 hours after ingestion of psoralens (dose, vide supra). Initial exposure 2 minutes, increased gradually to maximum of 15 minutes (as tolerated). Topical therapy, psoralens (0.01–0.1% solution of 8-MOP; usually 1% solution is diluted 30–40 times in propylene glycol) applied ½ hour before sun exposure—for 1 minute initially, gradually increasing to 5 minutes (as tolerated). Repeat every alternate day.

Indications: as for PUVA therapy. Effective, cheap, home-based ecofriendly treatment, if patient can expose conveniently. When compared with PUVA for psoriasis, it is more cost-effective with almost similar efficacy. When compared to PUVA for vitiligo, it is slower in repigmenting, less efficacious and produces less improvement in quality of life parameters.

Bath PUVA and Bath Suit PUVA/PUVA Sol

A variation in topical PUVA/PUVA sol. In bath PUVA, solution prepared by mixing 50 mL of psoralen solution (8-MOP) with 100 liters of water. Patient soaks in this solution for 15 minutes followed by sun-exposure or UVA chamber. In bath suit, 0.8 mL of 8-MOP solution added to 2 liters of water and bathing suit soaked in it. After squeezing out excess water, suit is worn for 15 minutes, then it is removed and body is exposed to sun or UVA. Advantages—no systemic psoralen side effects, ease and uniformity of application, and less UVA/sun-exposure dose required.

Turban PUVA/PUVA Sol

Modification in which a cloth is soaked in diluted 8-MOP solution and worn as a turban on scalp followed by sun-exposure/UVA. Helpful in case of scalp psoriasis, may help scalp vitiligo.

Turbo PUVA

Modification of oral PUVA studied for psoriasis. Sunless tanning agent dihydroxyacetone (DHA) is applied all over body. And usual course of oral PUVA started. DHA was noted to peel off later from the normal skin than psoriatic plaques, hence protecting the normal skin. Thus UVA could be given at high doses leading to quicker remission and better skin tolerance than in those patients who did not use DHA.

TARGETED PHOTOTHERAPY

Implies the use of various technologies which deliver the phototherapy only to the lesion and sparing the uninvolved skin. It includes: excimer laser, photodynamic therapy, intense pulse light therapy, low-level laser and light emitting diode therapy.

Excimer Laser

Delivers a specific wavelength (308 nm) of UVB radiation. Focused excimer laser/ light over localized lesions. Xenon chloride is lasing medium. Usual spot size of 1x1 cm, energy of around 3 mj/cm^2 per pulse at frequency of up to 200 Hz. Able to treat small lesions or large lesions over multiple sittings. Found useful in both vitiligo and psoriasis, in previously resistant lesions as well. Tested useful in other dermatoses like oral lichen planus, alopecia areata, topic dermatitis, mycosis fungoides, etc. But lesions at poorly responsive sites do not respond as well. Fairly expensive machine and not so impressive response. Only advantage is sparing of normal skin thus reducing long-term risk of malignancy in fairer skin types 1–3. Side effects include-local erythema, crusting, blistering.

Photodynamic Therapy (PDT)

A new therapeutic modality for malignant and non-malignant disorders. Requires a photosensitizing compound in presence of VL and oxygen.

Method: photosensitizers (porphyrins, 5-aminolevulinic acid, phthalocyanines, chlorin derivatives and porphycenes) administered topically, intralesionally or systemically, accumulate in target cells. Site selectively irradiated with VL in presence of oxygen. Peroxides, superoxide ions, hydroxyl radicals and singlet oxygen formed —result in direct as well as indirect cell damage (due to initiation of free radical chain reaction). PDT effectively combined with surgery and chemotherapy.

Indications: premalignant and malignant conditions (actinic keratosis, actinic cheilitis, Bowen's disease, keratoacanthoma, basal cell carcinoma, squamous cell carcinoma , malignant melanoma, mycosis fungoides, cutaneous metastasis from breast and Kaposi's sarcoma). Also in non-malignant conditions (psoriasis, common and genital warts, herpes simplex infection and port-wine stain). Advantages: selective damage, good cosmetic result.

Side effects: insignificant; erythema, edema, burning sensation, stinging or itching—limited to the illuminated site. Systemic PDT—occasionally long lasting generalized cutaneous photosensitivity.

EXTRACORPOREAL PHOTOPHERESIS

Extracorporeal exposure of blood fractions like plasma and blood cells to UVA light in presence of psora lens. To treat Sezary syndrome (erythrodermic cutaneous T-cell lymphoma). Also effective in atopic dermatitis, pemphigus vulgaris, chronic graft vs host disease and connective tissue disorders (systemic sclerosis, systemic lupus erythematosus, rheumatoid arthritis and dermatomyositis). Treat for 2 consecutive days, every 2–4 weeks. Advantage: good safety profile.

BALNEOPHOTOTHERAPY

Consists of bath with concentrated sodium chloride solution (as of Dead Sea) followed immediately by UVB exposure. Acts by elution of leukocyte elastase from skin surface. Or by anti-inflammatory effect of magnesium ions. Used mainly in psoriasis.

24

Cosmetic Dermatology

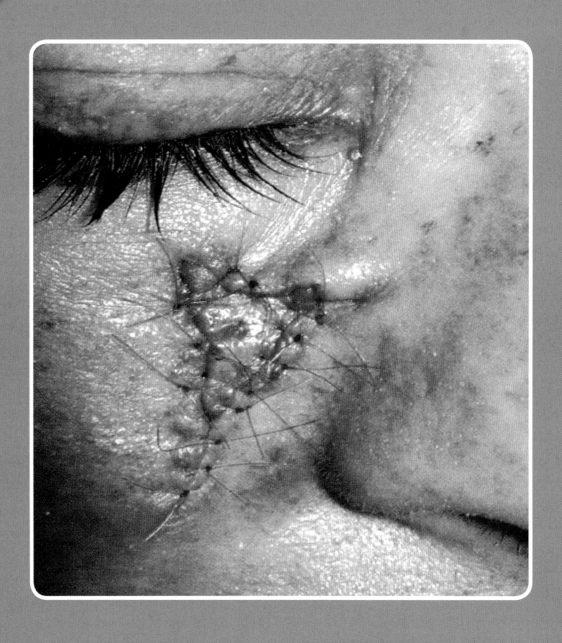

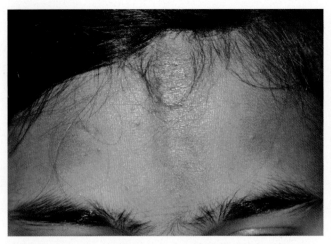

Linear morphea on forhead (en-coup-de-sabre) at baseline

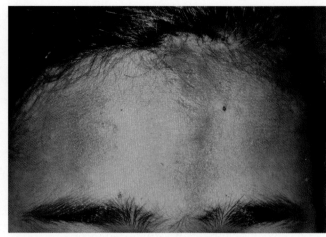

Linear morphea immediately after intradermal calcium hydroxyla-petite injection. Note the filling of defect and reduced pigmentation in the plaque.

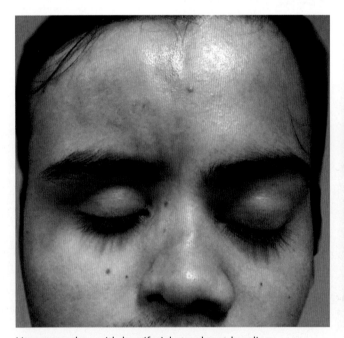

Linear morphea with hemifacial atrophy, at baseline.

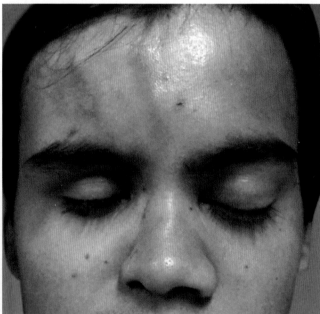

Linear morphea with hemifacial atrophy, 7 days after autologous fat injection. Note filling of the forehead defetcs and fullness of the medial right cheek which was depressed at baseline.

Cosmetic products (cosmeceuticals): substances or preparations applied on skin, mucosae, hair, nails, teeth or external genitalia to clean, perfume and protect or enhance appearance and maintain in good condition. Some products purely decorative, do not alter physiological state; *e.g.* hair dyes, lipsticks, nail polish and perfumes; part of proper cosmetology and do not directly fall in domain of dermatologist's work. Dermatologists need to be familiar to deal with their cutaneous adverse effects (irritant/allergic contact dermatitis or photoallergic/phototoxic reactions or contact urticaria).

Other products or procedures remedial; intentionally used to alter appearance and physiological state: to reverse effects of aging, improve quality of skin, augment facial structures and appearance in general. One of the most important part is vehicle. It may improve the efficacy of the active ingredient, inactivate the active ingredient, improve the skin barrier or cause allergic contact dermatitis. Common active ingredients in cosmetic products include: Alpha hydroxy acids, antioxidants, botanicals (herbals), depigmenting/demelanizing agents, exfoliants (keratolytics), moisturizers (emollients), peptides, vitamin derivatives (retinoids, vitamin C and E) and sunscreens. Evidence of efficacy exists for AHAs, demelanizing agents, exfoliants, moisturizers, retinoids and sunscreens. But majority of the cosmetic products contain above substances in inappropriate (usually lower, occasionally higher than normal) concentrations.

PROCEDURES IN COSMETIC DERMATOLOGY

Chemical Peeling

Indications

- *Superficial and medium chemical peels:* facial rejuvenation, melasma, mild acne, mild acne scars and post acne pigmentation, oily skin with dilated pores, rosacea, photoaging.
- *Deep chemical peels:* not recommended in skin types IV to VI (hence in Indian skin) because of high risk of prolonged or permanent pigmentary changes.
- *Other uses:* post inflammatory hyperpigmentation, freckles, lentigines, facial melanosis, fine wrinkling, superficial scars, seborrheic keratosis, actinic keratosis, warts, milia.

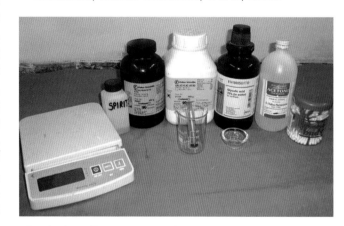

Chemical peeling start up: Cleaning agents (acetone, spirit), peeling agents (glycolic acid, trichloro-acetic acid, salicylic acid), equipment for making solutions (beaker, syringe, bowl, electronic weighing balance), applicators (ear buds).

Classification of common facial rejuvenation/cosmetic procedures				
Degree of Invasion	Fillers	Relaxation of muscles	Resurfacing	Re-suspending of loose tissue/re-orientation of scars
Non invasive	–	–	Topical Retinoids Topical Glycolic acid	Radiofrequency
Minimally invasive (superficial and mid dermal injection)	Collagen based Hyaluronic acid based	Botulinum toxin injection	LED Photomodulation Intense pulse light Microdermabrasion	Sculptra/Juvederm Voluma (cross-linked hyaluronic acid) Aptos/Contour thread lifts Blepharoplasty Lifts
Invasive (subcutaneous or deeper injection/harvesting and injection, surgical)	Synthetic fillers Fat autografting Fat autograft muscle inj Platelet rich plasma inj	–	Light chemical peel Pulsed diode/Nd YAG laser Non-ablative laser	Scar revision S-lift Neck liposuction Full rhytidectomy

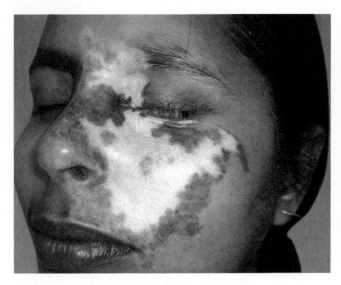

Segmental vitiligo: left side of face, at baseline.

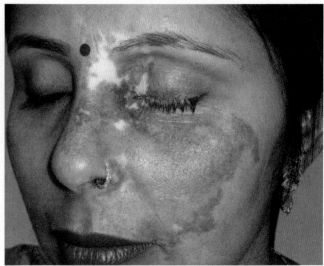

Segmental vitiligo: 1 year after a combination of sequential suction blister grafting followed by non cultured epidermal cell suspension.

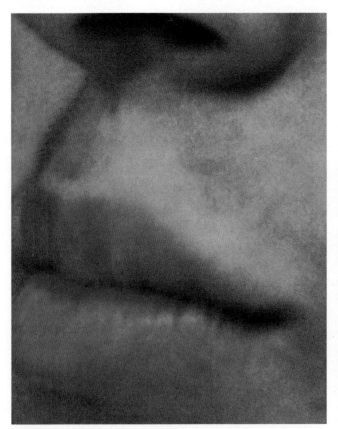

Vitiligo: pre-treatment photograph.

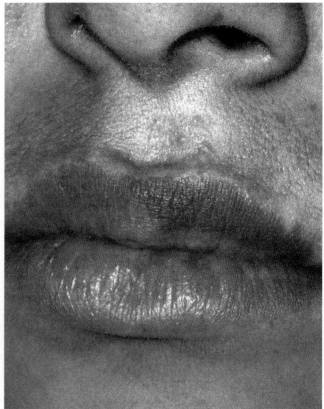

Vitiligo: after treatment with combination of blister and punch grafting.

Mark Rubin's classification of peeling agents based on depth and examples of agents achieving the depth	
Depth of penetration	Chemical peeling agents
Very superficial/stratum corneum exfoliation	Glycolic acid 20–50%
	Salicyclic acid 20–30%
	Resorcinol 20–30% (5–10 min)
	Jessner's solution (1–3 coats)
	Trichloroacetic acid 10% (1 coat)
Superficial/epidermal necrosis	Glycolic acid 50–70% (5–20 min)
	Jessner's solution (5–10 coats)
	Resorcinol 50% (30–60 min)
	Trichloroacetic acid 10–35% (1 coat)
Medium-depth/papillary dermal necrosis	Phenol 88%
	Glycolic Acid 70% (5–30 min)
	Trichloroacetic acid 35% in combination with:
	Glycolic acid 50–70%
	Solid CO_2
	Jessner's solution
Deep/reticular dermal necrosis	Pyruvic acid 40–70%
	Modified Baker's peel (2 drops croton oil)
	Baker-Gordon phenol peel

Pre-peel priming (with topical retinoic acid or glycolic acid for 2–3 weeks) and post peel care important for optimum results. Glycolic acid neutralized with water or sodium bicarbonate, TCA (frosting) and SA (pseudofrosting) washed with water.

Complications: infection, milia, pigmentary alteration, telangiectases, contact dermatitis, delayed healing and scarring.

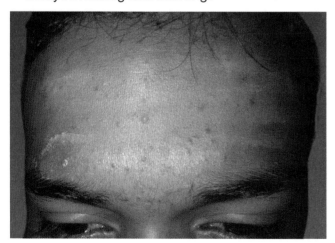

Salicylic acid peel: 'Pseudofrosting' seen as a fine whtitsh coating over the forehead in a patient of acne.

Botulinum Toxin Injections

Toxin A and B commercially useful. Type A more commonly used as type B injection is more painful and shorter acting produces temporary chemical denervation by blocking the presynaptic release of acetylcholine at the neuromuscular junction; has proven efficacy and excellent safety. Knowledge of facial anatomy and physiology of muscles, *a* must. Use cautiously in neuromuscular disorders like myasthenia gravis. Muscle paralysis takes 24–48 hours to develop fully and full effect lasts around 90 days.

Uses: upper and lower face wrinkles, palmoplantar or axillary hyperhidrosis, facial contouring, neck rejuvenation.

- *Non-dermatological uses:* include blepharospasm, torticollis, tension type headache, migraine. New uses-finger tip ulceration in scleroderma, epidermolysis bullosa erosions.
- *Complications:* transient swelling, brusing, ecchymosis, undesired muscle weakness (ptosis, quzzical brow, diplopia), dry eye (if injected periorbitally).

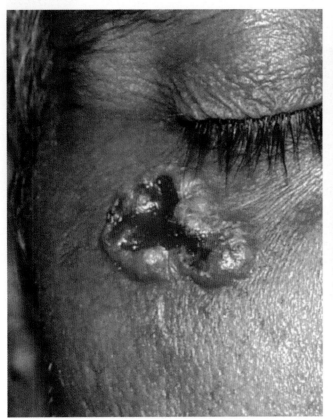

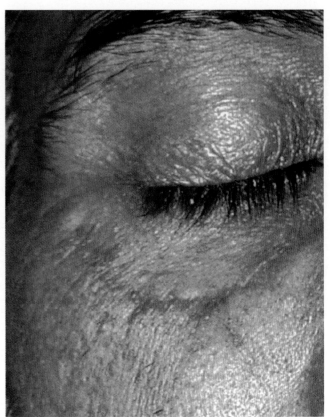

Noduloulcerative basal cell carcinoma: before excision with 2 mm free margin.

After 3 months of excision.

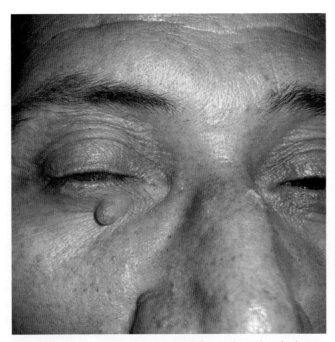

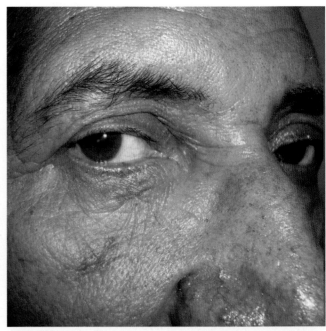

Neurofibroma, right lower eyelid: pedunculated lesion, 0.8–1 cm sized.

Neurofibroma, right lower eyelid: 10 days after complete excision.

Soft Tissue Augmentation

Fillers injected into dermis or sub-dermally to replace lost volume or increase existing volume. Also increase volume by imbibing dermal water. Also classified as temporary and permanent. The examples of US FDA approved fillers (except autologous fat) include: temporary (full effect lasting less than 1 year)—collagen, hyaluronic acid; permanent (full effect lasts more than 1 year, usually many years)—polymethyl meth-acrylate, poly-L lactic acid. Autologous fat can be permanent if injection procedure is right.

Classified according to Origin

- **Autogenic:** dermis, fat, plasma, cultured fibroblasts, collagen.
- **Allogenic:** cultured collagen, cadaveric collagen, cadaveric fascia.
- **Xenogenic:** bovine collagen, avian-derived hyaluronan, bacterial-derived hyaluronan.
- **Synthetic:** hydrogels, calcium hydroxylapatite, polymethyl methacrylate, dextran, silicone, expanded polytetrafluoroethylene.
- **Indications:** acne or surgical scars, mainly the fixed age related wrinkles (mainly mid face like nasolabial folds, mentolabial folds, but useful in upper and lower third of face as well), lip augmentation, shaping jaw line, filling facial defects, nose tip reshaping, etc.
- **Complications:** pain, swelling, redness, bruising, infections and hypersensitivity reactions.

Dermabrasion

- **Motorized resurfacing:** using wire brushes or diamond fraises, attached to rapidly rotating motor (@18,000–35,000 rpm).
- **Microdermabrasion:** with sterile micronized aluminium oxide crystals.
- **Indications of dermabrasion:** reduction of wrinkles, revision of traumatic or acne scars, treatment of comedones, photodamaged skin, rhinophyma, adenoma sebaceum, Bowen's disease and superficial basal cell carcinoma.
- **Complications:** scarring, keloid formation, hyper- or hypopigmentation and infection.

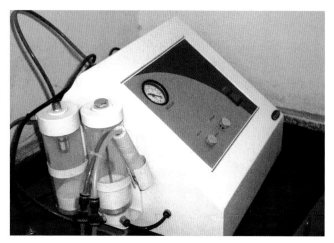

Microdermabrasion machine. Note: two see through containers partially filled with white powder (aluminium oxide crystals)—one of these is source of crystals when they are nozzled out and other is the reservoir in which they are aspirated and collected.

Management of Alopecia

Indicated in advanced androgenetic alopecia (Hamilton type 4 and beyond). May be done in female patients of androgenetic alopecia also. Occasionally done in scarring alopecia, but results are not impressive.
- **Surgical:** hair transplantation using follicular units, micrografts or minigrafts.
- **Medical:** minoxidil and finasteride.
- **Platelet rich plasma:** is recent technique. Takes advantage of several growth factors in present in platelet rich plasma. 'Cocktail' of growth factors is injected intradermally or subdermally (deep dermis to dermis-subcutaneous junction). These factors probably augment and induce hair growth. Under study, shown encouraging results in trial on alopecia areata and few series of androgenetic alopecia. But technique variable and not standardized.

Removal of Hair

Hair removal or reduction: temporary or permanent.
- **Temporary procedures:** shaving, epilation, plucking, waxing and threading.
- **Permanent procedures:** electrolysis, thermolysis. Contrary to popular belief, hair removal lasers

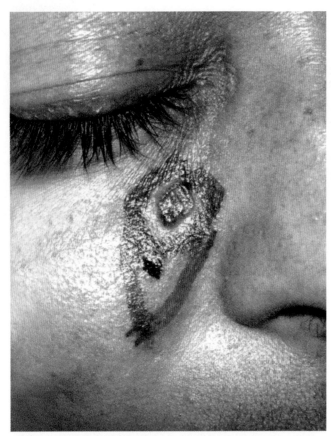

Island pedicle flap for basal cell carcinoma on cheek: excision margins outlined.

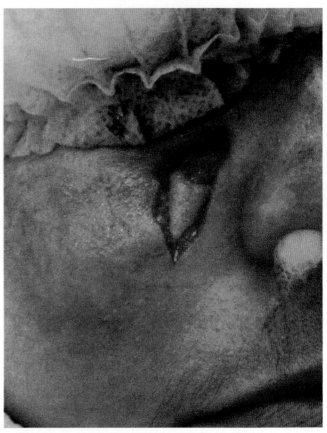

Island pedicle flap ready after excision of tumor.

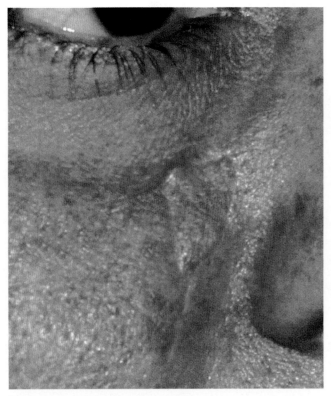

Final outcome 3 months after surgery.

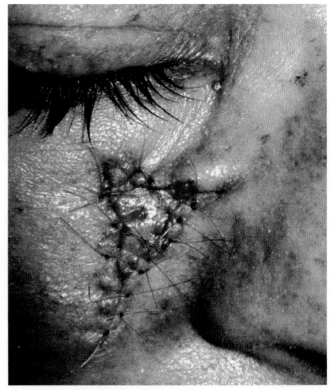

Island pedicle flap sutured in place.

do not give permanent results. Follow-up laser sittings always needed every 3–6 months.

Vitiligo Surgery

Variety of surgical procedures conducted for vitiligo patches on cosmetically concerning areas. Common ones include-micro-punch grafting, suction blister grafting, non-cultured epidermal cell suspension, ultra thin split thickness skin grafting. A new technique of follicular outer root sheath cellular suspension has been developed with encouraging results. Surgery performed only if lesions have been stable for at least 1 year.

Tattooing and its Removal

Indications for tattooing:
- *Medical:* camouflaging burns by micro-pigmentation. Producing permanent dots for radiation therapy.
- *Non-medical indications:* esthetic reasons, peer pressure, to provoke and enhance sexuality. Dermatologists approached for tattoo removal.

- *Methods:* excision, dermabrasion, infrared coagulation, salabrasion, grafting, cryosurgery and Moh's surgery.

Liposuction

Safe and effective technique to improve body's contours and rearrange distribution of adipose tissue without altering skin surface. Tumescent technique: infiltration of large volumes of vasoconstrictive anesthetic solution and removing adipose tissue through tiny holes using cannulas.
- *Indications:* lipomas, lipodystrophy and axillary hyperhidrosis. *Not a treatment for obesity.*
- *Complications:* ecchymosis, hematoma and infection.

Reconstructive Surgical Pearls

Aim to produce esthetically pleasing ideal scar that blends imperceptibly with natural creases and folds. Techniques: placing subcuticular sutures, punch and blister grafting, reconstruction using flaps (*e.g.* island pedicle flap) and scar revisions using W-plasty, Z-plasty and V-V plasty.

25

Lasers in Dermatology

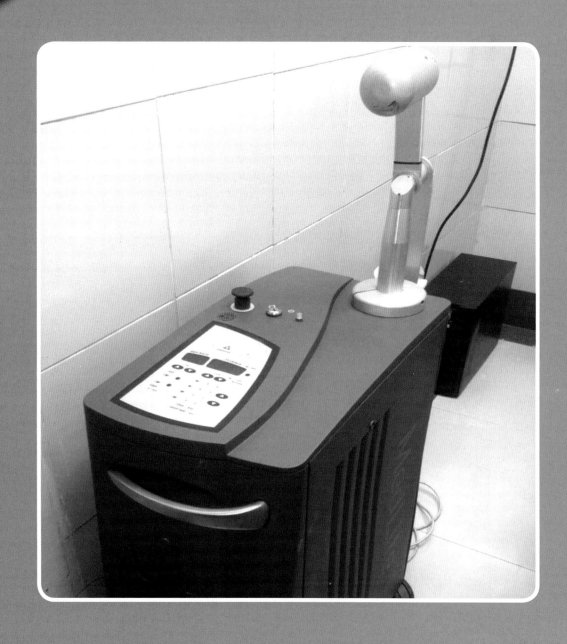

Laser, an acronym for *light amplification* by *stimulated emission of radiation*. First laser developed in 1959. Laser surgery first-line treatment for several congenital and acquired dermatological conditions.

PRINCIPLES OF LASER SURGERY

Based on—unique properties of laser light and complex laser-tissue interactions. Lasers—either absorbed, reflected, transmitted or scattered. Depth of penetration depends on absorption and scattering. Only absorbed light produces clinical effect. Amount determined by chromophore wavelength. Endogenous chromophores are water, melanin and hemoglobin. Tattoo ink, an exogenous chromophore. Laser energy produces photothermal, photochemical or photomechanical effects; destroys tissues.

Scattering minimal in epidermis; greater in dermis due to collagen; amount inversely proportional to wavelength of incident light. Upto mid-infrared region, depth of penetration increases with wavelength; thereafter, in longer-infrared range, penetration restricted by tissue water; forms basis of ablative skin resurfacing. Terms used in practice of lasers summarized in Table on page 477.

LASERS USED IN DERMATOLOGY

Lasers—vascular-specific lasers, pigment specific lasers, ablative lasers, non-ablative lasers, epilation lasers and lasers for scars and striae.

Vascular lasers (pulse dye, copper and bromide, KTP, krypton) target intravascular oxyhemoglobin (absorption peaks 418, 542 and 577 nm).

Pigment-specific (Q switched lasers-Nd:YAG, ruby, alexandrite) *lasers* target melanin.

Ablative lasers (high energy pulsed and scanned CO_2 lasers, Er:YAG laser or combination of these two) used for facial rejuvenation.

Non-ablative lasers (Q switched and long pulsed Nd:YAG, diode, KTP, pulse dye, Er:glass lasers), produce cutaneous resurfacing by collagen remodeling (without disruption of epidermis); results inferior to that of ablative lasers. Advantages—short down time (no leave required from work place), no or minimal analgesia needed.

Epilation lasers (long pulsed lasers like Nd:YAG, diode) target melanin within the hair shaft, hair follicle epithelium and heavily pigmented matrix. Melanin in epidermis competes for laser energy. Unwanted epidermal injury especially in darker skin types, can be minimized by using active cooling devices.

Fractional CO_2 laser (10600 nm).

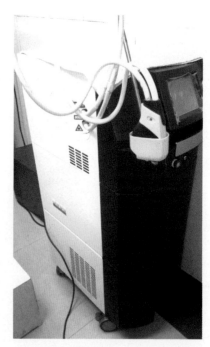

Long pulsed diode laser (810 nm).

Terms used in cutaneous laser surgery	
Monochromatic light	Light of single discrete wavelength.
Coherent light	Light traveling in phase with respect to both time and space.
Collimated light	Narrow intense beam of light emitted in parallel fashion to achieve its propagation across long distances without divergence.
Fluence/energy density	Energy absorbed in joules/cm^2.
Grotthus-Draper law	Only absorbed light produces clinical effect; transmitted or reflected light does not.
Thermal relaxation time	Time required for the target tissue to cool to half the peak temperature after laser irradiation.
Anderson and Parish's theory of selective photothermolysis	Controlled destruction of targeted lesion possible using a wavelength preferentially absorbed by chromophore and exposing it for a period less than the chromophore's thermal relaxation time.
Continuous wave (CW) lasers	Emit continuous beam with long exposure durations; result in non-selective tissue injury.
Quasi-CW mode lasers	Continuous wave beam shuttered into short segments producing interrupted (450 μs–40 millisecond) emissions of constant laser energy.
Pulsed laser	High energy light in ultra short pulse durations (0.1–1 second) with long interrupted time periods.
QS lasers	Quality switched lasers; electro-optical shutters permit stored energy to be released in short high-energy bursts.
Superpulsed lasers	Modified CO_2 laser; very short pulses in repetitive pattern, reducing thermal damage to adjacent tissue.
Fractional photothermolysis	Creation of columnar zones of thermal injury, called microthermal zones, in skin. Hence, minimizing the collateral damage to the adjoining epidermis and dermis. Collagen necrosis is followed by remodeling. Used more for ablative lasers.
Non-ablative laser	Damage to the dermis with relative or absolute sparing of the epidermis.
Selective photothermostimulation	Ability to stimulate adipocytes and mesenchymal cells of the subcutaneous tissue. New concept, may be useful in postliposuction, fat sculpting/grafting.

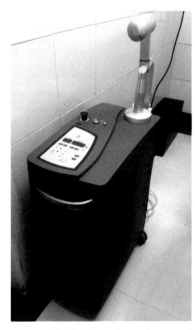

Q switched Nd:YAG laser (1064 nm).

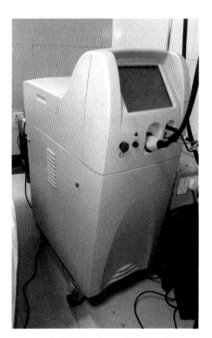

Pulse dye laser (595 nm).

Common lasers used in dermatology		
Laser type	*Wavelength (nm)*	*Application*
Argon (CW)	418/514	Vascular lesions
Argon pumped tunable dye (Quasi-CW)	577/585	Vascular lesions
Copper vapor/bromide (Quasi-CW)	510/578	Pigmented and vascular lesions
Potassium-titanyl-phosphate (KTP)	532	Pigmented and vascular lesions
Nd:YAG, frequency doubled	532	Pigmented lesions; red/orange/yellow tattoos
Pulsed dye	510 585–595	Pigmented lesions Vascular lesions, hypertrophic/keloidal scars, striae, verrucae, non-ablative dermal remodelling
Ruby QS Normal mode	694	Pigmented lesions; blue/black/green tattoos Hair removal
Alexandrite QS Normal mode	755	Pigmented lesions; blue/black/green tattoos Hair removal, leg veins
Diode Long pulsed	800–810 1450	Hair removal, leg veins Non-ablative dermal remodeling
Nd:YAG QS Normal mode Long-pulsed	1064 1320	Pigmented lesions; blue/black tattoos Hair removal, leg veins, non-ablative dermal remodeling Non-ablative dermal remodeling
Erbium:glass	1540	Non-ablative dermal remodeling
Erbium:YAG (pulsed)	2490	Ablative skin resurfacing, epidermal lesions
Cardon dioxide CW Pulsed	10600 10600	Actinic cheilitis, verrucae, rhinophyma Ablative skin resurfacing, epidermal/dermal lesions
Intense pulsed light source	515–1200	Superficial pigmented lesions, vascular lesions, hair removal, non-ablative dermal remodeling

INDICATIONS FOR LASER THERAPY

Indications for lasers in dermatology listed in Table on page 469.

SIDE EFFECTS AND COMPLICATIONS

- *Vascular-specific lasers:* Purpura, erythema, vesiculation, crusting, hypopigmentation, hyperpigmentation and scarring.
- *Pigment-specific lasers:* Transient pigmentary alterations, permanent depigmentation, guttate depigmentation, darkening and scarring; allergic reactions to the pigment liberated from tattoo.
- *Epilatory lasers:* Pain, perifollicular erythema, blister formation and scarring.
- *Ablative lasers:* Acne, hypertrophic/pigmented scar, post inflammatory hyperpigmentation, milia formation, contact dermatitis, pruritus and bacterial and viral infections.

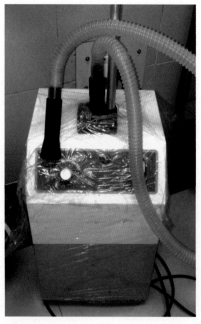

Smoke evacuator: with flexible goose-neck suction pipe, a must accessory for CO_2 laser.

Indications for laser therapy in dermatology		
Indications	**Laser specifications**	**Comments**
Port-wine stain	Flash lamp pumped pulsed dye (585 nm, 595 nm) (0.45–>10 millisecond pulse)	Treat > 1 year; central forehead most responsive
Capillary hemangiomas	Flash lamp pumped pulsed dye	Used for ulcerated lesions or if vital structures compromised or causing cosmetic morbidity; controversial for uncomplicated superficial lesions
Telangiectases	Flash lamp pumped pulsed dye Green light lasers	—
Pyogenic granuloma	Flash lamp pumped pulsed dye (585 nm) CO_2 laser, combined CW/pulsed	Small flat lesions
Angiofibromas	CO_2 laser, flash lamp pumped pulsed dye	Early small lesions
Lentigines	All pigment specific lasers	—
Nevus of Ota	QS-ruby, QS-alexandrite, QS-Nd:YAG 1064 nm	Best results with brown lesions
Congenital melanocytic nevi	Normal ruby, QS-ruby, QS-Nd:YAG (532 nm)	Controversial
Café-au-lait macules	QS-ruby, QS-Nd:YAG (532 nm), copper vapor	Variable response
Nevus spilus	Normal ruby, normal alexandrite, QS-ruby, QS-Nd:YAG (532 nm)	Variable response
Acne	Narrowband blue light (410–420 nm), Infrared laser	Approved by FDA
Acne scarring	CO_2, Er:YAG (585–1540 nm), flash lamp multiwavelength	Prolonged healing and erythema. Use with dynamic cooling
Psoriasis	Excimer (308 nm), flash lamp pumped pulsed dye (585 nm)	—
Vitiligo	Excimer (308 nm)	—
Tattoo Black Blue-green Yellow-orange-red	QS-ruby, QS-alexandrite, QS-Nd:YAG (1064 nm) QS-ruby, QS-alexandrite, Nd:YAG (1064 nm) blue only QS-Nd:YAG (532 nm), pulsed dye (510 nm) (green)	—
Hypertrichosis	Long pulsed ruby (694 nm), intense pulsed light Long pulsed alexandrite (755 nm), diode (810 nm), millisecond QS-Nd:YAG (1064 nm)	Used for darker skin
Keloids/hypertrophic scars	Flash lamp pumped pulsed dye (585 nm)	Reduce pruritus, may need adjunctive corticosteroids, dysesthesia
Striae	Flash lamp pumped pulsed dye (585 nm) Nd:YAG (1320 nm), fractional CO_2	—
Warts	CO_2, flash lamp pumped pulsed dye (585 nm) KTP	Variable response No local anesthetic needed
Epidermal nevi and other tumors	CO_2, Er:YAG (585–1540 nm)	—
Cellulite removal and body contouring	Nd:YAG laser (1064 nm)	Laser lipolysis

RECENT ADVANCES IN LASERS

New lasers under study—1720 nm for sebaceous glands (better hair removal), several non-ablative fractional lasers (1927 nm thulium, 1927 nm CO_2, 1940 nm thulium-alexandrite, etc.), 755 nm alexandrite picosecond laser for tattoo removal. In addition, home based devices like hand held non-ablative diodes (1410 nm, 1435 nm fractional) have been developed for fine facial rhytids.

Glossary and Clinical Examination

CLINICAL TERMS

Macule: a circumscribed area of change of color, not raised above or depressed below the surface of adjoining skin

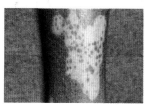

depigmented and brownish hyperpigmented macules

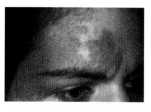

erythematous macule

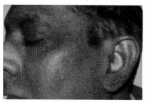

slate-grey hyperpigmented macules

Papule: a solid lesion, (< 1 cm), elevated above the surface of adjoining skin

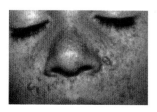

dome-shaped papules

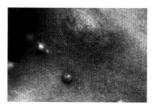

umbilicated papules

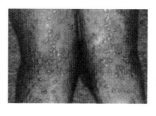

lichenoid papules (note Wickham's striae on the larger lesion)

Burrow: a linear tortuous papule; pathognomonic of scabies

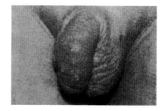

Comedo: a papule sometimes surmounted with a black punctum in the middle; pathognomonic of acne

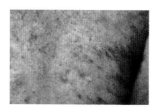

open comedones

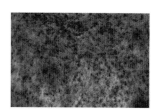

closed comedones (also some pustules)

Nodule: a deep-seated, large papule (> 1 cm)

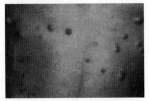 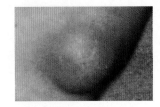

papules and nodules   a nodule

Tumor: a large, almost rounded, nodule

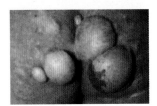 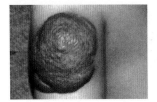

Plaque: a flat, indurated lesion, usually elevated above the surface of adjoining skin, with horizontal dimensions much more than the vertical

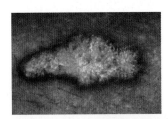

lichenified plaque

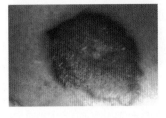

edematous plaque

Vesicle: a small, circumscribed lesion elevated above the surface of skin containing clear fluid

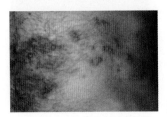

herpetiform configuration

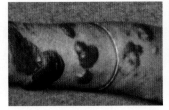 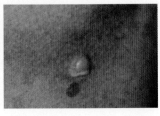

tense and hemorrhagic   hypopyon

Pustule: a circumscribed, elevated lesion containing opalescent, purulent fluid

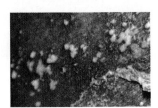

follicular pustules   lakes of pus

Bulla: a large vesicle

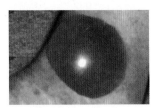 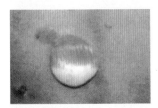

tense bulla   flaccid bulla

Crust: a layer of dried-up inspissated secretions

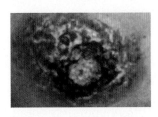 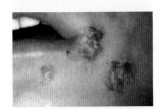

hemorrhagic crust   honey-colored crust

Scale: a sheet of adherent epidermal cells

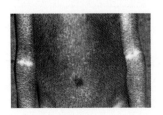 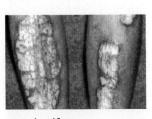

ichthyosiform   psoriasiform

Ulceration: a break in the continuity of skin

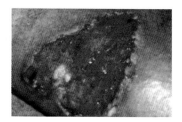

Lichenification: triad of skin thickening, increased skin markings and hyperpigmentation.

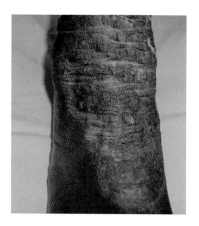

Telangiectasia: Dilated capillaries visible as thin, red, straight or branching lines.

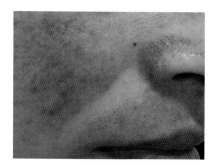

Purpura: Area of reddish purple discoloration secondary to bleeding in the skin or mucosa.

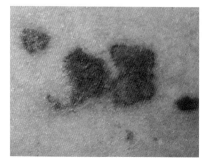

Eschar: Thick adherent crust covering an underlying ulcer.

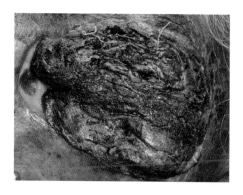

Poikiloderma: triad of atrophy, telangiectasia and altered pigmentation.

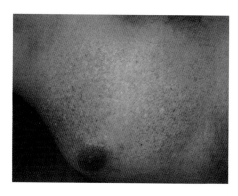

Wheal: flat patches or edematous plaques which are reddish or skin colored, transient by nature (subsiding in < 24 hours)

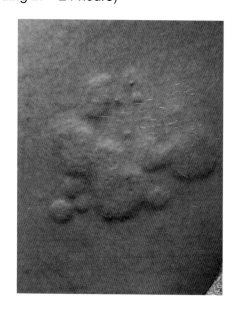

Index

Page numbers followed by *f* refer to figure and *t* refer to table